EFFECTIVE COMMUNICATION FOR HEALTH PROFESSIONALS

EFFECTIVE COMMUNICATION

FOR HEALTH PROFESSIONALS

Second edition

ELSEVIER

Elsevier
3251 Riverport Lane
St. Louis, Missouri 63043

EFFECTIVE COMMUNICATION FOR HEALTH PROFESSIONALS,
SECOND EDITION

ISBN: 978-0-323-62545-6

Notice

Practitioners and researchers must always rely on their own experience and knowledge in evaluating
and using any information, methods, compounds or experiments described herein. Because of rapid
advances in the medical sciences, in particular, independent verification of diagnoses and drug
dosages should be made. To the fullest extent of the law, no responsibility is assumed by Elsevier,
authors, editors or contributors for any injury and/or damage to persons or property as a matter of
products liability, negligence or otherwise, or from any use or operation of any methods, products,
instructions, or ideas contained in the material herein.

Previous edition copyrighted 2016.

Library of Congress Control Number: 2019945358

Senior Content Strategist: Linda Woodard
Director, Content Development: Ellen Wurm-Cutter
Content Development Specialist: Melissa Rawe,
    Kathleen Nahm, John Tomedi
Publishing Services Manager: Deepthi Unni
Project Manager: Haritha Dharmarajan
Designer: Brian Salisbury

Printed in the United States of America
Last digit is the print number: 9 8 7 6 5 4 3 2

Working together
to grow libraries in
developing countries

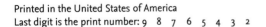

www.elsevier.com • www.bookaid.org

CONTRIBUTORS

Linda Boyd, BS, RDA, CDA
Professor Emeritus
Registered Dental Assisting Program
Diablo Valley College
Pleasant Hill, California

Sharon Campton, MA
Spiritual Care Counselor
Hope Hospice and Home Health
Dublin, California

Judy Frain, PhD, RN
Associate Professor
Goldfarb School of Nursing at Barnes-Jewish
    College
St. Louis, Missouri

Jaime Nguyen, MD, MPH, MS, BA
Director of Allied Health
Penn Foster Education
Scranton, Pennsylvania

REVIEWERS

Nicole Anderson
Professor
Ultimate Medical Academy
Tampa, Florida

Teresa Avvampato, OT Reg. (Ont.), MSc (OT)
Program Coordiantor and Occupational Therapist
Durham College
Oshawa, Ontario
Canada

Nancy Daley
Instructor
New Brunswick Community College
Miramichi, New Brunskwick
Canada

Daisy Deng, PhD
Program Director
Ohio Medical Career Center
Dayton, Ohio

Holly Dennis, PhD
Manager, Curriculum and Instructional
   Design
Ultimate Medical Academy
Tampa, Florida

Kimberly Head, BA, BS, DC
Director of Healthcare Programs
CE Health Sciences, Collin College
Plano, Texas

Lisa O'Bradovich, BS, MS
Health and Human Services Program Director
Ultimate Medical Academy
Tampa, Florida

Julie Pepper, BS, CMA (AAMA)
Instructor
Chippewa Valley Technical College
Eau Claire, Wisconsin

Lisa Rigs, CPC, CPC-I
Curriculum and Instructional Design Specialist
Ultimate Medical Academy
Tampa, Florida

**Bobbi Steelman, BS. Elem Ed, MA Ed, and Rank 1
School Administration CPhT**
Director of Education/Pharmacy Tech Program
   Director
Daymar College
Bowling Green, Kentucky

PREFACE

Welcome to *Effective Communication for Health Professionals*, 2nd edition. We hope this text will make it easier for you to interact and communicate in the medical field. We have revised the first edition of this book to present the communication strategies used every day by successful health care professionals.

We designed this text to approach communication in an easily understandable and interesting format. Communication is a learned skill. This book will help you to improve your communication skills with your patients and coworkers. You will read about various communication theories and challenges followed by suggestions and guidelines to help you work your way to effective communication. Grounded in practice, *Effective Communication* is loaded with vivid examples depicting real-world patient interactions. Our goal is to provide the reader with communication know-how that will be applicable to any patient care setting.

The text has been thouroughly revised to present the most up-to-date overview of communication in the health care field. Chapter 1 outlines the concepts of the communication exchange itself, as well as the basics of communicating professionally. Chapter 2 introduces the patient interview, offering best practices for gathering the clinical information needed to provide quality care. Chapter 3 addresses health literacy, presenting techniques to assess and evaluate patient education and improve patient compliance. Chapter 4 is devoted to awareness of the diversity of patients and their experiences, providing a strong foundation for respectful communication across cultures, genders, orientations, beliefs, and generations.

In Chapter 5, the reader learns how to recognize and overcome many barriers to communcation, such as language barriers, sensory impairments, and patients in distress. Chapter 6 details the communication issues unique to caring for patients with mental and physiologic illnesses. Chapter 7 is an overview of the grief process, containing the most current thinking on communcation related to loss and terminal illness.

The text introduces concepts related to communication in the health care workplace in Chapter 8. Here the reader learns the basics of patient privacy and the Health Insurance Portability and Accountability Act (HIPAA); the workings of staff meetings and case conferences; communicating with providers and coworkers; and professional use of the telephone and email. Finally, Chapter 9 presents the importance of proper documentation in the health record, including a discussion of the electronic health record (EHR) functions and benefits.

We filled the text with features that we hope will make the topic of communication as interesting to you as it is to us. These include the following:

- Communication Guidelines boxes summarizing best practices for the effective exchange of information in many situations.
- Words at Work dialogue boxes demonstrating conversations between health care professionals and clients.
- Taking the Chapter to Work boxes, which are case scenarios, to give you examples of compassionate, caring health care professionals working through everyday interactions.
- Spotlight on Success boxes containing information to remind you that the foundations you establish as a student will help you build a rewarding career.
- Legal Eagle boxes reinforcing the private and confidential nature of medical information and the ethical and legal responsibilties for users of this information.
- Learning Objectives alerting you to the skills or knowledge you should gain from each chapter.
- Key Terms introducing you to words or concepts that may not be familiar.
- Test Your Communication IQ boxes highlighting areas of communication in which you might be weak.

At the end of each chapter, Checking Your Comprehension will direct you back through the chapter to points you may need to reinforce.

Critical Thinking exercises aim to expand your mind with probing questions that have no clear-cut, black or white answers.

As you work your way through this text, keep in mind that the skills you gain now will make health care a rewarding career for many years to come.

EVOLVE RESOURCES

Users of Effective Communication for Health Professionals can access many additional resources on the Evolve Web site for this text. With the access code provided, students can watch videos that illustrate many of the communication concepts explored in the book, such as active listening and conflict management. For extra practice, students can work through a set of scenario-based quizzes that are directly related to the content in each chapter. The Evolve site also houses a unique Audio Practice asset, in which students listen to patient voicemail messages and interactions between patients and health care professionals, applying what they have learned to a series of challenging situations.

For instructors, the Evolve site houses TEACH Lesson Plans with reading and review assignments, ideas for classroom activities, and structured assessments to ensure student comprehension of the materials. These lesson plans delineate the ancillary materials and resources available by chapter and learning objective, so instructors can be sure they are utilizing all the assets that accompany this text. Also on Evolve, instructors may download PowerPoint presentations tailored to each chapter, student handouts for extra practice in preparation for exams, and a 200-question test bank. Each test bank question is assigned a Bloom's taxonomy, answer rationale, and page reference to check answers in the text.

CONTENTS

EFFECTIVE COMMUNICATION FOR HEALTH PROFESSIONALS

Communicating in Health Care

Judy Frain

CHAPTER OUTLINE

LEARNING OBJECTIVES

Upon successful completion of this chapter, you will be able to:

1. Discuss the importance of maintaining rapport and confidentiality with patients.
2. Discuss the elements of communication.
3. Differentiate between verbal and nonverbal communication.
4. List the steps in effective communication.
5. Discuss the responsibilities of both the health care professional and the patient in the communication process.
6. Explain the purpose of maintaining a professional distance and using empathy in patient care.

KEY TERMS

channel the means of transmitting the message
clarification the removal of confusion or misunderstanding
colloquialism informal speech, usually relying on regionally accepted terms and pronunciations
compliance the act of a patient following the instructions of the health care team
disclosure the sending of patient information
dynamics the psychological background and inner workings of interpersonal relationships

empathy the condition of experiencing the feelings of another

feedback the return of information solicited during an exchange; usually used to verify that information was received

Health Insurance Portability and Accountability Act (HIPAA) United States federal legislation protecting the privacy and security of health information

idiom an expression specific to a certain population that cannot be translated literally

incongruence incompatible, not in agreement, inconsistent

jargon specialized or technical language of a trade or profession

kinesics the study of body positions and movement in relation to communication

message a communication transmitted by spoken or written word or other means from one to another

paralanguage vocal expression involving rate of speech, tone, pitch, etc.

protected health information (PHI) under the law, any health information, such as medical history or current status, that can be linked to an individual

proxemics the study of personal spatial distances and their effect on interpersonal behavior

rapport a relationship, usually of mutual trust and regard

receiver in the communication process, the person or persons for whom the sender's message is intended

sender in the communication process, the individual who creates and transmits a message

slang informal words and phrases used around friends, family, and others in our social group

spatial pertaining to a space and its relationship with things found in it

sympathy understanding that another is in distress

verification the process of checking the accuracy of a statement

TEST YOUR COMMUNICATION IQ

Before reading this chapter, complete this short self-assessment test. Decide which statements are true and which are false.

1. The health care worker should maintain control of the conversation to keep communication brief and to the point.
2. Using the patient's first name makes the patient more comfortable and promotes rapport.
3. Nonverbal communication is often as important as verbal communication.
4. Effective communication is the key to good patient care.
5. Saying, "You'll be just fine," is reassuring to patients and is a good therapeutic response.
6. Using proper medical terminology will impress your patients and should be used whenever possible.
7. Tapping your patient on the shoulder for good luck is an appropriate use of touch.

Results

Statements 3 and 4 are true; all others are false. How did you do? Read the chapter to find more information on these topics.

THE IMPORTANCE OF COMMUNICATION IN HEALTH CARE

Communication is vital to our survival. It fills the practical need of transmitting our wants and needs to those who can fill them for us, and helps us respond to the wants and needs of others. Good communication also helps meet our social needs; it gives us pleasure and relief from stress and forms bonds with others in our group to increase our sense of belonging. Communication is easier for some people than for others, but with practice, everyone can learn the steps to better communication. Because we typically spend more than half of our waking hours communicating with others, this skill should be practiced and refined to be more effective, pleasurable, and rewarding.

The ability to communicate and interact effectively is a critical skill for all allied health professionals because of the many barriers and challenges unique to the profession. In this text, we describe ways to serve your patients and your health care career through therapeutic communication. We will help you to understand and to be understood in the many areas of health care and in the difficult and puzzling situations that you will confront during your career. Many of the tips and suggestions are helpful for purely social conversations and interactions, but you will find that communicating with persons who are ill, or who are stressed by caring for those who are ill, requires skills far more advanced than those we use in everyday social interaction. Even patients visiting the provider for nothing more than a routine physical examination frequently need help communicating in a stressful and potentially difficult situation. Patients usually spend more relaxed time with you than with the provider and, in most instances, they see you as more approachable and more open to communication. A positive attitude, pleasant presentation, and good communication skills establish rapport, a relationship of trust and understanding, for future interactions with patients. These skills also help maintain the flow of communication back and forth among health care professionals.

The information you receive while talking with patients must be transmitted accurately to providers and other health care professionals. You must also translate information from providers and other staff members in a manner that patients can understand. Because patient information is private and confidential, ethical and legal standards require that you communicate this information to appropriate persons in a secure manner.

Patient Confidentiality and HIPAA

The importance of patient confidentiality has been an issue in health care since the earliest concept of one person caring for another. The 2000-year-old Hippocratic Oath (or Oath of Hippocrates), a part of the graduation ceremony for physicians, emphasizes the importance of guarding patient information with the following statement:

"All that may come to my knowledge in the exercise of my profession or outside of my profession or in daily commerce with men, which ought not to be spread abroad, I will keep secret and will never reveal."

Throughout the centuries, those who provided health care understood that maintaining secrecy about a patient's health and treatment was central to the patient's trust in the physician. The patient's privacy is so important that it is included in every specialty's code of ethics. For most of medical history, however, a breach of confidentiality was not punishable by law unless it resulted in damage to a person's reputation, which is called defamation of character.

The Health Insurance Portability and Accountability Act of 1996, or HIPAA, is a federal law developed to ensure health coverage when an individual changed employment. It addressed the problem of guarding patient data in systems with multiple points of access, which became critical with the electronic transmission of sensitive patient information. Insurance companies, health maintenance organizations (HMOs), and other interested parties now needed access to health information that most of us would prefer not to share. This sending of health information is called disclosure. To address these concerns, HIPAA protects patients from disclosure of medical information without the patient's expressed permission.

HIPAA limits the communication of all protected health information (PHI), defined as health data that can be identified with an individual. If you work anywhere that PHI is created or maintained, it is your responsibility to protect patient privacy by ensuring no one has access to PHI unless the patient allows it. The law states that unless authorized by the patient, PHI may not be accessed by the patient's family or friends, insurance companies, or even other medical professionals and doctors. HIPAA protections apply to any information in the patient's medical record, as well as all information about the patient's condition. For example, consider the following scenarios, all of which are unauthorized disclosures of PHI:

- The medical assistant leaves a patient's medical record at the nurses' station where anyone walking past can see it.
- The nurse logs into the patient's medical record on the computer, then neglects to log out when leaving the area to ask the provider a question.
- Within earshot of a crowded waiting room, the nurse assistant says to a colleague, "The doctor thinks Mr. Jackson has Lyme disease."
- A patient's mother, who is a physician, calls the hospital to ask about her daughter in the emergency department, but the patient has not yet signed any forms allowing the release of her information. The medical receptionist assures the mother that her daughter is there and in a stable condition.

- The nurse's neighbor was seen at the urgent care center today and, although the nurse was not involved in his treatment, she checks his medical record just to make sure everything is alright.

As a health care professional, it is your responsibility to safeguard patient information, communicating to colleagues only the minimal amount necessary for the care of the patient, and releasing information only to those individuals designated by the patient. Even those closest to the patient, such as a spouse, parent, or child, may not receive health information without the patient's consent, with some exceptions for patients who are minors.

Each of the unauthorized disclosures of PHI above—and many more such examples—constitute a breach of confidentiality under HIPAA. Betraying patient confidentiality will result in termination of employment, and that individual betraying confidentiality may also be prosecuted. Any successfully prosecuted breach of confidentiality is punishable by a variety of fines, ranging from $100 for each violation to $250,000 for selling or using information for improper purposes [Sections 1176(a)(1) and 1177(b)(3) of Public Law 104-191]. Imprisonment ranges up to 10 years for the maximum penalty.

Clearly, keeping your patient's health care information confidential is not just an ethical issue; it is a matter of federal law. Employers are required to provide HIPAA training to all employees.

HOW WE COMMUNICATE

Communication at any level forms a bond or connection with another person or persons for an exchange that should benefit at least one of the participants. Ideally, all participants should be equally involved in the message for the best outcome. If one of the participants is not interested in the information, or does not place a value on it, the process of communication will not be complete. For example, think about times you needed to talk to a friend about a problem you hoped she would understand. If she was distracted or did not care to listen, she would not fully understand your problem or point of view. You probably were understandably hurt and frustrated and may not try to confide in her again. Patients feel the same way if they suspect we do not value their concerns.

Elements of Communication

To be effective, we must determine the information to transmit, choose the best way to send the message, and receive and interpret the responses in the exchange. All forms of communication require the following elements:

- A *message* to be transmitted in a form understandable to the receiver
- A *sender*, usually a person, to initiate and transmit the message
- A *channel*, the method for transmitting the message—verbal, nonverbal, or written
- A ready and receptive *receiver* to accept the message
- *Feedback*, a response indicating whether the message was received and understood

The message is the idea or information we wish to convey. This information must be in a form that the person for whom it is intended can understand. For example, if you say something in English to someone who speaks only another language, the message will not be understood and there will be no communication. Similarly, if you speak above the patient's comprehension level, such as using certain medical terminology, or if the message is not clear or well-defined, the exchange is more difficult. If you speak to a person who is physically unable to hear spoken words, that person will not receive the information or ideas you are transmitting. In all these examples, the message was not transmitted in an understandable form and the communication process is incomplete; the message must be in a different format, one understandable to the person for whom the message is intended.

The sender is the person who initiates and transmits the message. In other words, the sender begins the communication. The sender decides how to put a message in a form that will be understood by its intended audience.

The channel, or the way the message travels, may be a variety of methods. It can be *verbal*, either spoken or written: talking with someone in person or on the phone, hearing the radio, reading an email, a letter, or text message—or even reading this book!—are all verbal communication channels. Communication happens through *nonverbal* channels as well: it may be through body language, or even a simple facial expression. Verbal and nonverbal communication is explored in more detail below.

The receiver is the person for whom the message is intended. The receiver listens, reads, or sees the message, and decodes it to understand the ideas transmitted by the sender. For the message to be received as transmitted, the receiver must be ready and able to accept it. A distracted patient, for example, may not be capable of receiving a message. Consider a patient consumed by worry or stress over his diagnosis: an attempt to communicate may fail because the receiver is not ready. Another patient may not have learned to trust you yet, or may be in denial about her condition, and has decided to ignore or dismiss what you have to say. Attempting to communicate under these circumstances is like sending emails that go straight to the junk folder without being read by the recipient. If the patient is not ready to accept the message or cannot receive it because of the patient's physical or emotional state, the transmission is incomplete. In Chapter 5, we cover how to determine when the patient is "ready to receive," and how to communicate if he or she is not ready but you need to talk with the patient about his or her health care at this time.

 TAKING THE CHAPTER TO WORK

Distracted Patient

Mary is working on a busy surgical floor at the hospital. One of her tasks this morning is to change the dressing on the surgical wound of Mr. Clancy's lower left leg. After knocking, she enters Mr. Clancy's room to inform him of her plan. She will have him observe the dressing change today, and have him perform the dressing change himself tomorrow while she observes, making sure he performs the procedure correctly. Mary further explains that he will need to do this dressing change daily when he is discharged to his home in a few days, and she wants to be certain he can perform the procedure correctly.

Mary sees that Mr. Clancy keeps looking up at his television as she is talking, and she is concerned he is too distracted by the television to learn the dressing change procedure. Mary knows that communication is not possible if the receiver is not ready to receive the message.

Mary gets Mr. Clancy's attention. "Mr. Clancy, what I am about to do is very important. If you can perform this dressing change correctly at home, you will heal much faster, and decrease the risk for infection. I need your undivided attention for 10 minutes. We can either do this now, or I can come back in 1 hour and we can do it then, the choice is yours."

"I'm expecting visitors later this morning, let's do this now." Mr. Clancy turns off his television. He appreciates that Mary has given him some control in deciding when to do the dressing change. Mr. Clancy pays close attention to the procedure, asking questions as Mary explains what she is doing.

In this case, Mary realized that her message was not being received by her patient. By being flexible in when she completed the dressing change, Mary effectively taught Mr. Clancy this important task, and now feels confident that he will be able to perform this dressing change correctly on his own once he is discharged.

After a message has been transmitted, we determine whether it was received through feedback responses. Feedback tells the sender whether or not the message was understood with a verification. Recognizing these responses may be as simple as interpreting the receiver's body language, facial expression, or a head nod that the message was received. We may simply see it in the patient's eyes. The verification response may also be as complex as a lengthy and involved written or verbal response. Often, a receiver will respond with a type of feedback called clarification, which asks a question for more information to better understand the message.

WORDS AT WORK

In this example, the patient's response is *clarification*, which both offers feedback that the message was heard and asks the sender for more information about the message:

Medical assistant: We want to see you again for a follow-up.
Patient: When?
Medical assistant: Two weeks.

When the message is in the verbal or spoken form, the sender and receiver alternate roles as they transmit their part of the information needed in the exchange and look for responses in the form of feedback and verification. The process of message exchange, a *conversation*, is like a game of catch, with the message, like a ball, passing from person to person. Figure 1.1 illustrates the flow of oral communication with its common components.

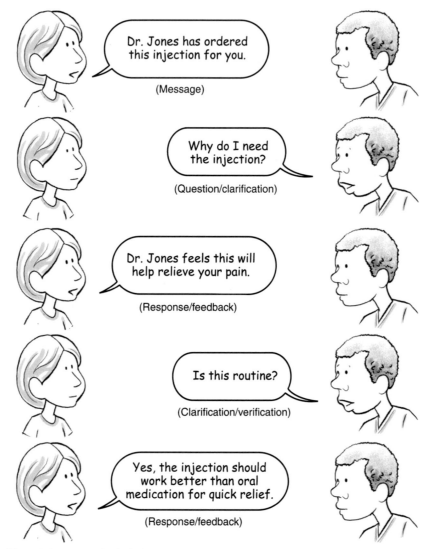

Fig. 1.1 A conversation includes a message, a sender, a receiver, a channel, and feedback.

Verbal Communication

Verbal communication exchanges messages using words or spoken language. It includes both oral and written communication. Good verbal communication skills are vital when performing such tasks as instructing, caring for, and educating patients or caregivers, sharing information with the provider or other members of the health care team, and documenting in medical records.

Oral Communication

We send and receive oral, or spoken, communication in health care more often than any other form of communication. Whenever we say hello to a coworker, tell patients that we will take their blood pressure, ask a provider for clarification about an order, or call a pharmacy to find out if a certain medication is in stock, we are using oral communication. The message is in the form of speech and spoken words. In the United States, the language we use most often is English.

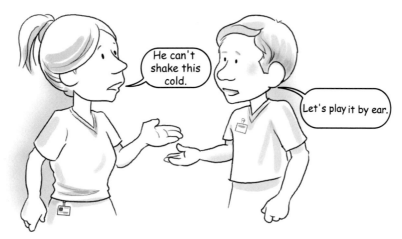

Fig. 1.2 Our speech contains idioms that convey meanings separate from a literal translation of the words.

Although we all generally share a common language, as individuals, we each have our own unique vocabulary, along with varying levels of understanding of the words others speak. The language we recognize and the words we choose are based on the speech of others; ultimately they are determined by our educators, the places where we live, and our culture. Furthermore, our language is constantly changing: new words are added, old words fall out of use, and existing words take on different or additional meanings.

Commonly, our everyday speech contains slang, the very informal words and phrases used around friends, family, and others in our social group. One type of slang is an idiom, a well-known phrase or sentence with a meaning completely different from its literal translation. These include sayings such as, "Let's play it by ear," or "He can't shake this cold" (Fig. 1.2). These expressions do not refer to anatomic ears or physical shaking. Idioms, by definition, do not mean what they say, they usually do not translate into other languages; they must be memorized by foreign speakers. If you think about the words literally, you can see just how confusing our idiomatic expressions can be.

Whether or not we are aware of it, we also use colloquialisms, regional phrases or terms spoken in informal settings by people living in a specific geographic area. One example of a colloquialism is the way people greet each other. "Hello" is preferred for formal occasions, whereas in some places people say "howdy," "hey," "hi," "how's it," "what's up," or simply "'sup." Another example of a colloquialism is the term people use to refer generically to soft drinks, like Coke or Pepsi. In the Northeast United States, someone might ask you if you want a "soda," whereas people in the Midwest call it "pop," and in parts of the South it is commonly called "coke" no matter what brand is served. Of course, colloquialisms and slang can appear often in the health professions, particularly among sensitive topics and among younger patients. Depending on her geographic region and social group, for example, a girl or young woman may refer to menstruation as cramps, period, flow, monthlies, or many other terms.

WORDS AT WORK

In this example, a woman calls to make an appointment because her mother has shortness of breath, referred to in medicine as "dyspnea." Note the way the caller uses common speech to describe her mother's condition.

Caller: Hi, I'm calling for my mom, a patient of Dr. Evelyn's. I just came to visit and it seems like mom is always winded.

Medical receptionist: Okay, is your mother alert? Is she able to speak?

Caller: Oh yes, it's just that she's huffing and puffing a lot. Like she just ran up the stairs. She can't even talk to me without stopping to catch her breath.

Medical receptionist: I understand. And she doesn't usually experience shortness of breath like this?

Finally, our speech may contain jargon, a type of language used within a particular profession and often unknown by those outside the work environment. Nearly all professions and trades use a special vocabulary in communication as a shortcut to convey certain meanings, and medicine is no exception. For example, "coding" is medical jargon for a patient who needs emergency resuscitation when used in the phrase, "The patient in room 234 is coding." This is short for saying "code blue." "Cabbage" is a term for a heart bypass procedure, a way to pronounce the abbreviation CABG, which means *coronary artery bypass graft*. Many abbreviations are used in speech among health care professionals. Some common abbreviations you may have heard are UTI, meaning *urinary tract infection*, SOB, meaning *shortness of breath*, CBC, meaning *complete blood count*, and CC, meaning *chief complaint* (Fig. 1.3).

Aside from jargon, the field of medicine itself uses an entire vocabulary unique to its profession. Developed specifically to eliminate confusion over language changes, slang, and regional terms, medical professionals use a distinct vocabulary to refer to human anatomy and physiology, diseases, and procedures. This terminology is based mostly on ancient Greek and Latin words and is used to standardize communication. Think back to the elements of communication discussed earlier in this chapter. When medical professionals use standard words in the message known by both the sender and the receiver, the communication process is complete. Medical language improves patient care, increases efficiency, and reduces potentially fatal errors.

 COMMUNICATION GUIDELINES

Verbal Communication

As a health care professional, your manner of speaking is important in any exchange. The language you use in the workplace must be pleasant, polite, and grammatically correct. Slang and other informal phrases may be fun to use at home or with friends, but *usually* are not appropriate in health care. Speaking in slang and jargon to patients is disrespectful to some and may not even be understandable to others. On the other hand, with some patients, using slang words may be the best or only way to help them understand their health and wellness.

For example, you may ask yourself, "Will this patient understand 'cerebrovascular accident' or should I use 'stroke'?" Patients with higher levels of education will understand and expect correct medical terms; other patients may be confused by the same phrases. Patients from some socioeconomic classes may be intimidated by medical personnel and find it hard to communicate openly; conversely, highly educated patients may intimidate you and keep you from communicating effectively. Knowing this information helps gauge the appropriate questions, responses, and explanations. Chatting with your patient as you establish rapport gives you clues that will help you through the interaction. Listen to your patient's grammatical structure, pronunciation, and general manner of speaking to determine her knowledge, and then use terms she will understand. By listening carefully to a patient, for example, you should be able to determine that patient's regional or cultural background. You may find that colloquialisms

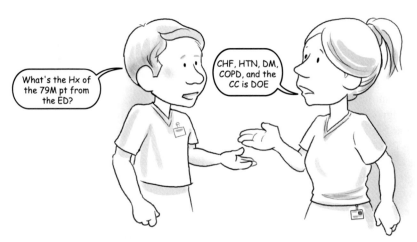

Fig. 1.3 Health care professionals commonly use jargon and abbreviations. In this exchange, one person asks, "What's the history (Hx) of the 79-year-old male (79M) patient (pt) from the emergency department (ED)?" The other person answers, "Congestive heart failure (CHF), hypertension (HTN), diabetes mellitus (DM), chronic obstructive pulmonary disorder (COPD), and the chief complaint (CC) is dyspnea on exertion (DOE)."

are a necessary means of communicating with certain patients. Remember, medical terminology is literally a foreign language, based on Greek and Latin. You would not presume that a Spanish-speaking patient understands English; do not presume that an English-speaking patient understands medical terminology. Are you trying to communicate with the patient or impress the patient with your education? Phrase your communication appropriately without talking down to the patient. Pay attention to non-verbal cues that your message is being received. Your patients may be embarrassed to admit that they do not understand everything you are telling them. Even highly educated patients can struggle to understand medical terminology, and the shorthand we so often use. When patients are under the stress of illness or injury they may find it harder to focus on the message you are trying to send.

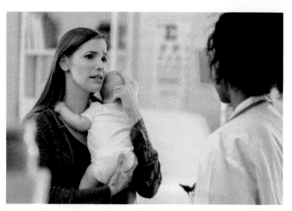

Fig. 1.4 Facial expressions and body language send messages as effectively as spoken words. What is this patient telling us? (iStock.com/Steve Debenport.)

Written Communication

Written communication encompasses all forms of communication that use written language to exchange messages. This includes exchanges between health care professionals, such as in medical record notes and memos, business letters and faxes with other offices, supply vendors, and insurers, as well as patient portal communication between patients and clinical care professionals. Because words are used in the exchange, written communication is considered verbal communication. Clear, concise, accurate communication in any form is important in all areas of health care. Patients generally receive instructions first as verbal communication, as you or the provider explain points of concern regarding health care. Written instructions then reinforce and remind patients of instructions and explanations. If your patient has poor reading skills or has any barrier to communication, verbal or written, and the instructions are not clear, the meaning may be misinterpreted. This in turn may interfere with treatment and delay recovery. You are responsible for making sure that information was received and understood as it was intended.

Nonverbal Communication

Body language—exchanging messages without words—is a form of nonverbal communication. We have all transmitted messages to someone across a room using only significant looks and body language (Fig. 1.4). A range of behaviors is included in the nonverbal categories of *paralanguage*, *kinesics*, and *proxemics*.

Paralanguage

Nonverbal components of an exchange affect the meaning of oral communication. These include non-language sounds and paralanguage, or paralinguistics. Non-language sounds include sighing, humming, chuckling, or laughing. These are sounds in addition to the spoken word. Paralanguage includes quality, volume, pitch, and tone of voice and is applied to the spoken word. Paralanguage and non-language are frequently more important than the verbal exchange. We have less conscious control over paralanguage and non-language (Box 1.1). For example, our voices tend to rise in pitch

BOX 1.1   COMMUNICATING WITH BOTH SIDES OF THE BRAIN

Although we use both halves, or hemispheres, of our brain to communicate, the left side of our brain is responsible for language and logic, and the right side processes emotions. We know that the left side of the brain is linked to the right side of the body, and the right side of the brain is linked to the left side of the body. Therefore, the left side, or language/logic side, seems to have better control of the facial expression on the right side of the face. Conversely, our right brain, or emotional side, controls the left side of the face. Theoretically, in an emotional situation, we are less able to control the muscles on the left side of our face. Observing the whole person—posture, gestures, paralanguage, non-language, etc.—is very important, but if the message seems incongruent, check the left side of the face for the most uncensored message.

when we are tense or upset, no matter how hard we try to appear calm. Our voices may tremble when we are sad or angry, or the quality may sound harsh, even if we try to cover our emotions. Our patients will be equally conflicted in words and underlying emotion and can give us clues to concerns they are reluctant to share during the conversation. If nonverbal cues are inconsistent with the message—called incongruence—there is a breakdown in communication. A patient may not be filling her part of the mutual agreement to exchange truthful information. You will need to spend more time and effort with this patient to determine what she is trying **not** to tell you. We cannot help our patients if we treat only the obvious signs and not the underlying concerns that may not be shared (Fig. 1.5).

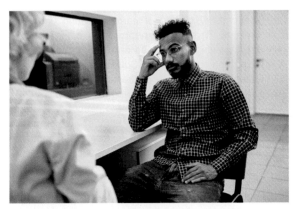

Fig. 1.5 Paralanguage is frequently more truthful than the words we use. If your patient states one thing, but body language shows another, the message is incongruent. This patient tells us he is fine; should we believe that this is true? (From iStock.com/mediaphotos.)

SPOTLIGHT ON SUCCESS

Paralanguage: Tone of Voice

To understand the influence of paralanguage, consider how a patient might interpret a simple statement such as "I'll be with you in a minute" when you vary your voice tone. For example, an impatient tone—with short, clipped speech patterns—implies that you are impatient and far too busy to listen to the patient's concerns. In contrast, a soft, low-pitched voice projects a calm and soothing acceptance and attitude. Try the phrase with emphasis on different words and see how communication is affected by the words or phrases you choose to emphasize. Using paralanguage appropriately increases your communication skills in all areas of interaction and leads to better personal and professional success and satisfaction.

Kinesics

Kinesics involves body movements, such as gestures, posture and body cues, eye movements, and facial expressions. Kinesics reveals inner feelings, such as sadness, happiness, fear, or anger that may not be apparent in the spoken word. In fact, many emotions are expressed best by nonverbal language. Emotions, such as anger, fear, and surprise, usually are projected first and best without words, before we have time to hide our emotions. Gestures also have many meanings. Squirming, shrinking away, and fidgeting may mean intense discomfort, perhaps with your line of questioning, if your patient does not appear to be in obvious physical discomfort. Nodding your head, a common gesture, communicates a positive response and lets patients know you are listening.

With straight posture, heads up, and eyes forward, patients indicate good health and self-esteem; slumped posture with restricted movements and eyes downcast may project pain, ill-health, or poor self-esteem.

Eyes often hint at what we think and feel. Maintaining friendly eye contact with patients shows interest, warmth, and concern. Patients who do not maintain eye contact may be impatient, may lack interest in the topic, or may be overwhelmed by information. As you observe your patients during the communication process, watch closely for messages you read in their eyes. "Eye messages" are hardest to hide and may be easier to read. That being said, keep in mind that this is not a definitive means of communicating. Moreover, patients from cultures other than North America may feel that maintaining eye contact is rude, challenging, or even sexually suggestive. Be careful as you maintain eye contact if your patient seems uncomfortable. Eye contact maintained for too long is inappropriate and disturbing and may be interpreted as staring.

Because some patients try to mask their feelings, nonverbal communication may carry more meaning than verbal communication. Pay attention to what may be unspoken, as well as what is spoken. Remember that facial expressions (Fig. 1.6) are so important in medicine that tribal doctors used elaborately carved facial masks in their healing rituals for more years than current traditional medicine has existed.

Patients also are very aware of your facial and nonverbal reactions to what they say. Watch your body

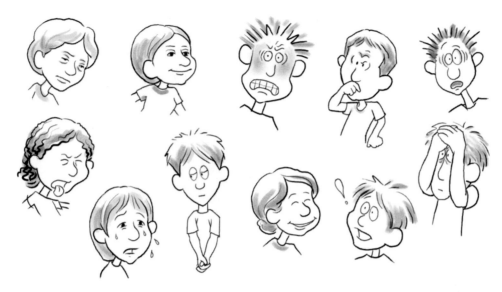

Fig. 1.6 Facial expressions are an important means of communication.

language to resist transmitting closure (i.e., arms crossed over your chest), distance (i.e., leaning away from the patient or turning your back), or rejection (i.e., frowning, looking away). Facial expressions also may cue patients to the response that you expect or would prefer to hear, such as a report that the treatment is working, whether or not this is true. For example, you ask Mrs. Smith if the latest prescription is working and she responds that she does not think it is. If you look surprised, she may change her answer to please you. Many patients try to anticipate what they think you want to hear and will alter their responses to satisfy you. If you register shock or rejection, you may immediately close all channels of communication between you and the patient, and it may be difficult to reestablish a working relationship. Conversely, listening closely, leaning toward the patient during conversation, and smiling improves the communication experience. When used appropriately, smiles are almost universally accepted as a gesture of good will and a means of establishing a friendly rapport.

Proxemics

Proxemics is the study of the physical closeness tolerated by most people, or our spatial relationships with each other. How near or far we place ourselves from others transmits strong messages (Box 1.2). Our dominant culture usually considers the space within approximately 3 feet as personal space, although this varies

---

BOX 1.2 PHYSICAL REACTIONS IN PROXEMICS

Think about how you react as you stand in a line or ride in an elevator. Americans typically step back when a stranger, or even an acquaintance without permission, steps into our personal space. If personal space is reduced for too long, symptoms of stress increase. These include a rise in blood pressure and heart rate, an increase in respirations, and feelings of panic. For the patient who is already stressed by illness or worry, it is important that we restore personal space as soon as possible after care. Proxemics varies significantly among ethnicities, geography, ages, and even religions.

---

among individuals. This space also varies greatly with our relationship to those around us—from a small space for close family members to a wider space for strangers. Stress levels rise significantly and measurably when personal space is invaded without permission.

In the medical setting, our physical distance from patients may be affected by odors, such as poor physical or dental hygiene, decay, or odors associated with certain illnesses. Patients may be upset by smells in the medical setting, such as disinfectants and medicinal scents, particularly if they bring back unpleasant memories of previous medical experiences. Use caution with your own hygiene. Patients may object to the smell of cigarettes or food on you and your clothing and may be uncomfortable with the perfume or body lotion that smells good to you. All of these factors have an impact on interaction with patients in the close-up, hands-on, medical environment.

In certain cases, physical distance may be limited for infection control. For example, if your patient has a communicable disease, direct contact may be limited. Many communicable diseases require physical barriers, such as masks and gloves, which may interfere with facial expressions and with using touch as a communication tool. Methods for overcoming these communication barriers are covered later in Chapter 6.

Even with our highly technological medical environment, we usually need to enter patients' personal space to deliver care. Because some people are uncomfortable when their personal space is invaded, and our patients are already stressed, it is important to develop a therapeutic rapport early in the relationship. Approach patients in a confident and professional manner, introduce yourself, and tell them what you plan to do. Explain the purpose of each step of the procedure. If patients shrink away or act fearful, reassure them that you will allow them to direct the interaction, and that you will stop at any point they indicate discomfort or need more information. *Patients have a right to self-determination and may accept or refuse any contact or treatment if they choose.* Patients do not have to submit to an invasion of their space. Back away when you are finished, unless the patient signals a need for closeness. Be alert to positive or negative signs that let you know the patient accepts you in his or her space. Signs of fear and increased stress usually indicate patients are uncomfortable and that you need to step back; leaning in your direction and maintaining eye contact may mean that they prefer that you offer comfort by staying near. These actions, and a professional attitude, help relieve patients' anxiety regarding care and the manner in which it is provided. Remember, it is important to allow patients to make decisions regarding their personal space and to respect their preferences. If in doubt, seek verbal clarification.

Touch as a Communication Tool

Proxemics, and the concept of spatial relationships, includes touch. Touch is required for procedures related to health care. You may use touch with patients to indicate emotional support or to show concern (Fig. 1.7). There is no better way than touch to demonstrate caring

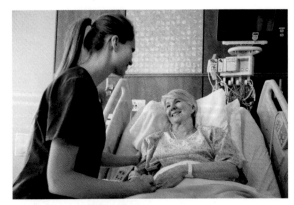

Fig. 1.7 If your patient is receptive, a caring touch helps calm the stress of medical care. (From iStock.com/MonkeyBusinessImages.)

and compassion to those who are "starved" for contact. Remember that some elderly patients are not touched by anyone for long periods of time, which increases their feeling of isolation when their hearing and vision are failing and moves them further away from social interaction. Although some patients welcome a caring touch, others may not be comfortable with physical contact. Touch is personal and cultural; some patients prefer that you not touch them except for treatment purposes. Many feel that touch in a medical setting signals that something unpleasant is about to happen. If you feel the patient will be receptive, offer a comforting touch when nothing invasive or painful is planned.

There is an increased need to use therapeutic touch with a warm and caring hand in our technologically advanced medical setting. However, before using touch as a means of showing concern and compassion, determine by watching the patient whether your touch is welcome. Without permission being granted, touching implies a certain intimacy and establishes power to the one who is touching over the one who is touched. Patients may feel that you will withhold your care and concern if they are honest about not wishing to be touched except for therapeutic care. In certain situations, an unwelcome touch may be considered assault. Therefore, either implied or explicit permission must be granted. For example, a patient who responds to your comforting touch by covering your hand with hers or by leaning toward you, welcomes your touch; conversely, a patient who stiffens, leans away from you or crosses her arms and legs is sending messages that your touch is not welcome (Box 1.3).

BOX 1.3 THERAPEUTIC TOUCH

In medieval Europe and England, the "royal touch" was thought to cure many illnesses. Sick people lined the roadways when the royal procession was scheduled to pass, hoping to touch the hem of the king's robe, or, if one was lucky, to have the king actually reach out and touch a hand or face. It did not seem to matter that the cure rate was understandably extremely low.

We no longer believe in the royal touch, but we do know that babies are more likely to die if they are not held and stroked, and that the elderly have measurably decreased levels of stress and pain if they are stroked and touched gently. Today, many religions, including that of the Navajo and Christianity, practice faith healing through "the laying on of hands." In Islam, the *ruqyah* are performed by placing the right hand on the painful area or on the forehead. The ancient healing practices of touch (reiki) and therapeutic massage are gaining favor in holistic medical practices. The theory holds that the body produces life energy, or "prana." When patients feel prana through touch, healing energy is produced. This energy provides emotional, physical, and spiritual comfort. Some hospitals and practices use these techniques to reduce pain and promote wound healing. A simple, caring touch may be the most therapeutic procedure you can perform for any patient.

▷▷ TAKING THE CHAPTER TO WORK

Using Nonverbal Communication
Jessica is working in a family practice office. She has just walked a young female patient into an examination room. The patient is 15 years old and has an appointment for a Pap test and gynecologic examination. While Jessica takes the patient's blood pressure and pulse, she notices that the patient does not maintain eye contact and is fidgeting and squirming in the chair. Jessica recognizes these kinesics as possible signs of anxiety and nervousness. To help alleviate these feelings, Jessica sits down in a chair next to the patient and begins to communicate with her. Jessica uses touch as a soothing technique. After a few minutes, the patient appears less anxious. Jessica knows that many patients are anxious about undressing, so she decides to have the patient stay dressed and sit in the chair until the physician comes in to talk to her. Jessica communicates her observations to the physician. Working as a team, they are able to reassure the patient and complete the examination without problems. The outcome of this situation would have been very different if Jessica had ignored or not noticed these signs.

COMMUNICATING WITH PATIENTS

Depending on your staff responsibilities, your relationship may be as short term as greeting patients for a one-time visit, or it may be an established relationship for long-term care. In either case, or in any health care situation, the dynamics of communication—how communication works—and the need for exchange remain the same.

Therapeutic relationships are established to benefit either the physical or mental health, or both, of our patients. The relationship is maintained by appropriately focused and respectful interaction and communication that leads to a full understanding of our patients' needs and concerns. Without fully understanding the needs of our patients, we cannot address and work toward correcting their concerns. To obtain an honest and full disclosure, patients must expect that their information will be held in the strictest confidence and will be used only to design a plan of care for their benefit.

Furthermore, there is a strong connection between the quality of patients' relationship with their health care providers and their compliance with prescribed treatment. Patients must respect those in charge of their care. If they do not feel that you have their best interests at heart, they are less likely to follow prescribed care. Communication is the key to the therapeutic relationship.

Steps in the Communication Process

Communication is conducted in steps (Fig. 1.8). The first is the *preparatory, introductory,* or *orientation* step. This step introduces the participants to each other and helps form a mutual agreement to exchange information. Roles and responsibilities are established within the first few moments, usually by implied agreement. There is usually no formal agreement that each participant will perform certain functions in the exchange, but by founding the relationship, each participant agrees to fulfill his or her part of the exchange until the situation is resolved or the interaction comes to an end. For example, if a patient makes a health care request that you can help resolve, the guidelines are implied that the patient will give you all of the information you need to help her or him. By coming to the patient's aid, you imply that you will do everything reasonable to fill the patient's needs. The two of you have reached an informal agreement, which completes the introductory phase.

The second step is the working, or *maintenance,* step. The conversation is focused on the task at hand

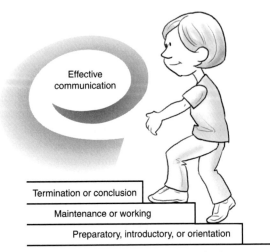

Effective communication

Termination or conclusion

Maintenance or working

Preparatory, introductory, or orientation

Fig. 1.8 The three steps to effective communication.

and works to meet the needs of each participant. Each participant observes the responses of the other for communication cues to determine that all messages are properly received. The health care worker usually directs, or leads, the interaction but should not control it. It is your responsibility to keep the exchange on track—to keep the patient from rambling—but *controlling* the flow interrupts the free and open exchange needed to determine all of the patient's needs. Today, the patient may need to talk about personal problems rather than participate in an intense and comprehensive health history, and you must respect that need while balancing your duties to that patient and to other patients. Helping the patient talk about personal problems may be as therapeutic as any clinical procedure you may perform, but gentle, tactful, probing questions (covered in Chapter 2, Gathering Information) may help guide the patient back on track to direct the conversation toward the patient's immediate health care needs.

The final step is the *termination* or *conclusion*. If the exchange was effective and successful, each party is satisfied that messages were transmitted and received as intended. At the conclusion of the exchange, goals should have been reached, such as determining the patient's current need for care, or, if you are working in an intermediate position, the relationship is transferred to another worker.

All of the steps listed above are involved in any exchange, from a brief conversation as you greet your patients to a complicated transfer of complex medical information over an extended period. If the relationship is long-term, well established, and pleasant for both the patient and you, at its eventual end you may feel a sense of loss, but you should also feel pride in the independence and growth you have helped your patient achieve.

Your Responsibility to the Patient

Before you can communicate effectively with anyone else, you must first communicate with yourself and understand who you are. Every culture, every age, every person you come in contact with will sense whether you genuinely care for his or her welfare, or if your interest is insincere. Box 1.4 outlines a number of questions to ask yourself to help determine whether you are ready for the demands of working in health care. When you can answer these questions honestly and selflessly, you have reached a level of self-awareness that puts the patient's needs before your own.

As you interview or interact with patients, you are responsible for the maintenance step, keeping conversations focused on the topics at hand. Patients should be allowed to talk about any concerns related to their health, but if they begin to ramble from the subject, you should gently move them back to the main concern.

BOX 1.4   ARE YOU READY?

To determine whether you are ready for the demands of health care, ask yourself these questions:

- Do you genuinely like who you are?
- Are you convinced you have made the right career choice?
- Do you mind being up close and personal with people of all ages, races, ethnic groups, and socioeconomic levels?
- Can you accept differences in cultures, religions, races, and morals and see these as interesting alternatives, not as threatening or inferior?
- Are you distant and detached?
- Do you give too much and have nothing left for yourself?
- Can you be firm but gentle when you need to be?
- Can you help your patients find their inner strength and then let go?
- Can you keep your personal life and concerns to yourself?
- If the relationship and rapport break down, can you work to resolve the problem, and then recognize and apologize for your part in it?
- When you find yourself disliking a person, can you determine why and rise above it?
- Do you resent taking orders or submitting to authority?

COMMUNICATION GUIDELINES

Your Responsibilities to the Patient

Your other responsibilities for ensuring good communication include the following points:

- Be familiar with the patient's history and current condition to determine what information is needed with the background already available. You need answers to questions such as: Is this simply an annual examination, or is the visit in response to a life-threatening situation? How ill is the patient now? Is he too sick for effective communication?
- Before you begin, know the goal of the communication—that is, asking about current concerns, offering educational material, transferring information—but be flexible. The patient may have other needs that you discover only after the exchange has begun.
- Check the patient's history for possible barriers to communication, such as English as a second language, hearing impairment, and so on. Do you need an interpreter? Do you need a notepad for a written exchange?
- Be aware of the patient's communication needs. Use common sense and good judgment. Does the patient need to talk today to relieve stress and anxiety, or is a casual conversation enough for today? Is superficial chatter a cover for more important information? If so, can you determine what the patient is trying **not** to tell you?
- Demonstrate courtesy and compassion. Even a brief encounter requires good manners and a caring attitude.
- Phrase your message so that patients can understand. Are you using terms above or below the patient's understanding? Are you trying to interact professionally, or are you trying to impress?
- Remain objective regarding personal and cultural differences. It is not necessary to agree with patients to understand their needs or to provide excellent care. Use your personal differences as a learning opportunity.
- Provide feedback and ask for it in return to be sure the messages were clearly received. Can the patient repeat your instructions satisfactorily and demonstrate understanding them? Did you understand what the patient was trying to tell you? Clarify the message for understanding. Ask or answer as many questions as needed for clarification.
- Validate the patient's feelings. The patient has a right to feel as he or she does: sad, angry, frightened, and so forth.
- Encourage good health care choices and independent care. It is our goal to turn the patient's care over to him or her when the patient is able to care for self. Did you use every opportunity to educate the patient in proper wellness measures?
- Provide learning tools, such as pamphlets (Fig. 1.9) or written instructions for self-care, and be sure they are designed for the patient's needs (see Chapter 3, Educating Patients).

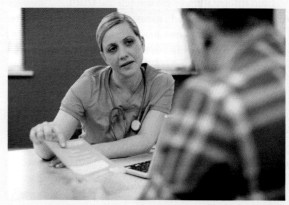

Fig. 1.9 Provide learning tools designed for the patient's level of comprehension. As you go over pamphlets and brochures, check for questions and make sure the patient understands his or her part in recovery. (From iStock.com/Daisy-Daisy.)

LEGAL EAGLE

Communication between patients and health care workers must be honest, ethical, and legal. The following points will help keep you within the proper limits:

- Discuss information only within the guidelines set for your scope of practice. You do not have the training and knowledge for in-depth explanations of complex medical information. Many of the patient's concerns must be handled directly by the provider. Formal procedures through training and common sense should help you determine what you can and cannot discuss with your patients.
- It is not within your scope of practice to inform patients of their diagnosis or prognosis. If patients ask you these questions, refer them to the provider.
- Patient education must follow the provider's instructions and guidelines and may begin only at the provider's direction.
- Diagnostic testing results (i.e., radiology or laboratory) may not be given to patients without the direct permission of the provider.
- Absolutely no patient information can be shared with family members, or with anyone else, without specific patient consent in accordance with regulations.

The Patient's Responsibility to You

Patients should be active partners in any communication or exchange. Each participant shares responsibility in keeping lines of communication open and clear of interference and misunderstanding. Our goal is to include patients in as many decisions as possible to help them feel in control of their health. Passive patients, who simply sit and listen, rarely make a conscious effort to restore or maintain health; they rely on their health care providers to do it for them. Active participants feel at least partially in control and are more likely to follow directions. Active participation begins with a truthful and in-depth interview (see Chapter 2, "Gathering Information"). The patient's responsibilities include the following:

- Being truthful and open regarding concerns. We cannot treat patients effectively and safely if they withhold information or do not tell the truth.
- Providing a full medical history regardless of how reluctant they may be to share potentially embarrassing information. Hiding parts of the health history may result in improper treatment. Health care professionals cannot force information that patients refuse to give, but the provider must be informed of areas that you feel need to be discussed further.
- Participating in independent care as much as possible. Most health care should be self-care.
- Complying with health care directions designed to promote wellness. Patients must do their share to maintain health or to ensure a return to an acceptable level of wellness.

Addressing Your Patient

How you approach your patients gives them clues to observe about you, just as you are observing them. They know quickly how professional you are by your poise, your physical appearance, and your actions. They hope that you will work for their trust and confidence, and that if you do not have answers to all of their questions, you can search for the answers together.

Patients frequently have preformed opinions of health care workers that may interfere with establishing an initial rapport. Some think all health care professionals, except the physician, are there to fill a servant-like role, and these people will look down on anyone other than the physician. Also others are in awe of all health care professionals and expect you to know all of the answers. Work for a balance in your interaction with both types of patients; do not be either overly friendly nor distant and inaccessible. Stress that we are in the health care field for patients, but that our scope of practice does not give any of us all of the answers. Speak respectfully and maintain your professionalism during all interactions to help establish and maintain positive patient relationships.

As you greet your patients, use a proper form of address, for example, "Mr. Green, how are you today?" or "How may we help you, Mrs. Brown?" Never address a patient by his or her first name unless requested to do so by the patient, and **never** use pet names, such as "Honey" or "Sweetie." Children, of course, will not expect to be addressed by their surname, but all adults should be treated with the respect that we show by using surnames. Certain cultures will be offended by familiarity that North Americans see as being friendly. Patients who insist on communicating with you on a first-name basis may not understand the therapeutic nature of the patient–health care professional relationship. This is not a friendship, although you may be genuinely fond of your patients; this is a professional relationship. It may be flattering to have patients try to establish a more personal relationship, but this may interfere with your ability to administer proper care. Try to determine why the patient needs to be addressed on a personal level and wants to move the relationship to a friendship, but maintain your professional distance (Fig. 1.10).

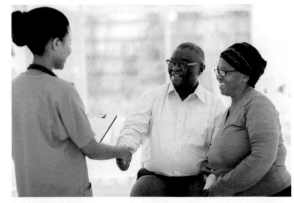

Fig. 1.10 Establishing an open and professional relationship with our patients is essential to proper care. (From iStock.com/michaeljung.)

Never refer to your patient as a medical condition, for example, "the fracture in the treatment room" or "the post-op in Room 3." Patients are understandably stressed and anxious in the health care setting and are sensitive to everything they see and hear (or overhear). If you refer to patients simply as a medical condition, anyone who overhears you will presume you do not care for your patients as individuals.

Maintaining a Professional Distance

Interaction and communication are affected by our emotional involvement with others. For example, we interact differently with our parents, our significant other, our children, and our friends, and each interaction is more intimate on many levels than our response to acquaintances and persons in the workplace. Communication and interaction in the health care setting must be conducted on a level that allows us to work closely with patients, observe their care and condition effectively, and provide opportunities for patient teaching. Professional distance allows us to work with patients while maintaining a therapeutic relationship. The focus must be on patients, not on our concerns; never share confidences with patients about your personal life that might shift the dynamics of the relationship to a more personal level. Patients have their own concerns and should not be burdened with yours. If your patient tries to engage in a personal exchange, briefly, politely, and truthfully (if appropriate) answer just that question—never answer rudely—but quickly and firmly turn the topic back to health care. If you find yourself trying to establish friendships with patients, step back and determine why you are searching for friendship among your patients, rather than in a more proper social environment. Recognize that it would be extremely difficult to give effective care to a friend, and search for your friends outside of the medical setting.

Sympathy, Empathy, and Compassion

Closely linked to the concept of professional distance are the expressions of *sympathy* and *empathy*. Sympathy implies that you care and that you are concerned for another; empathy means experiencing the same feelings as another person. In other words, sympathy usually means feeling sorry for someone. Sympathy does not require that we identify with the patient and is usually an expression of sharing the pain. Empathy means understanding at a deep level what the patient feels usually because we, as individuals, have experienced the same or very similar circumstances.

Empathy is the suspension of our own perceptions and, at least for a time, feeling what the patient feels. We may feel sorry for or sympathize with a patient who is dying and may distance ourselves. When we empathize, we imagine how it would feel to *be* the patient. To achieve or develop an empathetic character, set aside preconceptions and open your mind to personal differences and perceptions. We each react differently to pain, loss, sickness, and suffering. We do not have to change our firmly held beliefs and values to genuinely care for our patients, but we must understand that differences do exist and work around these differences.

Empathizing helps us recognize a patient's fear and discomfort so that we do everything possible to provide support and reassurance in the form of compassion. When we are compassionate, we feel a deep need to relieve the concerns of the patient. Because we feel the same pain, or know the patient is suffering, we do all in our power to provide comfort and care. Compassion means taking action to reduce the patient's distress. We must be sincerely committed to the need to relieve suffering to put ourselves in the position of caring.

Sharing a patient's suffering may open us to pain, and can be exhausting. It is possible to experience "compassion fatigue" when we are off-balance with the care we provide to others and the care we provide to ourselves. This can have both physical and emotional consequences, affecting our physical and mental health. Compassion fatigue is discussed in detail in Chapter 7, Communicating through the Grief Process.

⏩ TAKING THE CHAPTER TO WORK

Sympathy and Empathy

Jamie enters Mrs. Quinn's room planning to help her with her morning bath. Jamie noticed that Mrs. Quinn had been crying. Jamie knew that earlier that morning Mrs. Quinn had been told her cancer, which had been in remission, had returned, and she would have to undergo a new course of chemotherapy. Jamie set her bath supplies down on the chair and sat on the bed next to Mrs. Quinn. Because she had cared for her for several days Jamie felt comfortable putting her arm over Mrs. Quinn's shoulder and comforting her.

"I can appreciate this has to be a very difficult time for you. You beat cancer once and now you have to try and do it all over again. I can only imagine how difficult that must be to hear, and I am very sorry this has happened." Jamie then simply sat with Mrs. Quinn for a few minutes while Mrs. Quinn quietly wept and spoke of her fear of the long and difficult road ahead. Jamie responded with encouragement, but was cautious not to offer false assurances. "You know you won't be going through this alone, your family will continue to be a great source of support, and we will do everything possible to help you get through this. Please let us know if you feel overwhelmed, or if you have questions about your care." Mrs. Quinn smiled and thanked Jamie for her encouragement and kind words. Jamie and Mrs. Quinn continued talking as she changed her bed and helped her with her bath.

Learning From Communication Failures

If problems developed during your communication and your efforts to help a patient were not effective, mentally review the exchange. What could you have done differently? Were there factors in the interaction that blocked the communication flow, or disrupted the communication agreement with the patient? Or did you form a bond that was not appropriate for proper health care?

🔒 COMMUNICATION GUIDELINES

Learning From Communication Failures

To establish a better working relationship or rapport with the patient, try these suggestions at each contact:

- Avoid clichéd statements. "You'll be just fine" sounds false, diminishes the patient's concerns, and may sound suspiciously like a guarantee, which could lead to legal action.
- Do not offer false reassurance. Explain the health care plan and its possible benefits, but do not offer unrealistic hope. Again, the patient may assume this promises that he or she will improve, when this may not be the case.
- Avoid using idioms.
- If patients need to talk about themselves and their situation, do not change the subject immediately, even to redirect it to the topic at hand. You may discover issues that are affecting their health and that need attention. You might miss these concerns with tightly focused questioning. However, if patients begin to ramble too far from the need for health care, gently nudge them toward the current problem.
- Do not moralize. It is not our place to impose our values on our patients. Try to understand patients even if you do not agree.
- Avoid leading questions that suggest the answer that you want, such as, "You are taking your medicine, aren't you?" Many patients want to agree with you and will give you an answer they think you expect.

- Do not cue patients by your facial expressions or other kinesics. If they sense that the direction of the message is uncomfortable for you, they may stop trying to communicate.
- Control your tone of voice to convey sincerity and compassion without overdoing it. Sugary, flowery tones and language sound false (see Spotlight on Success box).
- Allow patients to make suggestions for their care; they know their situation better than you and may have good ideas. If you have self-esteem and a solid self-concept, you should not be threatened by changes in health care plans to meet your patients' needs.
- Sequence your questions from less complex or general, to more complex and specific. "How are you today?" should progress to questions such as "Can you describe the problem?" (This is covered in Chapter 2, Gathering Information.)
- If you cannot answer a question, be truthful. You will be more credible and professional for admitting that you do not have all of the answers than if you try to respond to a question for which you have no answer.

Observing these factors in communication and genuinely caring for your patients should result in relationships that lead to better health and that challenge and reward you as a professional.

⟩⟩ TAKING THE CHAPTER TO WORK

Avoiding Assumptions

Joe worked in a cardiac catheterization laboratory. His new patient was a nurse, which he found to be a little intimidating. When Joe went in to meet his patient for the first time he was very careful to present himself professionally, and discuss the plan of care using sophisticated medical terminology. His patient nodded as if she understood, so Joe continued his highly technical explanation. When at the end of his explanation he asked if she had any questions and she shook her head no, Joe assumed she had understood everything that was to be done. He left the room satisfied he had done a good job explaining the procedures.

When the physician went in to begin treatment, he realized the patient was confused about what procedures he was going to perform, and did not have a firm grasp of the plan of care. Joe knew he had gone over all of this with the patient, but realized when he listened to the patient and physician discussing the treatment that he had assumed a level of understanding that the nurse did not possess. The nurse had been working in a pediatrician's office for the last 20 years, and was not at all familiar with what was involved in cardiac catheterization. The patient had been embarrassed to admit to Joe that she did not understand what he had told her. He had assumed because she was a nurse she should understand his explanation, so she had simply nodded her understanding.

This was a great learning experience for Joe. He no longer assumed that just because a patient was another health care professional that patient would know all about his particular area of expertise. In future interactions with patients he made sure to ask about their familiarity with specific procedures, and gauged his explanations on their responses, rather than on their title.

Except in cases of a terminally ill or declining patient, independence in health care is the purpose of therapeutic interaction. When the patient can get better, avoid establishing a dependent relationship with the patient; your goal, and the patient's, should be independence and self-care. The patient should be free and competent to make proper health care choices and perform his or her own care independent of your skills. You must have a strong self-concept and be able to let go of your need to encourage the patient's dependence on you. If your interaction with the patient did not establish a therapeutic relationship, learn from it for the future.

CHECKING YOUR COMPREHENSION

Write a brief answer for each of the following assignments.

1. Define rapport and explain its importance to health care delivery.
2. Why is confidentiality important in health care?
3. What are the five elements of communication discussed in this chapter?
4. What are slang and jargon, and why should these terms be avoided in health care communication. Can you think of any occasions when either should be used?
5. Define and compare the terms kinesics and proxemics. Give two examples of each.
6. What is meant by the phrase therapeutic touch? How is touch used in the medical profession?
7. Explain the three steps to effective communication.
8. List five of your responsibilities in the communication process.
9. List four of your patient's responsibilities in the communication process.
10. How does sympathy differ from empathy? What is the relationship of sympathy and empathy to compassion?

EXPANDING CRITICAL THINKING

1. You explained to Mr. Brown how to collect a first voided specimen, but the next day you received a stool sample in the urine container. Why do you think Mr. Brown misunderstood your instructions? Was the message received as intended? Was the message in a form he could interpret? How could you have made sure that he understood? How should you respond to him when he presents you with the wrong specimen? Whose fault is it that he misunderstood?
2. Mrs. Simmons is in a moderately advanced stage of Alzheimer's disease and has very limited responses

to conversation and stimulus. You know, however, that you must talk to her as if she understands, as you would with any patient. You explain to her what you must do for her at each step of the procedure.

Response A. Her eyes follow your movements with mild interest, but she makes no other response.

Response B. You receive no response from her throughout the procedure, even to fairly unpleasant stimuli.

Which component of the communication flow is missing in Response B? Is more than one component missing? Can Response A be considered verification that she received your message?

3. List 10 examples of nonverbal communication you experienced today. Examples may include a smile from a friend, a message on a T-shirt, a yawn from your spouse. Next to each of these items, indicate the following:
   a. Did you respond positively or negatively to the communication?
   b. Do you think the sender of the message intended for you to have that response?

4. Body language and nonverbal cues carry as many messages as the spoken word. Read the following and identify the cues the person is sending, then answer the accompanying questions. "Fie, fie upon her! There's language in her eyes, her cheek, her lip. Nay, her foot speaks; her wanton spirits look at every joint and motive in her body." (William Shakespeare in "Troilus and Cressida")
   a. How has communication changed in the past 400 years? 100 years?
   b. How do you think it will change in the next 400 years? 100 years?
   c. What do you think Shakespeare meant by the above description?
   d. Rewrite the description in today's terms.

5. List five common idioms that you hear or say frequently. Write the literal meaning and then the intended meaning. Draw a picture or cartoon illustrating the idiom.

6. Do you consider yourself a positive or a negative personality? Name five of your positive and five of your negative traits. Have a family member or good friend make a list for you and compare the two.

7. Write a brief paragraph describing how you think others see you.

8. List ways to increase your self-esteem. Now list ways to increase someone else's self-esteem.

9. Plan an initial interaction as you get to know the following patients. What will you talk about to establish rapport?
   a. An elderly widower who lives alone with no close family.
   b. An HIV-positive former drug addict who has been drug free for more than a year.
   c. An HIV-positive prostitute in the early stages of AIDS.
   d. A young mother of four who suspects she is pregnant again and does not want another child.
   e. A 5-year-old Hispanic boy who speaks very little English and is clinging to his mother who speaks almost no English.
   f. A 45-year-old woman whose latest breast biopsy indicates that her cancer has returned.

10. Considering proxemics, should there be a difference between the professional distances of men to men, women to men, women to women? How do you feel when a male doctor stands close to you? Or a female doctor? Are you comfortable standing close to the opposite sex in a professional situation? How do you seal yourself off in a public place—with books, bags, folded arms, etc.? Do you sit in the same seat each class session? Do you look for a seat near or far from other students?

Gathering Information

Jaime Nguyen

CHAPTER OUTLINE

LEARNING OBJECTIVES

Upon successfully completing this chapter, you will be able to

1. Define the patient interview and explain its purpose.
2. List practices to prepare for a successful patient interview.
3. Contrast subjective and objective information.
4. Differentiate between open-ended questions and closed-ended questions and give examples of both.
5. Discuss the tools used to gather patient information.
6. Discuss active listening.
7. List the types of responses that support effective communication.
8. Discuss the importance of summarizing patient information.

KEY TERMS

acronym a word formed by the initial letters of a series of words

active listening a communication technique using the full attention of the listener to comprehend, respond to, and remember what the speaker is communicating

algorithm a step-by-step procedure for solving a problem using a logical progression

chief complaint a statement made by a patient describing the most significant or serious reason for concern

clarify to remove confusion

closed-ended question a question with a limited set of possible answers

cuing inadvertently eliciting an answer by giving positive or negative feedback that signals what the questioner expects or wants to hear

gate, gating to consciously block the reception of sensory stimuli, such as hearing or pain

leading question a question that encourages or expects a certain answer

objective in the patient interview, observed and measurable information

open-ended question a question for which the respondent must give a longer, freeform answer

paraphrase to restate in other words than originally transmitted, usually to make a meaning clear

reflective response a statement confirming that you received the message and leaving room for the patient to complete his or her thought or sentence or to explore it further

subjective the which is known or experienced only to the individual

summarize to restate in a briefer form

---

⑦ TEST YOUR COMMUNICATION IQ

Before reading this chapter, take this short self-assessment test. Decide which statements are true and which are false.

1. It is important to review the patient's medical history before beginning an interaction.
2. Patient responses give you subjective information.
3. The chief complaint is always the first thing a patient brings up at the time of the interview.
4. "Do you have nausea, vomiting, and diarrhea?" is the best question to ask a patient with abdominal pain.
5. "You are taking your medicine, aren't you?" is a good method in evaluating patient compliance.
6. Periods of silence may help a confused patient gather his or her thoughts.
7. Gating is an essential skill to develop when interviewing patients.

Results

Statements 3, 4, and 5 are false. All other statements are true. How did you do? Read the chapter to find out more about these topics.

THE PATIENT INTERVIEW

The patient interview is one of the most common tasks a health care professional has, and it is also one of the most critical steps in the patient care workflow. The patient interview is a conversation between a health care professional and patient with the goal of obtaining important and relevant patient information to improve the well-being of the patient. The information compiled during the patient interview is used to help diagnose any diseases and conditions, manage current diseases, provide treatment plans, and address any questions and issues the patient may have.

A comprehensive patient interview often includes inquiring about the patient's past and current medical history, medications, and family and social history. Although a patient interview may vary based on the patient's condition and the clinical setting, the basic components are

- Chief or presenting complaint
- History of presenting complaint, including any treatment and referrals
- Past medical history, including previous diseases and surgeries
- Medication history, including over-the-counter medication and any known allergies
- Family history, including those of parents, siblings, and children
- Social history: smoking, alcohol, drugs, accommodation and living arrangements, marital status, and occupation
- Review of systems: cardiovascular system, respiratory system, gastrointestinal system, nervous system, musculoskeletal system, genitourinary system

Having a thorough and accurate patient interview will lay the foundation for the patient examination, what the next steps should be, and the subsequent treatment plan.

Additionally, how we ask questions is often more important than what we ask. A health care professional's tone of voice, facial expressions, and body language will play a critical role in the patient interview. The clinical setting must also make the patient feel comfortable and safe to share personal information.

For students beginning their clinical experience, conducting the patient interview may be one of the most difficult skills to master. It often takes practice and patience, and it will take years of experience to ultimately master. On average, health care professionals conduct more than 200,000 patient interviews over the lifetime of their careers (Davidoff, 1996). It also takes flexibility and critical thinking because the line of questioning must change based on the patient's answers.

This leads to the question: "How will I know what to ask?" Unfortunately, there is no single best answer. The questions needing to be asked in a patient interview are as different as the presenting illnesses and the patients themselves. For example, you ask Mr. Martin, "How may we help you today?" and he answers, "I think I have the flu." This simple response should lead you to a line of inquiry that will help you confirm the diagnosis and what the treatment plan will be. However, the line of inquiry or type of questions asked would be different if Mr. Martin is young and healthy compared with whether he is elderly with chronic diseases, such as hypertension and diabetes mellitus. Every question and every response will be as individual as each patient's history and current concern. A health care professional skilled in patient interviews learns to follow a logical progression from the simplest "What can we do for you?" or "What brings you here today?" to the most probing, in-depth evaluation of the patient's problem.

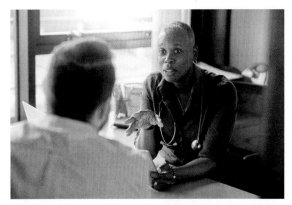

Fig. 2.1 Sitting comfortably face-to-face with your patient helps create a more open and friendly interaction. (iStock.com/sturti.)

SETTING THE STAGE

Although patient information may be gathered based on various patient contacts, such as by phone or by written communication, most are based on direct patient interactions. Thus, this text presumes that you and the patient are meeting face-to-face and sharing a verbal exchange.

As discussed earlier, the health care setting should be professional and friendly, not cold and sterile. Warm, bright colors and a comfortable setting will help put patients at ease. The setting should be private to ensure confidentiality and should limit interruptions so as not to disrupt the flow of the conversation.

When you call patients back into the examination room or when you first meet your patients, you should warmly welcome them and greet them by their names. Always use your patient's surname and title, such as Mr. Smith or Mrs. Jones, unless expressed permission is given for first names. As a matter of respect, it is not a good idea to place the relationship on such a personal, first-name basis. Then, introduce yourself and identify your specific role. Watch your patient's body language for cues about whether to shake hands. Some patients are eager to shake hands and comfortable doing so; others prefer not to. At times a handshake is inappropriate because of the patient's physical condition, such as when a person is bedridden or very weak. In these instances, a touch on the arm or shoulder may serve the same purpose and go a long way toward establishing a therapeutic relationship. However, there are a growing number of health care professionals and organizations pushing to "ban" the handshake or any

unnecessary patient contact to prevent the spread of communicable disease (Sklansky, 2014).

Once you have greeted the patient, sit at the patient's level, face-to-face (Fig. 2.1). If it is culturally acceptable to the patient, maintain eye contact (see Chapter 4). Sit in a comfortably relaxed and open position, as your body language will speak even before you do. For example, crossed arms may communicate rejection and defensiveness; a rigid posture may be intimidating; and slouching may appear unprofessional. Show your interest by appropriate facial and nonverbal expressions, such as smiling and nodding. Throughout the patient interview, show an active interest in the patient, which will help establish trust and encourage honest and open communication. Practice good personal hygiene and proper grooming to make a good impression and to establish or maintain rapport and respect for your professionalism (see the Spotlight on Success box).

SPOTLIGHT ON SUCCESS

A Professional Appearance

You never get another chance to make a first impression and, unfortunately, a bad first impression is hard to change. If you are neat, clean, and organized, patients and other health care professionals are more likely to respect you and your professionalism. They will feel you are more knowledgeable compared with others who are disorganized and unprofessional. Patients tend to feel more relaxed and communicate more freely with someone they feel is professional. Professionals with these skills are more likely to be trusted with responsibility and to advance in their careers.

WORDS AT WORK

In this scenario, Nicole, the certified nursing assistant (CNA), properly greets the patient and introduces herself:

Nicole: Hello Ms. Zhou, my name is Nicole, I'm a CNA here on the floor.

Patient: Hi, Nicole, it's nice to meet you. Please call me Cynthia.

SPOTLIGHT ON SUCCESS

Limiting Patient Wait Time

An important part of creating a favorable setting for the patient interview is limiting wait time. Wait time is generally defined as the number of minutes from the time patients check-in and when they are taken back to an examination room. Although wait times may vary based on location and specialty, the average wait time is 18 minutes and 13 seconds. Studies have shown that long wait times negatively impacted patient satisfaction (Xie & Or, 2017). Of patients, 30% reported leaving their medical appointments and 20% of patients have switched physicians because of long wait times (Larson, 2018). Long wait times will also make patients more agitated and the health care professional more rushed during the patient interview, potentially missing crucial information that may aid in the patient's care.

GATHERING INFORMATION

Once a respectful, private, and welcoming environment is set for the patient interview, you must next ask the right questions to gather the information needed for diagnosis and treatment with the most efficient use of time. In the patient interview, it is your job to obtain from the patient the reason for seeking health care services. Why is the patient here? What problem(s) does he or she have?

A full assessment of a patient's current health issues involves two kinds of information: subjective and objective. Subjective information is open to personal interpretation and what is known or experienced only to the patient. What is fast or slow, large or small, will vary from person to person. One patient may describe a wound as very large, whereas another may think of it as small. The subjective information is the patient's symptoms and the current complaint, or why the patient is present today.

TABLE 2.1   Examples of Subjective and Objective Information

Subjective	Objective
Nausea	Blood pressure
Fatigue	Respiration rate
Pressure	Heart rate
Headache	Height and weight
Chills	Body temperature

Objective information measures or closely describes the situation with no room for interpretation or errors. Objective information is what we can see, measure, and determine for ourselves, such as vital signs, the size of a laceration, or the extent and appearance of a rash. For example, a patient complaining about a headache and the information regarding its duration is subjective information. The information from taking a patient's blood pressure is objective information. In objective terms, the patient's wound is not very large or small, it is three centimeters. Table 2.1 contains examples of subjective and objective information. Both subjective and objective components are necessary to reach a diagnosis and plan a course of treatment.

Often the patient interview begins with documenting the subjective information from patients. Subjective information is not usually something an observer can see, so we must rely on the patient for information. It may include itching or burning of the rash; how much the laceration hurts, how it happened, and what has been done so far; how the fever or hypertension feels, how long either has been elevated, and how he or she has treated it to this point.

The first and most important subjective information will be the chief complaint. The chief complaint, abbreviated as CC, is generally the reason why the patient presents or the reason for the medical visit. Before you begin, review your patient's chart and his or her chief complaint, if you have on hand the reason for the visit. Oftentimes the patient reports this before the patient visit, either when making the appointment or on arrival and during the patient intake. Knowing the patient's background and medical history shows that you are interested and concerned, and it gives you an idea of the kind of questions you should ask to address his or her current concern.

The chief complaint is the initial focus of the patient interview and should direct your opening line of questions. The depth and detail of the patient interview will vary depending on the patient's chief complaint. For many chief complaints, certain basic information should be obtained:

- Onset of the problem
- Location of the complaint
- Duration of the problem
- Quality of the pain, such as sharp, dull, or throbbing

Thus, the types of questions you ask should help you focus on the patient assessment and physical examination, narrow down the patient's diagnosis, and develop a treatment plan. In many situations, a patient may have scheduled an appointment for a specific concern (his or her chief complaint) only for you to discover during the interview that the patient's issue is more serious than what was initially presented. For example, your patient's chief complaint is a headache. We know that a headache can be the presenting complaint or symptom for many medical conditions. You may begin with a line of questions regarding the duration of the headache, how it feels (steady, throbbing, etc.), what he has done for it so far, what other symptoms the patient is experiencing. During the interview, you may discover that the patient is under a lot of stress at work and is not handling it well. Your assessment of his vital signs tells you that his blood pressure is dangerously high and may be a result of the work stress. Without a thorough and detailed interview and supporting health evaluation, you may miss the main reason that he is experiencing a headache. Keep an open mind as you conduct your patient interview to determine what may be the most important health issues.

In the patient interview, all the information we gather by observation and measurement is considered objective. For example, we document our observations regarding the appearance of a rash, the condition of a laceration, and the measurement of a fever or a blood pressure.

Sometimes patient information can be both subjective and objective at the same time. For example, a patient states that she feels chills (subjective) and you notice her shaking (objective). Or, a patient says he has abdominal pain (subjective) and he is crouched over and clutching his abdomen (objective).

Pain is reported as subjective, because health care professionals cannot observe or sense it for the patient. The only way to measure it is to ask the patient to assign a number on a pain scale (Fig. 2.2). However, there has been much discussion whether it should also be considered objective. In 2001, in an effort to better manage patient's chronic pain, the Joint Commission, the organization that accredits more than 21,000 health care organizations and programs in the United States, recommended that pain be considered a "fifth vital sign" with blood pressure, respiration rate, heart rate, and body temperature (Baker, 2017). The policy hoped to encourage health care providers to ask patients about their pain and to help them better manage it. However, since then, many organizations, including the American Medical Association, have recommended the removal of pain as the "fifth vital sign" in professional medical standards because it cannot be measured as blood pressure or temperature can (Frieden, 2016).

 WORDS AT WORK

Subjective and Objective Information

Nicole has reviewed the patient's chart and learns that Cynthia Zhou is in the office for neck pain. She wants to gather subjective information about the onset, location, duration, and quality of her symptoms.

Nicole: Can you tell me when the pain started?

Cynthia: About two weeks ago. I was having trouble starting the lawnmower with the pull cord when suddenly my neck felt like it got zapped.

Nicole: I see. Where exactly on your neck?

Cynthia: The left side, mostly. *(Cynthia points to the place where it hurts.)*

Nicole: Is the pain confined to the left side of your neck or does it radiate anywhere?

Cynthia: Mostly there. My left shoulder hurts a little as well.

Nicole: I understand, your left shoulder hurts a little too. Does it get worse with activity, or is it worse at different times of the day?

Cynthia: Yes, I think it's always worse in the morning.

Nicole: In the morning, alright. Is it a stabbing pain, or more of a burning, or…?

Cynthia: It felt like a shock at first, but not it's more like a severe ache.

PAIN MEASUREMENT SCALE

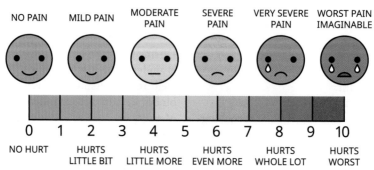

Fig. 2.2 Example of a pain evaluation scale. Because pain perception is subjective and varies significantly from one patient to another, pain assessment tools help simplify documentation. Although some patients tolerate high levels of pain with few complaints and highly reactive patients who confuse discomfort with pain, scales such as this one help maintain a level of consistency and conformity in recording pain. (iStock.com/lukpedclub.)

▶▶ TAKING THE CHAPTER TO WORK

Now, let's meet Sandra and see how she applies this chapter information in the workplace.

Mrs. Archer presents at her appointment complaining of feeling feverish, having body aches, and coughing. Sandra asks her a number of different questions, including any changes in diet and medication, when the symptoms began, and the pattern of the symptoms. Sandra documents Mrs. Archer's responses and her symptoms. She then proceeds to the physical examination where she takes Mrs. Archer's vital signs, which include body temperature, to better assess her feelings of fever, and respiration rate to hear if there are any issues with her ability to breathe. Blood is taken for laboratory work to perform a complete blood count. The vital signs and laboratory results are objective, measured information that better confirms the diagnosis of the flu.

✳ LEGAL EAGLE

Many highly sensitive and confidential conversations regarding patients occur throughout the day in the health care setting. Remember that patient communication, treatments, diagnoses, prognoses, and other communications must never be discussed outside of the medical facility or with anyone in the facility not involved in a patient's care. Patient information may be shared only with the patient's consent and on a "need-to-know" basis. Written consent is required before any information is released to anyone other than those directly involved in the patient's immediate care. Sharing information without the patient's expressed consent is illegal and may result in legal action against you and your employer.

Getting to the Point

The most direct way to gather specific information is to ask questions that require patients to structure their answers. These are called open-ended questions. Open-ended questions usually ask "what," or "how," which encourage the patient to fully express any possible concerns and does not restrict an answer to "yes" or "no" responses. They promote discussion between the health care professional and the patient. These types of questions also help patients organize their thoughts and relay them efficiently and effectively. Examples of open-ended questions are

- "*What* are your symptoms?"
- "*Who* do you live with?"
- "Describe *what* happened next."
- "*What* do you like about this treatment?"
- "*How* is school going?"
- "*How* did you feel when it happened?"

If possible, avoid questions asking "why?" "Why" questions may imply that the patient did something wrong and he or she may become defensive and stop trying to communicate. For example, do not ask, "*Why* didn't you take your medicine?" If you must ask "why" questions, phrase them so they do not sound like accusations.

Closed-ended questions are questions that elicit short, direct answers from a limited set of possibilities, such as "How many pills did you take?" or "What was the date of your last menstrual period?" These types of questions may be needed after a series of open-ended questions.

A combination of open-ended and closed-ended questions are needed to compile patient information (Box 2.1).

BOX 2.1 OBTAINING A HISTORY

Talking with patients to determine a current history requires many of the following questions:

- "How may we help you?"
- "Can you describe the....(pain, sensation, bleeding, etc.)?"
- "How long has this been bothering you (or going on, etc.)?"
- "What happened to cause you to ask for help? Did it get worse, bother you more, etc.?"
- "Has it happened in the past? What did you do about it that time?"
- "Does anything make it better or worse?"
- "Have you taken anything?" or "What are you taking?"
- "How much....?" "How many....?" "How often....?"

Remember that many responses are subjective, or experienced only by the patient and cannot be measured. For example, extreme pain to one patient may be simply discomfort to another. A small amount of blood to one patient may be profuse hemorrhage to another. Thus, closed-ended questions help clarify responses, such as exactly how much blood, or registering pain on a scale of 1 to 10 (see Fig. 2.2).

Leading the Way

If the conversation lags or if the patient seems to drift from the line you need to pursue, it is important to bring the focus back by using leads such as, "You were saying....", or "And then what happened?" Be careful about diverting the patient from a direction he or she feels the need to follow. Allow the patient to lead the conversation, within reason, and it may bring out information you may not have gathered by tightly focused questioning.

Leading the line of questions to gather specific information, however, is not the same as asking *leading questions*. A leading question is one that encourages or expects a certain answer. For example, "You are taking your medicine, aren't you?" probably will lead to a positive answer even if the patient stopped taking the medication some time ago. A more productive *sequence*, or order of questions, might be "What medicines are you taking now?" followed by "How are you taking these medicines?" This type of questioning may also uncover misunderstandings as patients explain their health care routine to you. If you assume that patients are following their treatment plans correctly and simply ask for assurance that they understand what is expected, you

may not discover that they do not understand important points about self-care or managing their medical care.

Be especially careful of leading questions based on your own biases. For example, avoid questions such as, "You have never had unprotected sex, have you?" or "You have never used IV drugs, right?" Instead, you might ask, "Have you ever had unprotected sex?" or "Have you ever used IV drugs?" When the questions are asked without preconceived notions or judgment, patients are more likely to answer truthfully. You have established a nonthreatening, accepting attitude that lets patients know that you will not judge them for their answers (see Legal Eagle box).

Some patients may be suggestible. If you must prompt the patient by offering leads, give him or her a wide range of choices. For example, you might ask, "Mr. Martin, how long have you felt this pain?" If he answers vaguely, "I don't remember." Offer suggestions such as, "Would you say several days, two weeks, a month, or longer?" Or you may ask, "Mrs. Jones, how much blood do you think you saw: a cup, a half-cup, a tablespoon, or a teaspoon, more or less?" If your choice range is too limited, patients may believe there are no other options, giving you an inaccurate answer.

Similarly, avoid cuing the patient's answers by inadvertently giving positive or negative feedback. For example, you ask the patient "Do you think the treatment is working?" and the patient answers, "No, I'm not any better." If you follow up with the question, "Are you sure?" the patient may presume the first response is not what you wanted to hear. As a result, the patient may change his or her response to whatever he or she thinks you want to hear.

COMMUNICATION GUIDELINES

Leading the Way

- Start with general questions, such as "How may we help you today?" and work toward more probing questions. Working from simple to complex gives you time to establish rapport and trust with the patient.
- Avoid compound questions or when more than one question is combined in what seems to be a single question. For example, instead of asking "Do you have nausea, vomiting, and diarrhea?" ask one question for each symptom. Otherwise, the patient may give a positive answer when the patient has only nausea and vomiting.
- Although you must lead the line of questioning to determine the reason for the patient's visit, avoid leading the answers.
- Listen attentively and stay focused on the conversation. Patients are aware when you are not listening or are distracted.

This is not effective, therapeutic communication and may lead to an inaccurate diagnosis and improper treatment.

If the patient's past and current history are not fully and accurately captured, vital information may be missed, which may require backtracking and a delay in diagnosing and treating the patient. Thus, the goal is to know as much as possible about a patient by gathering information effectively before any procedure begins.

Information-Gathering Tools

To make gathering information more effective and efficient and to ensure that all necessary points are covered, some specialties develop algorithms for specific complaints (Fig. 2.3). An algorithm is a process or, in this case, a series or path of questions to follow, depending on the patient's answer at each step. For example, if the answer to a specific question is "yes," a suggestion for the next question follows. If the answer is "no," the next question follows a different path. Algorithms works well in many instances, but may not allow for individual responses. An algorithm system may be too focused for individual patients or too general for a focused interview. However, an algorithm may, at least, prompt the health care professional down a general direction of questioning that may help in the patient interview.

Another effective tool to help in the patient interview is the use of acronyms. An acronym is a simple phrase or word formed from the initial letters or groups of letters of words in a set phrase or series of words. The purpose of acronyms is to simplify a series of words or to help us more easily remember the words. For example, Box 2.2 shows an acronym—MDVISIT—that is used for a routine medical visit with a health care provider. Although the acronym will help remind you of questions to ask, it is important to remember that even the best acronym or algorithm will not replace your responsibility to adjust your questions based on what you see or hear during the patient interview.

Listening to What You Hear

Listening is often more important than speaking in a patient interview. Additionally, hearing and listening are very different concepts. Hearing is simply the sensory perception of sound and is usually passive. Hearing requires almost no focused involvement. Listening, however, means paying close

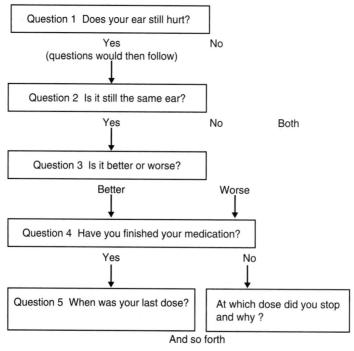

Fig. 2.3 Example of an interviewing or questioning algorithm for a check-up visit after an ear infection.

BOX 2.2   ACRONYM

This is an example of a common acronym used for a general visit.

Medications—Are you taking any prescribed medications or over-the-counter (OTC) preparations? Can you list them? How and when do you take each one? Do you need refills?

Diet—Describe your normal day's diet. How is your appetite? Have you lost or gained weight recently?

Visits—Have you visited another health care provider or been in the emergency department (ED)(or emergency room [ER]) since the last time we saw you?

Injuries—Have you had any injuries/falls/accidents recently? Describe what happened.

Symptoms—Are you experiencing any new problems/symptoms?

Information—Do you have questions regarding your medical care?

Treatments—How are you performing the treatments the provider discussed on your last visit?

attention to what is being said or heard (Box 2.3). Active listening is a communication technique using the full attention of the listener to comprehend, respond to, and remember what the speaker is communicating. It requires recognizing the significance of both verbal and nonverbal communication and it involves focused perception and attentive body language on the part of the listener. Although much of what we hear does not require that we listen actively, all that we hear during patient interaction requires that we listen with close

BOX 2.3   HOW WE LISTEN

How do we listen? There are different forms of listening for different situations:

- Directed—a specific transfer of information; may not require evaluation of cues
- Attentive—gathering information for careful consideration, as in taking a medical history
- Pleasurable—for no purpose except enjoyment; includes music and story-telling
- Courteous—because it is the right thing to do; may not be very attentive
- Passive—simply hearing sounds in passing and easily ignored

A patient who tries to communicate with you when you are not listening will soon give up, believing you are not interested in his or her health care concerns.

attention. As health care professionals, we must practice listening without an all-too-human tendency to filter what we hear through our preconceptions, prejudices, past experiences, and prior knowledge of the situation. An open mind and suspension of personal prejudices are vital to open communication.

In a quiet, private area, give the patient your full attention and keep interruptions and distractions to a minimum. The active listener learns to gate, or exclude, sounds not involved in the exchange. Other sounds in the hallway, other voices, or any other distractions are not your concern during the patient interview. Tune them out and concentrate entirely on the patient.

SPOTLIGHT ON SUCCESS

Gating

As you sit in your classroom, you are surrounded by sound, even during the enforced quiet of an examination... papers rattle, pens scratch, feet shuffle under desks, and noise continues in the hallway. If you concentrate on what you are doing, you can gate these sounds and can choose not to hear them. You may not be aware of this skill, but you use it any time you ignore or minimize sounds around you, and hear only the sounds you want to hear. Develop this skill; learn to ignore the ambient noise in the health care setting. Being able to gate is an important skill and is the foundation of focused interaction.

Focus on what is being said and on what is transmitted through paralanguage, body language, and other cues. Remember incongruence from Chapter 1? Look for cues that conflict with the patient's statements of concern. What is actually bothering the patient? Much more may be discovered than the initial or presenting complaint (Fig. 2.4).

If verbal messages are incongruent with nonverbal messages, search for the reason. For example, is the patient saying she is fine, while everything you observe—her facial expression, posture, tone, etc.—tells you she is not fine? If her nonverbal cues are conflicting and you still cannot determine the cause after questioning, talk with the health care provider about your concern. In some cases, it may be a good idea to have another colleague take over the care of the patient. It is important to do some self-evaluation to determine if there was anything you could have done to improve the situation with the patient.

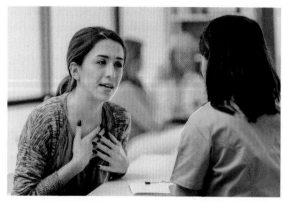

Fig. 2.4 This patient is concerned about something we have not yet addressed. How we progress through our interaction may help us determine the best way to help her resolve the issue (iStock.com/Steve Debenport.)

We all have trouble listening at times, such as when we are far too busy and are falling behind.

Rushed, hurried, unproductive situations are inevitable; however, active listening is a skill that must be developed over time.

COMMUNICATION GUIDELINES

Listening to What You Hear

The following are recommendations and best practice on improving your listening skills:

- Never complete the statement for patients. Your conclusion may not be what the patient intended to say and many patients will not correct you.
- Do not form your response or your next question until the patient is done speaking. You may miss valuable information and the patient certainly will know that you are not listening (Fig. 2.5).
- Let the patient set the speed and tone of the conversation, but do gently nudge the topic toward the necessary information. Review "Leading the Way," previously in this chapter, for examples.
- Sit with an open posture, face-to-face, and making eye contact, if appropriate.
- Be aware of attentive body language, such as facial expressions and leaning in when listening to the patient. These cues encourage the patient to respond to you.
- Consider your responses before proceeding with questions. Decide the best way to approach the patient in order to gather the most complete information.
- Provide affirmations to patients for productive exchanges. For instance, "This is very good information.

It will really help the physician." In this way, patients feel they have contributed and play a role in their medical care.
- Indicate when the exchange is over by stressing points that need clarification and by summarizing your impressions. Ask if the patient has additional questions or comments before moving to the next step.

Remember that the chief complaint is only one part of the patient's problems and may not even be the main reason for asking for help. Find out what changed in the health status to cause the patient to ask for help. Additionally, careful observation will help you determine what the problem is and what is causing the greatest concern for the patient. By observing cues and body language, you may discover there is more the patient needs to tell you, but may not know how. An in-depth, effective exchange often brings to light many of the patient's concerns.

RESPONDING TO THE PATIENT

Your responses to the patient are the feedback portion of the communication process, ensuring that the patient has communicated to you completely and accurately. This also provides the patient an opportunity to share additional information and ask any questions. There are many different tools and techniques that you can use that will enhance the patient interview.

Reflective or Paraphrasing Responses

Open-ended statements (not questions) that repeat or reinforce what the patient has said are called *reflective responses*. Reflective responses confirm that you received the message but leaves room for more information by allowing the patient to complete his or her thought or sentence. For example, you might say, "Mr. Smith, you were saying that you began to have this problem when you…."; the patient may then supply the missing information. This method encourages the patient to share pertinent information and may help bring the patient to the point if the conversation begins to drift.

Paraphrasing is when you reword what the patient stated while keeping the original meaning. This helps verify that you understood what the patient said. It also allows patients to clarify thoughts or statements.

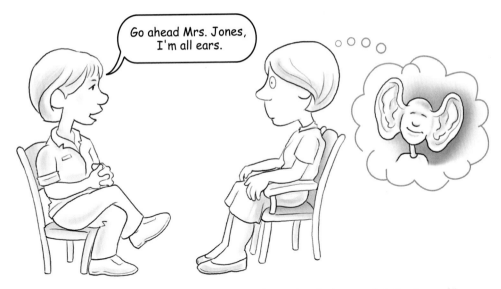

Fig. 2.5 Listen actively and let your patient know that she has your full attention.

A paraphrased statement or question may begin, "Did I understand you to say that…" followed by what you understood from the patient. For instance, the patient may say, "Nothing has any taste." Your paraphrase may be, "You are saying that your food does not taste as you feel it should?"

Reflecting and paraphrasing work well when gathering information and are effective tools during the patient interview. However, be careful not to overuse either as some patients may wonder if you are really listening.

Clarifying

Clarifying is essential for open and effective communication (Fig. 2.6). When we **clarify**, we make clear what patients say to us and what we say to them, removing confusion. You may need to clarify confusing statements for the patient regarding medical procedures or a medical diagnosis. Do not presume that all patients understand common medical terms or procedures. For example, consider the question, "Have you been fasting?" The patient may or may not understand what you are asking and why it is important. You may want to clarify your query to the patient, as in, "You are scheduled for fasting blood work today. When did you last eat or drink?" You may discover a misunderstanding about what "fasting" means, which could lead to a delay in diagnosis and treatment. Further, abbreviations can be very confusing. For instance,

"Mr. Smith in Room 3 has SOB." We know that "SOB" is a common medical abbreviation for shortness of breath, but other patients and family members may misinterpret it as a slang term.

> ### WORDS AT WORK
>
> In the exchange below, can you see how Manuela uses clarifying, paraphrasing, and reflecting responses when discussing Tania's dietary behavior?
>
> **Tania:** I love food, but I don't want to eat.
> **Manuela:** So, you are saying that you aren't hungry?
> **Tania:** No. I get hungry, but I usually try to get past that feeling.
> **Manuela:** I see. So, you feel hunger, but you decide not to eat.
> **Tania:** Right, I just don't want to eat.
> **Manuela:** Does the idea of food disgust you, like it seems gross?
> **Tania:** No, I love all kinds of food. I even cut recipes out of magazines and save them. I just don't want to eat. It's like I don't want to let myself eat.

Another use of clarification is asking patients to use examples. This may help you understand what the patient feels is the current problem and how he or she feels about it. For example, the patient may have trouble describing a certain pain. You can state, "Give me an example of what it feels like." The patient may say "It feels an ice pick scraping against

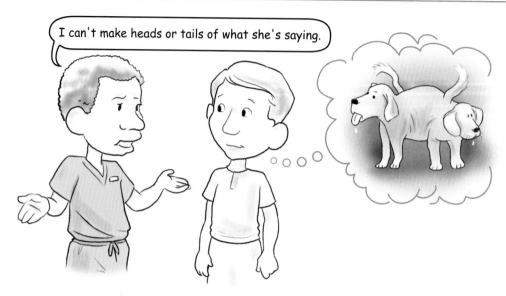

Fig. 2.6 Clarifying helps clear confusion for both you and your patient.

my bone." or "It feels like an elephant sitting on my chest." Using examples for clarification helps further explain a patient's feeling and experience during the interview.

Productive Silences

Although some people are not comfortable with silence, it can be a productive part of the interview process. Silences occur in most conversations. But some people are not comfortable with silences and will try to fill the quiet moments with words. However, well-timed and well-placed silences allow patients to form new thoughts and organize ideas, to remember events, and to summarize in their minds where they are in the conversation. Periods of silence also allow you to observe the patient without dividing your attention away from what the patient is saying. Encourage silence if patients seem particularly scattered and confused; it may be the break they need to gather their thoughts (Fig. 2.7).

SUMMARIZING THE INFORMATION

Summarizing, or restating information in a briefer form, helps to highlight the main points given by the patient. It also provides the patient with an

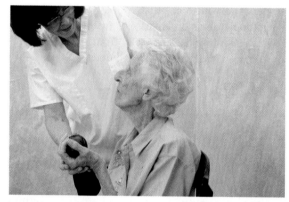

Fig. 2.7 This assistant is instructing a patient on a strength exercise. A moment of silence may help the patient gather her thoughts when she seems hesitant or confused. (iStock.com/Pamela Moore.)

opportunity to correct any information and to clarify central concerns. For example, you may summarize by asking, "You feel like you don't have the same energy that you use to have and that your appetite has not been as good for about a month. Is that correct?" Summarizing also helps to organize information into sequential events and to determine that you and the patient have covered every issue of concern at the time of the visit (Fig. 2.8). For example, you could summarize by stating, "So, you had pain in your stomach a

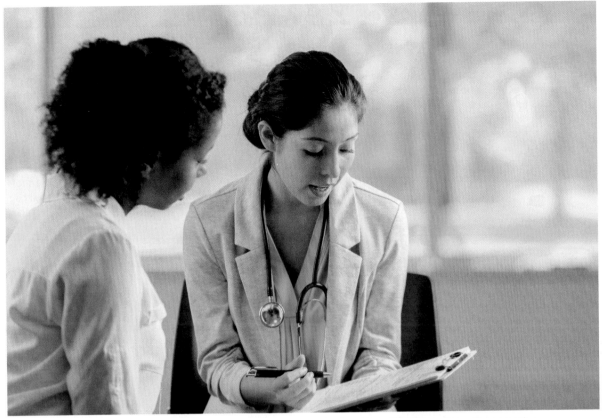

Fig. 2.8 Go back over any points of concern before closing the interview. (iStock.com/Steve Debenport.)

week ago and you started having bloody stool two days go. And, today, you started vomiting."

After establishing a proper rapport, these techniques, used appropriately, should help gather the pertinent information you need to assist the patient and the health care provider in resolving the patient's concerns.

Patient interviewing is a skill acquired with practice. With rising demands on the time allowed for each patient, information you discover during the interaction or exchange should suggest steps to follow and procedures to perform before passing the patient's care to the next member of the health care team. Knowing what to ask and what to do next will vary depending on the specialty. For example, consider a situation involving an elderly patient (Mr. Martin) who has chronic health problems (insulin-dependent diabetes mellitus) along with an acute illness, such as a virus (described at the beginning of this chapter). In addition to routinely checking his vital signs, you should also check his blood glucose level and question Mr. Martin to make sure he is following his health care routine.

However, if the patient is a younger, otherwise healthy patient, you would gather and record basic information, but measuring glucose levels may not be necessary. Thus, it is important to gather the appropriate information and perform the preliminary procedures for each patient to expand on the current health complaint. This will provide information to health care providers and allow them to make an accurate diagnosis.

As you assist the patient to the next step of care, make sure you review your documentation to ensure its accuracy and thoroughness. Your part in interviewing the patient and recording information helps direct the examination and treatment, establishes a foundation of rapport, and helps put your patient at ease. Additionally, remember that the patient's file is a legal document and your record of the interaction may be called into question.

▶▶ TAKING THE CHAPTER TO WORK

Questioning Skills

Now, let's meet Patsy and see how she has applied this chapter information in the workplace.

Patsy is working in an orthopedic clinic. She has begun to interview a patient who is 84 years of age who complains of aches and pains. The patient has been seen in the clinic on multiple occasions for arthritis. Patsy starts by asking the patient open-ended questions using the words "what," "where," "when," and "how." The patient states that she has had aches and pains for years. Patsy then clarifies this information by asking, "The aches and pains in your knees started at the same time as the aches in your back. Is that correct?" The patient states that the knee pains have been present for years, but the back pain started 2 days ago and that is why she made today's appointment. Patsy then directs her questioning about the back pain, and finds out that the patient also has trouble urinating and is experiencing burning and itching sensations after voiding. Patsy identifies these symptoms as a possible urinary tract infection and communicates this to the health care provider. A urinary specimen is obtained, and it shows signs of an infection.

Because Patsy took the time to clarify and reflect on the patient's answers, she was able to identify the root of the patient's problem. It is important to explore all patient complaints and to search for possible problems and not allow yourself to become complacent.

■ CHECKING YOUR COMPREHENSION

Write a brief answer for each of the following assignments.

1. In your future profession, describe your role and responsibilities in the patient interview.
2. Describe how you should prepare yourself and the setting for a patient interview.
3. Explain the difference between a sign and a symptom. Give two examples of each.
4. Explain the difference between an open-ended and a closed-ended question and give two examples of each type.
5. List and describe the different techniques used in patient interviews.
6. Explain the difference between hearing and listening. Discuss why active listening is so important.
7. Describe the difference between the terms paraphrasing and reflecting. Explain why each is important. Give an example of each.
8. Describe the purpose of summarizing when performing a patient interview.

■ EXPANDING CRITICAL THINKING

1. The following patients all have symptoms of nausea and vomiting. List five common questions you would ask these patients. Which questions are common to all patients? How would your questions differ based on the patient?
   a. A mother reporting about her 3-year-old daughter.
   b. A 20-year-old woman with no other symptoms and normal vital signs.
   c. An elderly woman with sharp pains in her upper right abdomen and stable vital signs.
   d. A chronic alcoholic with obvious jaundice and stable vital signs.
   e. A 30-year-old athletic man with a temperature of 102°F.
2. Using the patients in Question #1, list at least two questions that would be specific to that patient.
3. Select two patients in Question #1. Create an algorithm of questions for each patient.
4. Using your patients and answers from Question #3, which technique would work best for you in the patient interview process? Why?
5. Create an acronym for two different patient complaints.
6. Refer to the Legal Eagle box. It is important that patients disclose information to their health care professionals. However, some patient information and situations are more sensitive and personal than others. List five such topics. About which topics would you feel uncomfortable questioning patients? How could you overcome your discomfort in questioning patients about these issues?
7. Silence may make some people uncomfortable. How do you feel about silence during a conversation?

Experiment with a family member or classmate. How did each of you feel?

8. Describe the technique of gating in a patient interview. How can you improve your ability to eliminate distractions?

9. How would you address the following issues during a patient interview?
   a. A patient who does not speak English.
   b. A patient who arrives in a wheelchair with his caregiver.
   c. A patient who refuses to disclose information and only responds with "yes" or "no" answers.
   d. You are interviewing a patient and her husband keeps answering for her.

10. As you question Mrs. Brown about her current concern, she gives you answers that do not make sense. She lives alone and drives herself where she needs to go, but you suspect that her orientation and reasoning are impaired. What should you do?

3

Educating Patients

Jaime Nguyen

CHAPTER OUTLINE

LEARNING OBJECTIVES

On successful completion of this chapter, you will be able to:

1. List the goals and describe the function of patient education.
2. Assess the patient's learning needs, learning style, and health literacy.
3. Plan for patient teaching by creating learning goals and learning objectives.
4. Use various teaching aids in the implementation of the teaching plan.
5. Discuss the importance of and methods for evaluating patient education and improving patient adherence.
6. Recognize the importance of documentation in patient education.

KEY TERMS

adherence to carry out the care plan as directed

affective learning growth or change in feelings, emotions, or a mental state

assessment the collection of information about the patient's physical, mental, and emotional health

cognitive learning the acquisition of knowledge

continuity of care the communication and coordination of a patient's care among various health care professionals

evaluation the appraisal and review of the patient's learning progress during and after patient education

health literacy the patient's capacity to access and comprehend basic health information and services needed to make appropriate health decisions

holistic considering the whole of a person, including the physiological, intellectual, emotional, and social factors, rather than physical manifestations alone

implementation the act of setting a plan into effect

learning goal the purpose toward which the gaining of specific knowledge or skill is directed

learning objectives an observable or discernible outcome as the result of acquired knowledge or information

patient education the process of sharing information and instruction to allow patients to gain knowledge and skills to better address their health problems and improve their wellness

psychomotor learning the acquisition of a skill

❓ TEST YOUR COMMUNICATION IQ

Before reading this chapter, complete this short self-assessment test. Decide which statements are true and which are false.

1. You should do everything you can to help the patient, even if it is beyond your scope of practice.
2. Patients should be discouraged from using the Internet for patient education.
3. Sometimes changing a person's attitude is part of the patient education process.
4. Patient education often involves teaching the caregiver as well.
5. A patient who asks a lot of questions will probably not adhere to the care plan.
6. Some providers document patient education in the health record, whereas others do not.

Results

Statements three and four are true; all others statements are false. How did you do? Read the chapter to learn more about the topics.

FUNCTION OF PATIENT EDUCATION

Patient education is the process of sharing information and instruction to allow patients to gain knowledge and skills to better address their health problems and improve their wellness. Patient education continues to play a critical role in improving health outcomes.

In the clinical setting, patient education occurs between the health care professional and the patient and/or the patient's family or other caregiver. The information conveyed in the patient education depends on the patient's assessment, evaluation, diagnosis, prognosis, and the patient's ability and personal needs. Examples of patient education topics may include management and treatment options for the disease or injury, correct use of medication and any possible adverse effects, and preventative services (Fig. 3.1).

The primary goals of educating the patient are:

- To promote, maintain, and restore health
- To change health behaviors
- To improve patient compliance

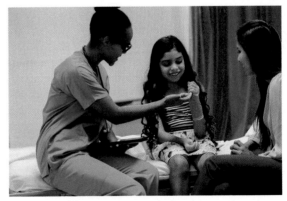

Fig. 3.1 A health care professional teaches a child and caregiver how to care for a cast. (iStock.com/Steve Debenport.)

By providing proper patient education, there will be clear communication between the health care professional and the patient, which will create more trust between the two parties. It will also allow the patient to be an active participant in his or her health care. Additionally, effective communication and patient education will increase the patient's compliance by improving patient motivation and morale, and the patient is more likely to respond well to the treatment plans, resulting in improved outcomes and fewer complications.

There are generally five steps in patient education:
- Assessment
- Planning
- Implementation
- Evaluation
- Documentation

Each of these steps is equally important in effective patient teaching. Knowing your patients is the key to successful and effective patient education.

ASSESSMENT OF PATIENT NEEDS

The first step in patient education should be assessment. The assessment should define the health care needs and concerns of the patient and family, and evaluate the patient's learning needs and readiness to learn. As the health care professional, you should determine what the patient currently knows, what he or she wants to and needs to know, what he or she is capable of learning, and what methods are best to provide that learning. To better assess the patient, you will need to:
1. Determine the patient's readiness to learn
2. Evaluate the patient's learning needs
3. Assess the patient's learning style

Understanding the patient's physical and emotional needs will prepare you to teach the patient. Being able to effectively assess your patient's learning needs also allows you to individualize the information for each patient. You may know most of the patient's background information, such as sensory barriers, education and comprehension levels, and so forth, from previous interaction with the patient or from the record. Consult other staff members and the patient's caregivers for additional information that will make education easier.

LEGAL EAGLE

It is very important for every health care professional to work within his or her scope of practice, which is composed of the terms and limits of one's job responsibilities, duties, and/or license. Exceeding your scope of practice can put your career in jeopardy and can endanger your patients. In certain cases, you may even lose your license or certificate, be fined, or even terminated from your position. If you are unsure of your scope of practice and responsibility in patient education or other tasks, get clarification from your supervisor.

Readiness to Learn

Many factors interfere with a patient's ability to learn what we need to teach. We speak a medical language unfamiliar to many of our patients, and the terms we use may sound frightening to them. Often patients may have just learned of their diagnosis and are in the acute stage of an illness. During this time, their readiness to learn may be low. But, as the patient begins to recover or learns to adjust to or accept his or her illness, his or her learning readiness will increase and will be more receptive for managing and preventing further problems.

When assessing the patient's readiness to learn, consider the potential factors that promote and hinder learning before beginning to teach:
1. Patients who are overwhelmed by pain, sedation, or emotional shock cannot learn. Relieve as many of these factors as possible and proceed when the patient is ready.
2. Patients who use sensory aids, such as hearing aids or glasses, must have them in place before they can fully understand what you are saying or demonstrating.
3. Trying to educate a patient in a hospital bed or on an examining table in a paper gown puts the patient at a disadvantage (Fig. 3.2). If possible, wait until the patient feels more in control and presentable before beginning an education session.
4. If you are not prepared with proper teaching tools or are unsure of the information, wait, if possible, until you have the necessary knowledge and educational materials before you begin.
5. If the patient does not speak English well and you do not have an interpreter, attempts at communication may be frustrating for both of you.

Chapters 5 and 6 of this text explore barriers to communication in detail.

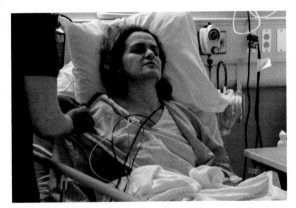

Fig. 3.2 This patient, who is in pain, is not ready for an education session. (iStock.com/Juanmonino.)

Health Literacy

An important factor when assessing a patient's readiness to learn is his or her health literacy level. According to the US Department of Health and Human Services, health literacy is "the degree in which individuals have the capacity to obtain, process, and understand basic health information and services needed to make appropriate health decisions." Unlike literacy levels, which may be the result of neurologic issues or education, patients who are educated and are high performing may still have health literacy issues. However, older adults, ethnic minorities, people with education level lower than a high school diploma, and those for whom English is a second language are more likely to have low health literacy levels.

Patients with low health literacy levels may not be familiar with medical terms, anatomy, or how the body functions. They may not be able to understand statistics and evaluate the risks of a treatment or a procedure. The lack of health literacy may also prevent patients from sharing pertinent personal and health information with their health care provider, and may create obstacles in navigating the health care system, such as seeking second opinions or referrals for specialists. Additionally, patients with poor health literacy may find it difficult to make lifestyle changes because they may not understand, for example, the relationship between smoking and cardiovascular and respiratory diseases. Thus, patients with higher health literacy levels are more likely to seek medical care earlier, and they more often utilize preventative services, such as mammograms, Pap smears, and immunizations, thereby promoting their wellbeing.

As the health care professional, it is your responsibility to effectively address your patients' health literacy issues. The patient education that you provide must not be too difficult for them to understand. It must add to the patient's knowledge and should result in improved behavior. To address health literacy issues, all patient education should

1. Be appropriate for the patient
2. Be easy to use
3. Be clear and easy to read and understand.

It is important to identify and understand the target patient population, specifically the demographics and their pattern of behavior, culture, and attitude. The patient information should be appropriate for the age group, culture, language, and literacy level. Use simple and familiar language, and avoid jargon and slang terms.

✴ LEGAL EAGLE

Prior to any medical treatment or surgical procedure, the patient must give *informed consent*, which occurs when the patient understands the purpose, benefits, risk, and alternative options and gives permission to proceed with a treatment plan. However, studies have shown that patients may sign over consent, but may not fully understand the risk of a treatment or procedure or may not even ask basic questions. To ensure informed consent, consent forms should be written in simple sentences in a patient's primary language. An interpreter or reader should be offered to patients, if needed. The health care provider must also engage patients in appropriate dialogue about the nature and scope of the treatment or procedure, and convey the risks associated with high-risk procedures.

Learning Needs

Once you assess your patient's readiness to learn, you will then need to assess his or her learning needs. A *learning need* is the difference between the desired level and lack of the knowledge, skills, behaviors, or attitudes required for patients to manage their own health care. When evaluating the patient's learning needs, you must find out what the patient wants and needs to know or do and what the patient already knows.

Determining how much the patient already knows and understands about the illness can direct how much and what type of information is needed in each situation. For example, diabetic patients who do not understand how nutrition works will not understand or retain information as well as those already actively involved in good dietary habits. Patients with a poor nutritional background may require a referral to a nutritionist or dietitian to help establish a basis for healthful nutrition. Likewise, a patient who understands exercise physiology will more likely continue a physical therapy routine than one who is set in an inactive lifestyle. Learning is easier when we already have an established knowledge base for adding new information.

WORDS AT WORK

Some questions you may want to ask patients to better assess their learning needs are:
1. "What are you most concerned about?"
2. "What do you feel you need to learn?"
3. "What are you most interested in learning?"
4. "What do you know about your disease or condition?"
5. "What specific problems are you having?"

Another effective technique for assessing a patient's learning needs is using a questionnaire or checklist. Patients may be overwhelmed, unsure of what to say, and may not know what they do not know. Thus, written material may help you better evaluate the patient's learning needs.

There may be times when the health care professional and the patient have a different view of how much and what kind of information the patient should know. The health care professional may consider the need for information when the patient may not. For example, the physician may schedule a colonoscopy procedure for a patient to evaluate a history of rectal bleeding. The medical assistant provides information on how the patient makes the necessary preparations for the procedure. The colonoscopy requires a clear digestive tract, so preparation for the procedure involves strict fasting and laxatives. If both the physician and medical assistant do not impress the patient of the importance of understanding and following the preparation instructions, the colonoscopy cannot be performed. This will delay the procedure, as well as potentially the diagnosis and treatment plan.

SPOTLIGHT ON SUCCESS

Patients and the Internet
According to a 2012 study, 72% of American adults use the Internet to look for information about health care, including specific diseases and treatments. In fact, the use of the Internet as a primary source of medical information is expected to grow. Half of Internet users (48%) who go online for health information say their last search was on behalf of another person. These percentages are even higher among people living with one or more chronic illness. Thus, it is unsurprising that you will have many patients and/or their families bring their own health information to appointments. Patients who use the Internet are more compliant, ask questions and are more active in their medical care, and have better medical results. There may be times when patients get health information from the Internet that is incorrect and may even use it to self-diagnose themselves. It is important to remind patients that information from the Internet should not be used as a second opinion or a substitute for their own health care provider. You may want to recommend some examples of reliable websites, if possible, such as those ending with ".gov" for government sites and ".edu" for educational sites.

Maslow's Hierarchy of Needs

Patients may have trouble complying with patient education and cannot learn if certain basic needs are not met. In the late 1960s, Abraham Maslow, an American psychiatrist, developed a theory to better understand basic human needs. Maslow's theory included that a need is essential if:

- Without its fulfillment or presence, illness results.
- Fulfilling the need restores homeostasis or wellness.
- We feel a sense of satisfaction when the need is met.

Before we can progress to higher needs and personal accomplishment, we must first have our basic needs met (Fig. 3.3). Our most basic needs are *physiologic needs*, which are essential for life and are the basis on which all else depends. This includes oxygen, water, and food. Without these physiologic needs, there are multiple barriers to communicating patient education. Once these are met, *safety and security* is the next level of Maslow's hierarchy, which includes shelter, financial security, and freedom from fear. The next hierarchy is *love and belonging*, which is having family and a strong support group or community network. Without a support system, people may feel isolated and depressed and may be less receptive

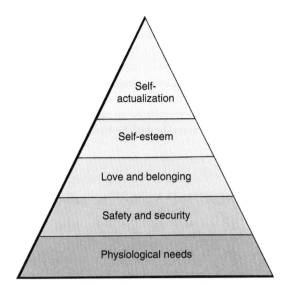

Fig. 3.3 Maslow's hierarchy as a pyramid.

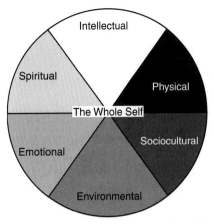

Fig. 3.4 A holistic view of the patient treats the whole self.

to receiving patient education and managing their health condition. *Self-esteem*, sometimes referred to as ego, is a need that provides us with pride of accomplishment and the respect of those we value. Even with all our more basic needs met, we often become restless if we do not earn or feel respected. This need may be compromised by a patient's disease and disability when his or her perception or role has changed. The final hierarchy is *self-actualization*, which is when we reach our full potential. We accept ourselves and others because we are fulfilled and all our basic needs have been met. At this level, our patients are at their most compliant and are able to seek and follow patient education.

Holism

Another approach to assessing learning needs is the holistic approach, which considers the needs of the person as a whole and not just focusing on one aspect. In addition to the patient's medical needs, the holistic approach includes the patient's spiritual, physical, emotional, sociocultural, and intellectual needs (Fig. 3.4). For example, when we have an illness, it impacts more than just our health. Will we have to miss days of work? Will we be able to care for our families? Will we be able to enjoy our hobbies? How expensive is the treatment? How will this affect our quality of life? It is particularly important that patients must be able to trust their health care professionals because this approach focuses on so many aspects of a patient's life, and patients should be involved in decision-making about their care.

SPOTLIGHT ON SUCCESS

Stay Informed

Publicity about new health concerns can be frightening and confusing to the general public. News programs and other forms of media can create panic very quickly. For example, in 2014 many people panicked when the Ebola virus afflicted health care workers in the United States. In 2016, the Zika virus, a mosquito-borne illness that can pass from mother to fetus and cause birth defects, captured the media's attention. When these types of health issues occur, your patients will turn to you for reassurance and clarification. Listen to the nightly news or read the daily newspapers and other news journals and develop a keen interest in health-related information. Seek guidance from your employer about how to communicate with patients about outbreaks, their true threats, and precautions to take. Taking the initiative to stay abreast of current trends shows your supervisor that you have the qualities looked for in a health care professional.

Learning Styles

During the assessment stage, determine the patient's best style of learning. This includes how patients learn best and when they learn best. Does the patient learn best by hearing, reading, or demonstration? In the 1950s, Benjamin Bloom's work categorized learning in three distinct domains

1. Cognitive: to acquire knowledge
2. Affective: to grow emotionally or change one's attitude
3. Psychomotor: to acquire a skill

Each of these domains is reflective of the goal of the learning process, but learning within all three domains helps us store information in more areas of our brain for better recall. The more places we store information—seeing, hearing, reading, reasoning, and demonstrating—the more likely we are to remember it. To retain information, we must receive facts, compare them to what we already know, store them in accessible memory banks, and value the information received enough to keep it for future reference, much as our computers do for us. We remember best those things we know are important. We also remember more easily those things that relate to something we already know and can add to our knowledge base.

Cognitive Learning

Cognitive learning style is composed of processing facts, forming conclusions, and making decisions by listening to or reading instructions or information. Examples of methods and techniques for cognitive learning are discussions groups, role playing, seminars, literature, and questions and answer sessions.

Most literate adults do well with self-directed, independent learning when they understand how important it is, especially if they feel that the learning experience is under their control. Most patients quickly and easily understand that learning how to handle an illness will help improve their health or, at the very least, help them cope with the changes they are experiencing. For example, patients who are active participants in their medical care will approach you with stacks of information from many various sources, some more reliable than others. They may even challenge you with information they find that contradicts what you are trying to teach them. If the information gathered by patients contradicts or disagrees with the physician's orders or the treatment plan, let the physician know so that more time can be set aside to explain the purpose of the order or the individual treatment plan.

Affective Learning

Affective learning appeals to emotions or feelings to change someone's beliefs or attitude and to reinforce the importance of the change in concepts. It is more difficult to learn new information if it goes against firmly held beliefs. However, once adults are convinced it is important to their health, most will adapt to new concepts. The new way of thinking and believing may need to be explained or approached from different viewpoints and by various means until the patient accepts the information. This may include recruiting family members to help convince the patient of its importance or introducing patients to support groups of those who have experienced or are experiencing the same type of health problems. For example, if a patient was recently diagnosed with cancer, she may greatly benefit from joining a support group with people who have experienced or are experiencing the same doubts and fears she may be having.

Psychomotor Learning

Psychomotor learning is the acquisition of a skill. If the new knowledge can be taught by the patient actively participating in a skill, it is more likely that the patient will understand and retain that skill. For example, the patient may have better compliance if he or she learns how to self-inject insulin to manage diabetes compared with if the patient just merely read how to perform the injection. Further, if the treatment plan includes the patient performing a task, such as an injection or using an asthma inhaler, you cannot be sure that the patient understands or will perform the task correctly until he or she demonstrates it with you.

PLANNING FOR PATIENT EDUCATION

Once you have assessed the patient, the next step in patient education is proper and effective planning. This step identifies a goal and utilizes all information gathered during the patient interview and the assessment process. The planning stage is the formal creation of learning goals and objectives, which help to define expected short-term and long-term results. Program goals and objectives establish criteria and standards against which to determine performance or outcome.

Learning goals are broad statements about the long-term expectation of a desired result. They are usually broad statements that are general in nature. Learning goals serve as the basis or foundation for learning objectives. Learning objectives are statements that describe the desired results and how they will be achieved. The objectives should be specific and measurable. In most cases, there will be multiple learning objectives for one learning goal. Learning goals and objectives should be created specifically for each patient and for each situation, and they should include a standard by which learning and achievement can be measured. Table 3.1 shows an example of learning goals and objectives for a patient managing her diabetes.

TABLE 3.1 Learning Goals and Objectives	
Learning Goal	**Learning Objectives**
A. Patient will understand that diabetes is a lifelong disease and will be able to manage her diabetes to avoid long-term complications of diabetes	1. Self-monitoring of blood glucose: Patient will check blood glucose daily—before each meal and 2 hours after largest meal. 2. A1C monitoring: Patient will have 3-month routine check-up with physician to monitor A1C levels.

IMPLEMENTING THE PLAN

The next step in patient education is implementation. This step puts the process in motion and it can be carried out in several ways to suit the patient's needs. In most cases, implementation will use a variety of resources and teach tools that will help patients better connect and understand. The types of teaching tools will depend on the patient's learning style and learning need, which were discussed earlier. For example, you may instruct patients through one-on-one meetings, group discussions, support groups, pamphlets, fact sheets, booklets, and videos.

Because our patients have varying education needs and preferences, the types of teaching tools in patient education cannot be a one-size-fits all or all-inclusive solution. Effective teaching tools must be from a variety of different resources and use multiple modalities, including traditional print material to highly technical interactive videos. The use of teaching tools in the implementation step in patient education improves patient engagement and allows patients to be more of a participant in their own health care. However, more teaching tools does not necessarily lead to better patient education. Once you determine how your patient prefers to learn and what that patient needs to learn, you can better select which implementation method to use.

Lecture

Lecture presents the basic information, but it does not require a patient's participation to reinforce or retain the information. This method may be enough for highly motivated patients who you know are generally compliant, but it does not work well for patients who need to participate in psychomotor learning or practice

for reinforcement. If written information is used, it should be available for reference, should questions arise. Follow-up appointments should be made to allow patients time to think and to ask questions later to prevent any misunderstandings.

Role-Playing and Demonstration

Role-playing and demonstration require that you perform a medical procedure as the patient watches, and then that patient performs it so that you can evaluate his or her understanding and practice (Fig. 3.5). When you demonstrate procedures for patients to perform at home, make the examples as realistic as possible so that patients can anticipate how to perform them when they are at home and without your guidance. Patients who do not understand important points, or those who cannot translate what they learned into their home environment, may delay recovery or may make their medical condition worse rather than better.

Have the patient demonstrate the process without your help until you feel the level of skill is appropriate for self-care. Additionally, written instructions should be available for reference as needed. Skills checklists work well at this point for reinforcement. Using this method, patients are more likely to retain the information.

Discussion

Discussion is a back-and-forth exchange of information and concepts. You present information and patients reply back to you what they understand and how this affects them. This reinforces affective or emotional retention of information. This type of implementation

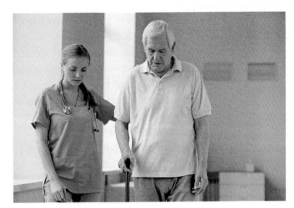

Fig. 3.5 The medical assistant teaches a patient to walk with a cane. (iStock.com/mediaphotos.)

method works best for patient education for lifestyle changes but is not as effective for medical procedures.

Discussion can be one-on-one or may be conducted in a group. Patients who are confident and assertive do well in either format, but may dominate the discussion. It is important to monitor the group to ensure that less vocal and assertive patients do not get lost in the discussion and group environment.

Patient Education Material

Patient education material (PEM) is any material that provides accurate and concise health information in a variety of formats, including pamphlets, fact sheets, booklets, posters, and videos. The American Medical Association has documented that a large number of adults have low health literacy levels, making it difficult to provide effective patient education using lecture or discussion alone. Further, patients often forget or misinterpret what was being said when meeting with health care providers in the clinic. Thus, having PEM to bring home or to be shared with family members or caregivers can be useful teaching tool.

Printed Material

Printed material and programmed instructions have been commonly used teaching tools in patient education. Examples of printed materials are brochures, pamphlets, patient instruction handouts, and posters, and most health care organizations have a variety of printed materials for their patients. Printed material can help introduce important and sensitive topics, reinforce medical information that was previously discussed with the health care provider, and may save time by addressing simple topics that the health care provider may not need to waste time on during the clinical visit.

These are simple, relatively inexpensive teaching tools that can be used to address a variety of diseases and conditions. However, printed material alone does not effectively address the patient's literacy or health literacy level, and requires a high level of patient participation. Before presenting any printed material for patient education, think about your patient population. Look at the overall visual appeal, the format, the illustrations, and the vocabulary level of the material.

Do you need Spanish or Vietnamese language aids? What about large print for the vision-impaired patient? Are the majority of your patients poorly educated with low reading skills, or is your facility more likely to attract highly educated patients? The average American adult reads at a 6th to 8th grade level and most of them have never had an anatomy and physiology course. So, ensure the readability, or the ease in which patients can read and understand the material, is appropriate for your target population.

Provide copies of any printed material for the patient to bring home and have him or her review it before the next scheduled information session. Ask the patient to mark any areas of concern or confusion and to write down questions to be addressed at the next session. If the patient has no questions or comments, it does not necessarily mean the patient understands the information. Thus, it is important to review the information in the printed material at the follow-up evaluation.

Multimedia Materials

Multimedia materials work well as an effective reinforcement and alternative to printed materials. Multimedia is any content using more than one format, usually including audiovisual formats that use sight and sound. Examples of multimedia materials are electronic booklets and websites, spoken audio files, streaming videos, and interactive videos.

Supplementing verbal instructions with easy-to-read written materials, videos, interactive computer programs, models, posters, and diagrams or pictures will contribute to the patient's interest and emphasize and reinforce health information. Being able to mix and match different types of materials and formats helps us individualize our patient education and responds more holistically to our patient's learning needs.

Support Systems

As Maslow theorized, we have a basic need to belong and connect to a group. If we have no support system, we have no safety net and we feel that we do not belong. Many studies show that patients with a strong support system have shorter recovery time and are better able to recover from illness. Many types of support systems exist in our lives, including our families, friends, social groups, and structured support groups.

Families and Caregivers

The traditional concept of *family* with two opposite-sex parents and 2.5 children has evolved now to mean many arrangements and assortments. A family, in any sense of the word, implies a mutually supportive relationship. The term family now loosely means a group of people living together or who are closely connected by bonds of interdependence. The members have common concerns and meet each other's needs for safety, security, love, and belonging. Illness for one affects the whole group. Families are affected differently, depending on the age of the patient and the extent of the illness. If the family is close and loving, everyone is affected by the illness of any one of its members. How the family reacts depends on how severely the illness affects the family dynamics. For example, a sick child is devastating to the whole family and may result in immense demands on the parents and other siblings. A sick parent cannot productively contribute to the family safety and security and is a source of anxiety rather than comfort.

As a result, you will often be caring for more than just the patient. Working with a family in the health care setting may require interaction with more than one caregiver or family member. Many viewpoints may have to be coordinated and considered. For example, for an elderly, dependent grandparent, one family member may feel that long-term care (such as in a nursing home) is more appropriate than home care, whereas another family member may feel that long-term care should be a last resort (Fig. 3.6). Some members may want a "do not resuscitate" (DNR) order signed, whereas others may strongly be against it. Families often need as much emotional support as patients do.

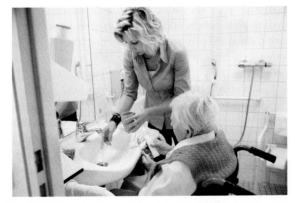

Fig. 3.6 This patient's granddaughter acts as her primary caregiver four mornings every week, and must be a part of the patient education process. (iStock.com/Silvia Jansen.)

Support Groups

Support groups bring together people with a common issue. Support groups are usually structured and formal; they regularly meet to share any concerns, experiences, and expectations with one another. Most support groups are composed of members and a facilitator or a group leader who helps motivate the group, keeps it on task, and assigns and coordinates the regularly scheduled meetings. Facilitators also help enforce boundaries and manage group dysfunction, such as aggression and dominating personalities. Examples of support groups are Alcoholics Anonymous, Reach for Recovery (postmastectomy), and Candlelighters (parents of children with cancer). Additionally, there are support groups for most common illnesses and life experiences.

Support groups are beneficial because they share how others are adjusting and how they handle the illness or problem. Seeing other group members doing well with an illness may encourage and offer support to other members who may not be coping with the illness so well.

There are many formats for support groups, including its size, how often it meets, for how long it meets, and who can join and when. For example, support groups may be open or closed. Open support groups allow people to join at any time. Closed groups may allow for more confidentiality and intimacy, and help members work more cohesively.

> ## TAKING THE CHAPTER TO WORK
>
> **Utilizing Support Groups**
>
> Jacob is working in a community clinic and is doing a patient intake for a 42-year-old man who has a cut that does not seem to be healing. He received the cut over 2 weeks ago when he fell while at his home. The patient interview uncovers that the patient has been depressed and going through a divorce, job loss, and has filed for bankruptcy. He states that he has been drinking more than usual over the last few years and barely eats anything. He has been feeling sad since his wife has left him and he feels lonely with no one at home. A physical examination and laboratory tests are performed. Jacob discusses with the patient how his depression and mental state, lack of family support, and poor nutrition are all affecting his current health. These factors are intertwined, resulting in poor wound healing of his cut. Jacob provides some information on local support groups in the area and a brochure on nutrition.

COMMUNICATION GUIDELINES

Implementing the Plan

After deciding which combination of the formats listed above works best for your patient, use all the appropriate communication skills you have learned to transmit the information. These suggestions will help reinforce the learning experience:

- Speak slowly and clearly. Repeat the information in a variety of ways for reinforcement. Use everyday language and define all medical terms.
- Allow time for questions and clarification. Patients who feel rushed may not have time to absorb the information and may be too confused and overwhelmed to think of appropriate questions.
- Build on the patient's knowledge base: What does she already know about what you need to teach? Add additional information in a simple-to-complex sequence.
- Keep up with current medical advances and make sure the information available in your agency is current. Some patients may need you to provide and interpret information on emerging medical technology for them.
- Help patients find community resources to continue complicated at-home care, such as home health agencies and medical supply companies. Many pharmaceutical and medical supply companies have well-written brochures, pamphlets, and websites that provide useful information regarding how to use their products.

Understanding Medication Administration

Following assessment and diagnosis, the provider may prescribe medication to the patient, which is one of the most common therapeutic interventions in health care. The United States spends more money on prescription medication per capita than any other country. According to the Centers for Medicare & Medicare Services, in 2015, the United States spent $328 billion on prescription medication, or 10% of the total national health expenditures (Centers for Medicare and Medicaid Services, 2018).

The provider's judgment of which medications to prescribe, the dosage of the medication, the route by which it is administered (Table 3.2), the frequency the patient should receive the medication, and the reason for taking it (e.g., when the patient is in pain) is individualized. The provider prescribes medicines based

TABLE 3.2   Routes of Drug Administration

Route	Description
Oral	Taken by mouth and swallowed
Sublingual	Placed under the tongue
Buccal	Placed between the gums and cheek
Intravenous (IV)	Injected into a vein
Intramuscular (IM)	Injected into a muscle
Subcutaneous (sc)	Injected under the skin
Intrathecal	Injected around the spinal cord
Rectal	Inserted into the rectum
Vaginal	Inserted into the vagina
Ocular	Placed in the eye
Otic	Placed in the ear
Nasal	Sprayed into the nose
Inhaled	Breathed into the lungs through the mouth
Transdermal	Absorbed through the skin

on many factors, including weight, health history and symptoms, other medications the patient is currently taking, and more. Often the provider schedules a follow-up appointment or monitors the patient to see how well he or she is responding to the therapy. Clearly, the patient's care plan requires the patient to follow the provider's medication regimen in order to evaluate its effectiveness. Health care professionals must teach patients not only how to take medications at home, but also the importance of following the providers instructions exactly.

If it is your responsibility to educate patients regarding medication administration, it is important to have a standard procedure or protocol when educating patients on how, when, and why they are taking their medication.

1. Ask the patient to demonstrate how he or she takes the medication. If the patient has a family member or caregiver who dispenses the medication, have him or her demonstrate as well.
2. While the patient is demonstrating, ask the patient about the dosage, time, and frequency of taking the medication.
3. If the patient takes multiple medications, ask the patient to explain when he or she takes each medication and what each medication is for.

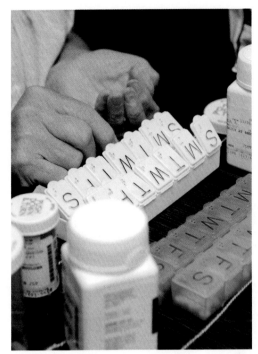

Fig. 3.7 Proper medication administration is so important that several forms of aids are available to help ensure that medications are taken on a proper schedule. This patient sorts pills by day, then uses the different colored boxes to indicate whether the pill should be taken in the morning, at noon, or at night. (iStock.com/Jorge Salcedo.)

If the patient is showing difficulty or confusion or does not have an established daily routine, you may want to discuss with the patient, family, or caregiver about creating a calendar, diary, list, or purchasing a pillbox that allocates the medication to be taken daily (Fig. 3.7). Another helpful hint is to label each medication bottle with the condition for which it is to be taken. If writing on the bottle, be sure not to obscure any important information on the prescription label, such as the drug's name, number of refills, and specific instructions.

When providing patient education on medication administration, additional questions to ask are

- Determine whether the patient is vision-impaired. Can he see the labels well enough to know which medication he is taking? Can you provide him with visual aids to make measuring and administration easier?
- Does she have the manual dexterity to draw up medications and self-inject? Is there a family member or caregiver who can inject it for her? Should she be

referred to a home health service if no one is available to help with administration?

- Can he understand which medication must be taken, at what time, and in what manner? Can the routine be simplified?
- Does he understand how important it is to take the medication as prescribed and what might happen if he does not follow the proper regimen? Does he know that he should not discontinue the medication without informing the physician's office?
- Should you demonstrate with special memory aids, such as divided dosage boxes to make it easier to remember dosage times?

Help patients and caregivers understand how medications affect the patient's health since the patient will primarily be responsible for properly taking the medication. Provide them with the necessary resources and information to be adherent; there are many available resources about the drugs prescribed in your facility. For example, the Physician's Desk Reference (PDR), the US Pharmacopoeia (USP), and several other good, brief reference books outline the properties of most current medications. The National Council on Patient Information and Education (NCPIE), a nonprofit organization in Washington D.C., also provides literature on the appropriate use of medicines for patients: http://www.bemedwise.org/. Other excellent resources are pharmacists, who are required to provide standard instructions with each prescription, and some pharmaceutical representatives, or "drug reps," may also supply patient-friendly information. Tell your patients about the medication, ask for questions, and have a report-back system in place for questions later.

EVALUATING PATIENT COMPREHENSION

Once the patient has been educated and provided information about his or her care, the next part of the education process is to determine the patient's progress and continued his or her understanding of the medical care plan. Evaluation is the appraisal and review of the patient's learning progress during and after the patient education. The goal of the evaluation step is to determine if the patient has learned what you taught. In a hospital setting or one with constant, direct patient care, evaluations of understanding and progress may be made more frequently. However, once the patient has been discharged or leaves the ambulatory clinic, the patient is then responsible for self-care. It is our responsibility as health care professionals to evaluate patient understanding and to report our findings to the health care provider responsible for coordinating his or her care.

Evaluation may be informal and casual and there may be multiple methods of evaluating. If the treatment plan involves a procedure, you can use the "teach-back" method. This is when you ask patients to demonstrate the procedure you taught them and observe if they performed it correctly. It is important to observe patients performing the steps at various times during their care. If the patient is doing it correctly, praise her and encourage her efforts. If the patient is not performing the procedure correctly, tactfully and without making her feel inferior, guide her in the correct performance. A performance checklist may help prevent further missed steps.

Another method of evaluation is asking specific and relevant open-ended questions to see if the patient can apply the information to their situation (Fig. 3.8). For example, to determine if the patient understands the significance of glucose levels, ask "Your glucose level is 164. What do you think that means?" If this is done in a non-judgmental manner, he may explain his misconceptions about how food affects his glucose level, giving you the perfect teaching moment.

⊞ WORDS AT WORK

Sheri is getting her patient Mrs. Benjamin ready to see Dr. Scaramucci. Although Mrs. Benjamin's appointment is a follow-up for her anticoagulant medication, Sheri knows that she also recently began oxygen therapy and takes the opportunity to evaluate her understanding of the equipment.

Sheri: I see you started using a portable oxygen concentrator. How are you adjusting to the therapy?

Mrs. Benjamin: It's nice not to be out of breath all the time. I'm less dizzy too. That was terrible, but it's better now.

Sheri: When your body doesn't get enough oxygen you can be short of breath, confused, and sometimes your heart rate can speed up. If that happens you might have hypoxia, so just call 911. Do you know about safe places to keep the portable oxygen concentrator?

Mrs. Benjamin: Yes, when they set me up at home, they said to keep it away from the drapes, the stove, and the fireplace.

Sheri: That's right, at least 8 feet from any open flames.

Mrs. Benjamin: And my husband can't smoke in the house anymore.

Sheri: That's right. Did you get a fire extinguisher?

Mrs. Benjamin: Yes, my son hung one up on the wall in the kitchen last week.

Even though Sheri's evaluation sounds casual, she has gathered information that suggests Mrs. Benjamin understands the safety precautions surrounding her equipment.

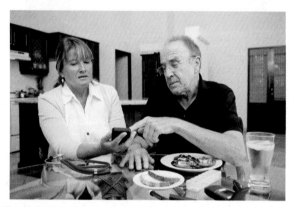

Fig. 3.8 The diabetic patient shows the home health nurse how he checks his blood sugar using a glucometer. (iStock.com/Fertnig.)

Based on the evaluation, learning goals and objectives may need to be reevaluated and restructured as the patient progresses through treatment. Is the patient's medical condition responding to treatment? Does the patient need additional support, such as a caregiver or a support group? If you find that he or she did not understand the care plan or is not complying, the health care team needs to evaluate why. Did she understand how following with the plan affects her health? Is he committed to whatever it takes to get well? You may need to schedule more in-depth education and evaluation if the patient is not following the care plan. If the care plan is too complicated or difficult, a home health agency may need to be contacted to help with home care.

Finally, do not forget to evaluate your own efforts at education. How do you think you handled the situation? What went right or wrong? How can you improve next time? How the patient learns is only part of the education equation; how you teach is equally important.

COMMUNICATION GUIDELINES

Evaluation

These suggestions will help you to evaluate the patient's comprehension:

- Answers to open-ended questions are more revealing than the patient answering with "yes" or "no." When checking for comprehension, instead of asking, "Did you understand what we just covered?" ask specific points such as, "Can you tell me when you should use Standard Precautions?" and "How will you dispose of your soiled dressings?"
- Offer to follow up with patients in the next few days to check if they have any additional questions or concerns (Fig. 3.9). Patients may be hesitant and reluctant to call you with what they consider a small problem, but a small problem may develop into a much larger health issue if not addressed in a timely manner.
- Schedule visits to the health care facility for evaluation and additional education as needed. Home health agencies are available to reinforce at-home care if the patient does not need to return to your clinic or if transportation is a problem.

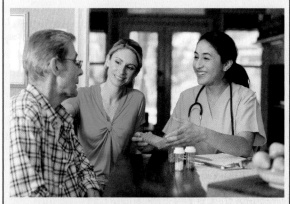

Fig. 3.9 After reviewing medication with the patient and caregiver, the home health nurse offers to schedule a follow-up appointment for further evaluation. (iStock.com/Steve Debenport.)

Patient Adherence

Despite all our efforts to understand our patient's learning styles, to create education material, and to provide the information, the patient may have trouble adhering to or complying with the treatment plan. Although the terms *adherence* and *compliance* are often used interchangeably, they are distinct and differ in their meanings. *Compliance* had traditionally been used to describe a patient's ability to take medications as prescribed or

comply with a health care provider's instruction, but recently this term has fallen into disfavor. Some have suggested that compliance implies a paternalistic relationship between the provider and patient, and that the patient is obedient to the provider's authority. On the other hand, *adherence* better represents the complex nature of the relationship between the patient, health care provider, and health care system. According to the World Health Organization (Adherence to Long-term Therapies: Evidence for Action, 2003), adherence is "the degree to which the person's behavior corresponds with the agreed recommendations from a health care provider." Adherence is more active and is a collaboration of all parties to improve the patient's health by integrating the health care provider's medical advice and patient's lifestyle, values, and preference for care. Thus, adherence is the preferred term in health care.

The results of not following the health care provider's care plan are poor productivity, increased disease morbidity, increased medical visits and hospitalizations, and increased costs.

COMMUNICATION GUIDELINES

Adherence

As we work toward educating patients we will find that we value the "good" patient, one who adheres to all we suggest, who does not question, who does not complain, and who passively follows any health care plan set for him, either for correction or for prevention. However, we may encounter the "difficult" patient. These "difficult" patients ask questions regarding their care, make suggestions that differ from ours, and make logical and healthful changes that work better for them than those we may suggest. Although this may annoy us and we may even feel resentful, this kind of patient is more likely to make healthier lifestyle choices than those who merely follow directions without questioning or understanding. The "difficult" patient is asking questions and is playing an active part in his or her health care, resulting in better adherence. The patient understands and agrees to the needed treatment, asks questions, and monitors his or her treatment to be sure it has the expected results.

Many factors influence adherence in health care, such as poor provider–patient communication, economic and social factors, treatment plan complexity, and health care disparities. For example, adherence may be affected by cost and access barriers if the physician prescribes a medication to a patient, but the patient never has the prescription filled owing to an inability to afford the medication. Patients may raise or lower medication dosages without consulting their provider or they may not take the full course of an antibiotic owing to miscommunication. A recent National Public Radio-Truven poll suggests that nearly one-third of patients stop taking their medication without informing their health care provider. Although affordability may be a factor, only 10% of people cited it as the reason they stopped taking their medication. Other reasons for the medication nonadherence were side effects (29%); a belief they did not need the drug any more (17%); that they were feeling better (16%); and that they felt the drug was not working (15%) (Hobson, 2017).

Studies have shown that a majority of patients misunderstand their physician's directions for treatment immediately after the medical visit (Jimmy & Jimmy, 2011). Thus, it is important for you to identify patients at risk for poor adherence as early as possible in their management. Despite innovative methods to improve medication adherence, such as electronic reminders and financial incentives, one of the best methods was training health care professionals to engage with and communicate with patients about their medications.

Many patients gradually become less compliant as time goes by. Therefore, frequent evaluations may be needed to make sure the patient continues to follow the plan and to evaluate the need for changes in procedures as the patient improves or the illness progresses. If treatments and lifestyle changes are long term and complicated, adherence to a health care plan is less likely. For example, adherence is usually hard to maintain if the disorder is chronic and does not have severe early symptoms, such as the early stages of hypertension or non–insulin-dependent diabetes mellitus, as compared with acute and painful disorders, such as a severe migraine headache. Patients will more likely follow the treatment plan if they receive immediate relief from pain or nausea.

Many patients also choose the parts of the routine that interfere least with how they prefer to live. For example, the physician's treatment plan instructs the patient to exercise more, stop smoking, and eat healthier. The patient may slightly modify his diet and cut down to three packs a day instead of four packs. Because the patient does not observe the immediate benefits from these lifestyle changes, adherence to the treatment plan is less likely. The goal is to help patients maintain adherence

for long-term changes as well as they do for short-term illnesses. Thus, use short-term goals with positive feedback to encourage patients to continue to progress. As you evaluate the patient's understanding and adherence, tell him how well he is doing on those points performed and how it is benefiting and improving his health. Most patients genuinely want to take charge of their health care. Try statements such as, "You understood (or performed) that quickly and well. Now let's go over the next point." Or, "Mr. Jones, you have done an excellent job keeping your dressing clean. The wound looks good. Now, it is time to begin to soak the area."

Determining the best method of improving adherence to patient education is a whole-team effort and will not rest on any single team member. Questions to help determine why the patient has poor adherence may include the following:

- How involved is the family, especially a spouse or parent? Adherence is far more likely if it is a collaborative effort that includes caregivers who are genuinely committed to and supportive of the patient's recovery.
- Were the patient and caregiver included in the planning process? Most people are more cooperative if given choices that include their individual needs.
- Have caregivers or family members lost patience with the patient? Have they found the changes and sacrifices too disruptive? Can these changes be modified to be more acceptable to the patient and caregivers?
- Is this nonadherence owing to poor communication from the health care team? Did the patient understand what he or she must do?
- Did the patient understand the importance of the directions given? Did the patient think the directions were optional?
- Do the directives go against the patient's cultural beliefs? Does his culture believe that illness and healing are divinely ordained and beyond his control? Will his culture continue to accept him in the group if the changes he must make are deeply prohibited?
- Finally, what is your relationship with the patient? Does he or she trust you? Can the patient share concerns without fear of reprisal or judgment?

It is important to remind patients that, if they do not adhere to the treatment plan, the health care provider may make unnecessary and possibly dangerous adjustments to their treatment. For example, Mr. Smith did not finish his full course of antibiotics for his urinary tract infection (UTI). He returns to the clinic because the UTI has not been resolved, but he does not mention during intake that he did not finish taking the antibiotics. His physician prescribes a stronger antibiotic for the UTI, thinking that the first antibiotic was not effective. This not only may lead to drug resistance, but Mr. Smith may experience more adverse effects because of taking the stronger antibiotic. If patients understand the importance of following directions, they are more likely to comply. Additionally, if they trust their health care providers, patients are more likely to keep them informed of their progress.

It is an important reminder that patients have a right to refuse or to discontinue treatment without asking for the health care provider's permission or approval. But we must try to determine why they have chosen to do this. Only in that way can we understand their reasoning and then try to persuade them to return to their treatment plan. Anytime that you feel the patient is not adherent, first check for understanding. If the patient understands the consequences and still refuses to adhere, this must be documented and brought to the health care provider's attention.

WORDS AT WORK

In this scenario, notice how the licensed practical nurse (LPN), Phil, uses open-ended questions to evaluate his patient's understanding and adherence.

Phil: It looks like your blood pressure is higher this visit than your last. Are you still taking your medication for high blood pressure?

Patient: Yes. I try to take it when I can.

Phil: So, remind me, what are you taking? And do you remember the dosage?

Patient: I think it's metoprolol and the pill is 100 mg.

Phil: And when do you normally take it?

Patient: I take it twice a day—one in the morning and another at night. But I don't always take the one in the morning because it makes me tired and my hands cold.

Phil: Well, I'm glad you told me that you're having some issues with your medication. But it's very important that you take your blood pressure medication as the doctor prescribed because we want to make sure we keep your blood pressure controlled. Otherwise, there are some long-term complications, such as heart attacks and strokes, with high blood pressure. We'll make sure the doctor knows and maybe you can discuss lowering the dosage or changing the medication with her.

▶▶ TAKING THE CHAPTER TO WORK

Medication Adherence

Joyce is performing a patient intake on a 20-year-old man who was diagnosed with insulin-dependent diabetes when he was 12 years old. He has come in for his annual check-up. He states that he usually meets with his certified diabetic educator once a year to manage his diabetes but missed his last appointment. Additionally, since he started college, he has been skipping meals and has not been good about checking his blood glucose levels. He states that it has been difficult for him to monitor his blood glucose level and to take his insulin injections as he should because of his busy and unpredictable schedule. Joyce documents this information in the patient's medical record and informs the physician, who discusses with him the long-term consequences of not controlling his diabetes. To help improve the patient's medication adherence, the physician recommends a new hybrid continuous glucose monitoring and insulin pump system, which will better accommodate his busy lifestyle. Joyce explains how the system works and how to care for it, and also provides a brochure on the system. She schedules a 3-month follow-up appointment and plans to call the patient in the next few days to see if he has any questions or is having any issues.

DOCUMENTING THE RESULTS

Documenting every patient encounter is critically important in ensuring quality of care and providing a legal record of that care. Patients are often seen by many different health care providers for a variety of medical issues who must know about the patient's health history and current treatments to provide care that is safe, efficient, and effective. Providers communicate with one another by recording patient information in the patient's medical record. Health care professionals review the patient's medical record to see relevant information from previous medical visits, including laboratory tests, treatments, procedures, and patient education (Fig. 3.10). This documentation maintains the continuity of care, which ensures the quality of patient care over time.

Documentation of patient education promotes communication between the patient and the health care provider on the patient's progress among the health care team. It ensures patient education was performed and prevents duplication of teaching. Documentation is also important for accreditation purposes, as a legal record,

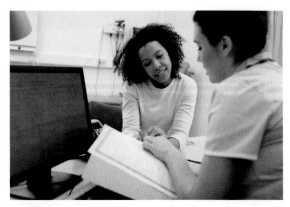

Fig. 3.10 A medical assistant and patient look over the patient's paper medical record from a different provider to be sure she has the correct information in her electronic health record. (iStock.com/bowdenimages.)

and for obtaining reimbursement from insurance companies for services rendered.

As you evaluate understanding and adherence, remember to record each contact. This includes encounters other than person-to-person with either the patient or a caregiver, such as telephone conversations and emails. At the end of each education session, each team member involved should sign the medical record to document the information covered and include his or her qualifications as a health care professional. If an interpreter was used for a patient who speaks English as a second language or if the education included caregivers, document this information.

In health care, it is presumed that any service that is not documented was not performed, which includes patient education. Each step of the education process must be documented and should include the following:

1. The patient's learning needs, learning style, and readiness to learn
2. The patient's knowledge of his or her condition and treatment options
3. The objectives and goals and what information was provided to the patient
4. How the information was provided to the patient, such as through discussion, demonstration, videos, or patient instruction sheet

5. The patient, family, and caregiver response to the patient education
6. The evaluation and effectives of the teaching
7. The date and time of the session if separate from regular care, such as over the phone. Include education given during routine patient care under the appropriate record entry.
8. A copy of the signed educational material provided to the patient, when appropriate. The patient keeps the original and signs that the information has been explained adequately.

An entry in the patient's medical record for instructions on a dressing change may look like the following:

Demonstrated and instructed on wound care and Standard Precautions for patient and wife. Wound cleaning and inspection of the site were explained, as well as how to dispose of soiled dressings. Patient and wife understood the importance of proper care and successfully demonstrated comprehension by repeating the procedure. Patient and wife received written instructions for home use and signed the Patient Education form. Next appointment for follow-up care is scheduled in 10 days.

▶▶ TAKING THE CHAPTER TO WORK

Patient Education Opportunities

Francine is working in a surgeon's office. She is caring for a patient who has multiple ulcers on her lower extremities. After the surgeon examines the patient, he asks Francine to apply gauze and compression stockings to the areas. Francine uses this opportunity to teach psychomotor skills to the patient. She explains why the dressings are important and then demonstrates how to apply them. She applies the dressing to the left leg and then has the patient apply the dressing to the right leg. While the patient applies the dressing, Francine is able to provide helpful hints and suggestions on caring for the ulcers. At the end of the teaching session, Francine asks the patient questions to ensure comprehension.

■ CHECKING YOUR COMPREHENSION

Write a brief answer for each of the following assignments.

1. Identify the five patient education steps. Write a short explanation of each step.
2. Describe the characteristics of a person who is "health literate."
3. Describe the three basic learning styles.
4. Differentiate the learning goal from the learning objective.
5. Give examples of the five most common implementation methods. Write a short explanation of each method.
6. Write six questions that you can ask to determine a patient's adherence.
7. List five key components that must be included in a patient's medical record after a teaching session.

■ EXPANDING CRITICAL THINKING

1. Look back at Maslow's Hierarchy of Needs. Where do you think the following people are on the pyramid? A young mother in a war-torn country; an artist at a showing of her award-winning sculpture; a young man in the initiation ritual into a gang in a dangerous inner city; a young event planner working her way up the corporate ladder. Does the communication level differ among these people? If so, how? With which person would you feel the most comfortable communicating and why? With whom would you feel least comfortable and why?
2. List three situations that may make you uncomfortable teaching patients. Would you be more comfortable if the patient were about your age and sex?

How would you feel if the patient is older than you? Younger than you? The opposite sex? How could you overcome your discomfort in each situation?

3. Mr. Carter is 85 and has recently suffered a cerebrovascular accident (CVA) and will need assistance at home with activities of daily living (ADLs), such as toileting, bathing, dressing, and eating, as well as range-of-motion exercises to increase his mobility. Mrs. Carter, who is his only relative, is a frail 83-year-old. In your opinion, do you think she is capable of his unassisted care? What should you do to help her to ensure that both patient and caregiver benefit during his recuperation? How would you communicate this need?

Communicating With Diverse Patient Groups

Judy Frain

CHAPTER OUTLINE

LEARNING OBJECTIVES

On successful completion of this chapter, you will be able to:

1. Recognize how the patient's perspective in the health care system differs from the perspective of the health care professional.
2. Describe how different cultural perspectives affect the delivery and receipt of health care.
3. Explain health disparities related to race and ethnicity.
4. Differentiate sex and gender and define key concepts related to gender identity.
5. Discuss health care and communication best practices when providing health care services to patients of diverse sexual orientations.
6. Discuss health care considerations regarding religious diversity.
7. Discuss health care considerations regarding treatment of patients across the lifespan.

KEY TERMS

asexual the characteristic of having no sexual feelings

bias a tendency to favor one way of thinking

cisgender a gender identity that aligns with the sex assigned at birth

concrete operational stage psychologist Jean Piaget's developmental stage from age 7 to age 11, during which children become more logical in thought, less egocentric, and begin to understand different viewpoints

culture the set of acceptable behaviors, beliefs, and material traits of a racial, religious, or social group

cultural imposition the tendency of a person or group to believe other cultures should adhere to its values and patterns of behavior

diverse the quality of being different

formal operational stage psychologist Jean Piaget's developmental stage from age 11 to age 15, during which children think abstractly and develop full autonomy

gender the psychosocial condition of being male, female, or neither of those gender expressions

genderfluid the characteristic of fluctuating between presenting as masculine, feminine, or neither, or both

gender identity one's conception of being male, female, or a non-binary gender

genderqueer having a non-binary gender identity

health disparity an unequal health outcome among disadvantaged populations

non-binary a category of gender identities that are not exclusively masculine or feminine, such as

identifying with both genders, neither gender, a third gender, or oscillating among genders

prejudice an opinion formed about a person, group or situation before facts and circumstances are known

preoperational stage psychologist Jean Piaget's developmental stage from age 2 to age 7, during which children tend to be egocentric and begin to use language

sensorimotor stage psychologist Jean Piaget's developmental stage from birth to age 2, during which children learn through their interactions with the environment

sex the biological aspects of being male or female

sexual orientation an individual's pattern of emotional, romantic and/or sexual attractions to others

transgender a gender identity or gender expression that differs from what is typically associated with the sex assigned at birth

transition process of altering one's sex from his or her birth sex

---

⚡ TEST YOUR COMMUNICATION IQ

Before reading this chapter, complete this short self-assessment test. Decide which statements are true and which are false.

1. When we use the term *diversity* we are referring only to persons of other races.
2. A person's religious traditions should have no bearing on his or her health care.
3. Sex and gender have the same meaning.
4. Recognizing our own personal biases can improve communication with diverse patients.
5. We should consider an adult patient's age when instructing them.
6. A child's developmental stage will always regress during an illness.
7. When caring for patients who are transitioning or transgender, always refer to them according to their sex at birth.

Results

Statements 4 and 5 are true; all other statements are false. How did you do? Read the chapter to learn more about these topics.

INTRODUCTION

The ability to communicate openly is vital to patient care. The exchange of thoughts, concerns, messages, and other important information eases stressful situations and environments and promotes health. When we engage with people who look like us, act like us, and share our values, we generally find that communication is simple; but as we engage with people who are **diverse**, or different from ourselves, both patients and coworkers, we may discover that communication is more challenging. Sometimes differences are easy to identify. Sometimes differences may be subtle and we may not be aware of them. When you hear the word diversity, what comes to mind? Initially you might think of cultural or ethnic differences, but diversity has many forms and layers. Consider, for example, that age, race, sex, sexual orientation, gender, gender identity, ability, socioeconomic status, and religion are among the many characteristics of diversity, and that multiple dimensions are present in every individual. Although differences present challenges, awareness of the diversity of our patients and their experiences provides useful information

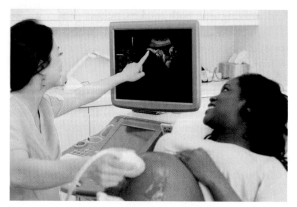

Fig. 4.1 Awareness of cultural diversity helps us understand our similarities and is central to providing the highest quality patient care. (iStock.com/MonkeyBusinessImages.)

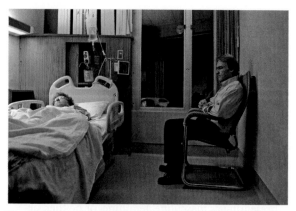

Fig. 4.2 Remember that an ordinary day for you is not a usual day for your patient and her family. (iStock.com/13Claudio13.)

for effective communication. As we practice awareness, we will begin to recognize not only differences but also similarities in "diverse" groups of people. This recognition and awareness will provide a strong foundation for effective communication (Fig. 4.1).

In patient care settings, you will often find that you and your patients have grown up with different values, views, and perspectives, and it will be important for you to pause and consider your own personal biases as you engage with those patients. It is your responsibility to listen to your patient's concerns and adapt your communication style to communicate effectively during each patient interaction. Remind yourself daily that the communication skills you bring can set the tone for a positive and effective experience for your patience.

This chapter discusses ways in which our biases may contribute to miscommunications and distrust. We will also consider care and communication issues among diverse patient dimensions such as race/ethnicity, sex, sexual orientation, gender, religion, and age.

THE DIVERSITY OF THE PATIENT EXPERIENCE

When health care professionals operate in the clinical workplace on a daily basis, it can be easy to lose sight of the patient's perspective (Fig. 4.2). What is a normal, average day for the certified nursing assistant, for example, can be an extraordinary life experience for the patient. To begin with, the health care system is intricate and often difficult to navigate. The flow of patients in the facility, the array of clinical and administrative personnel, and the details of billing and scheduling processes are second nature to the health care professionals who work in this environment, but can be daunting to many patients. On top of this, the stress of illness and the uncertainty of what the future might hold for patients and their families add to the difficulties. Consider for a moment that the assessments and other duties that you perform daily, such as taking vital signs, bathing patients, even taking health care histories, are not "routine" experiences for many of your patients. The presence of these stressors in conjunction with cultural differences and language barriers may make a clinic or hospital visit feel overwhelming to patients and their families.

Therefore, it is important to establish good communication with every patient. Take time to tell your patients and clients what you are doing and why, because this communication will plant seeds of trust. When trust is established, your patients and their families will be better able to absorb and consider information, follow medical advice and instruction, and adhere to medication and therapy regimens. In addition, patients will appreciate your efforts at recognizing and respecting their unique qualities, cultivating confidence in them that you are providing the best possible care. Making an effort to ensure that your patients understand what you are doing and why you are doing it may also provide a level of comfort, thereby reducing or alleviating some of the stresses on patients and their families as they deal with illness or injury.

As health care professionals, we are constantly shifting, moving from patient to patient, from one task to the next, all while prioritizing patient care. Most of us have experienced moments, maybe even entire shifts, when we feel we cannot devote time to learning to communicate with a patient who is different, who does not speak our language, or does not understand our body language. Be mindful, particularly in those busy moments, that effective communication can improve the patient's experience, shorten length of stay, reduce readmissions, and decrease health care costs. Effective communication in the health care setting, an art that can be developed with practice, contributes to better health outcomes for patients. Therefore effective communication is essential to providing the highest quality of care for every patient.

AWARENESS OF CULTURAL BIASES

As the world becomes smaller and more interdependent, it is common for health care professionals to care for and treat persons from a variety of cultures. A culture is the set of acceptable behaviors, beliefs, and material traits of a racial, religious, or social group. Therefore, a person's culture influences, at least in part, his or her perceptions of the world. Persons from diverse cultural groups may have their own views of health and illness, and their views may be very different from your own. As health care professionals, we must recognize that patients from different cultures may have different ideas about what it means to be sick or well, how to make decisions about treatments and care, who should be involved in those decisions, and what those treatments should be. It is important for health care professionals to be open to and accepting of cultural differences. Our inability to appreciate these differences may lead persons from diverse cultures to distrust the health care system and keep them from seeking care.

Cultural imposition is a term that describes when a person or group believes others should adhere to its values and patterns of behavior. Generally, when health care professionals impose their personal beliefs on patients, they decrease the chances of having a successful interaction with their patients. Patients may feel that their beliefs are not understood or respected. Feeling disconnected with care providers, patients may elect to

BOX 4.1 HEALTHY PEOPLE 2020 AND HEALTH DISPARITIES

Healthy People is a U.S. federal government initiative that sets 10-year goals and objectives to improve the overall health of the nation. Currently, national public policy operates under the framework of Healthy People 2020, with objectives to promote healthy behaviors and safe communities, and prevent and reduce diseases and disorders. Spanning 42 topic areas with more than 1200 objectives, Healthy People 2020 tracks progress toward a healthier life for all people. Thus, an overarching goal is the elimination of health disparities, or unequal outcomes among disadvantaged populations. To that end, Healthy People 2020 tracks rates of illness, death, chronic conditions, behaviors, and other types of outcomes in relation to race and ethnicity, genders, sexual identity and orientation, disability status or special health care needs, and geographic location (rural and urban) creating policy specifically to address social determinants of health (HealthyPeople.gov, 2019).

seek health care elsewhere, or disengage from the health care system entirely. Cultural imposition is one reason for the health disparities identified in Healthy People 2020, which has made eliminating disparities in health a priority (Box 4.1).

Culture also affects how patients perceive health care. A person's culture may have an impact on how they relate to and manage pain, illness, and injuries. Culture may also influence how patients feel about the health care profession versus traditional or natural healers, whether they feel they have control over their health, and whether they will follow our health care directives. Because our patient population is increasingly culturally diverse, we must strive to listen and learn as much as possible about the unique needs of each individual patient during the health care encounter. When we listen, we learn about other cultures and we tend to set aside our prejudices.

Now, take a few minutes to reflect on your own culture. Recognize how important your place in your community is to you. When you can do this objectively, you may become more aware of how alike we all are. Through awareness you develop respect for cultural differences and can better serve diverse patient groups.

TAKING THE CHAPTER TO WORK

A Diverse Clientele

Sue was orienting Bill, the new patient care associate, on how to interact with patients when meeting them for the first time. "How do you feel about working with patients who are different from yourself, with different attitudes, behaviors, and values?" she asked.

Bill responded, "It does not matter. I will treat all of my patients exactly the same; I will explain what I'm doing and educate my patients using the most up-to-date technical medical technology so that they have all the information possible."

Sue replied that although providing as much information as possible is a good rule to follow, not every patient will understand technical jargon and some may not even understand English. "We have to consider each patient individually and explain what we are doing using terms they can understand. Treating all your patients equally doesn't mean treating them all the same." Sue went on to explain further: "In this institution we see patients of all different ages, ethnicities and socioeconomic levels, with very diverse backgrounds. To communicate effectively we need to consider our audience, and tailor our messages to each individual patient. Your patients will appreciate that you took the time to make sure they understood what you were trying to communicate."

Personal Biases

Perhaps the most challenging obstacles to effective communication are our own biases and prejudices. Stated simply, a **bias** is a tendency to favor one way of thinking. You might hear of a newspaper being biased toward one political party, or a little league coach showing bias toward his own child when deciding who should play. Our personal biases can often reflect our own cultural norms about what is right or wrong, and inform our judgment about what is "good" or "bad." **Prejudice** means prejudging a person, group or situation, before facts and circumstances are known. Bias or prejudice may be formed through personal life experiences or lack of experiences. We may be unaware that some of our closely held beliefs interfere with communications more so than other obvious, superficial differences. The inability to recognize our personal beliefs and biases may lead to poor communication and present obstacles to beneficial patient care.

SPOTLIGHT ON SUCCESS

Looking Within

Be curious. Before each shift, or a few shifts a week, take a few minutes to take your own internal temperature. Notice, without self-judgment or self-criticism, a personal bias or strongly held belief—just notice it. At the end of your shift take a few minutes to assess whether and in what ways the simple awareness affected your interactions that day.

Diverse Patient Groups

In this text, we cover a lot of information about diverse patient groups. It should not be considered all-inclusive. As you enter the workplace, new situations will arise that you may feel unprepared to handle in a professional manner. You may find yourself unable to let go of some strongly held beliefs that could interfere with providing the best care to your patients. Remember, you do not have to agree with every view or choice your patient makes. You do not even necessarily have to understand the diverse views expressed by your patients. You do, however, need to be respectful of these differences and not let your personal biases interfere with caring for your patients in a professional manner. In every patient interaction, be honest, be flexible, be patient, and above all, **be kind**, without exception.

ETHNIC AND RACIAL DIVERSITY

Race and ethnicity are terms used for categorizing groups of people. Although these terms are sometimes used interchangeably, race concerns more of a shared ancestry and biological and genetic traits, whereas ethnicity refers to cultural characteristics, such as a common language, history, and shared traditions.

The United States is a racially and ethnically diverse country. The census recognizes five different racial categories: White, Black or African American, American Indian or Alaskan Native, Asian, and Native Hawaiian or other Pacific Islander. U.S. Census survey respondents may also report their race as "other," or select multiple races. The census categorizes ethnicity as "Hispanic or Latino," and "Not Hispanic or Latino." Hispanics and Latinos can be of any race.

As noted earlier, the world has become smaller and more interdependent, and the United States has become a more racially and ethnically diverse country. As a result, we, as health care professionals, now have opportunities

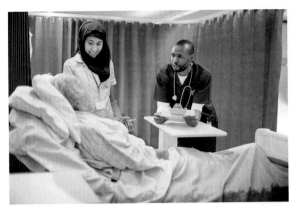

Fig. 4.3 As the world becomes smaller, we have the opportunity to work with and care for a variety of patients. (iStock.com/sturti.)

to treat and care for patients from many different races and ethnic groups (Fig. 4.3). It is therefore critical that we maintain a good awareness of how race and ethnicity can have an impact on a patient's access to health care, and his, her, or their experience within the health care system.

In the United States, racial and ethnic minorities including Blacks, Asians, and Hispanics have less access to health care services, primarily because they are less likely to have health insurance (Artiga, Foutz, & Damico, 2018). Lack of health insurance contributes to racial and ethnic health disparities in numerous ways. Without insurance, persons may delay or completely forgo health care, especially preventative and follow-up care. Persons who are seen regularly for health care may be diagnosed and treated earlier, precluding major health care problems and reducing health care costs. When uninsured persons do seek care, they are more likely to visit an emergency department for treatment, even for minor injuries or ailments. This can lead to further problems. Emergency departments are not designed to treat nonemergent health conditions. Emergency departments may not have access to a patient's medical history and, as a result, emergency physicians may order unnecessary tests. Emergency departments are not designed to provide follow-up care; patients are provided on-the-spot treatment for symptoms, but may have no access to follow-up care and treatment. Emergency departments are not capable of establishing and maintaining ongoing relationships with patients to promote continuity of care, making it more difficult to return the patient to

wellness. Therefore, this limited access to health care promotes health disparities among minority groups.

The Affordable Care Act (ACA) has led to a drop in the rates of uninsured persons across all races and ethnicities. Because minorities were less likely to be insured prior to the implementation of the ACA, uninsured rates dropped significantly more for Blacks and Hispanics than for Whites (Artiga, Foutz, & Damico, 2018). Whereas access to health care under the ACA has served to reduce health disparities in minority populations, persistent and significant gaps in health and access to health care remain. When comparing minorities and nonminority Medicare patients, a 2017 report published by the Office of Minority Health and the Rand Corporation found that Black and Hispanic men and women reported that it took longer to get health care appointments then it did for White men and women, and they were less able to get needed care. Asian and Pacific Islanders reported worse communication with their doctors than was reported by White men and women. Blacks, Asians, Pacific Islanders, and Hispanic men and women all reported more difficulty getting needed prescriptions than did White men and women (CMS Office of Minority Health and RAND Corporation, 2017).

COMMUNICATION GUIDELINES

Ethnic and Racial Diversity

When persons do seek access to health care at a clinic, urgent care, or private practice, be mindful that they may have never been treated outside an emergency department setting. How you treat your patients on their initial visit could have an impact on their decision to return for follow-up appointments and other subsequent health care visits. In some instances you may be the "face" of your health care facility. You may be the first health care professional to interact with the patients and you may spend more time with them than the physician or nurse practitioner. Your ability to relate well to all races and ethnicities will help to ensure a positive experience for your patient. A positive experience could open the way to developing a trusting and respectful health care relationship in which patients will return for regular visits, including check-ups, screenings, and preventative care. This could improve the quality of life for your patients by improving their overall health.

Health disparities can be noted in numerous health care measures, including access to prescription medications, prevalence of chronic conditions, and

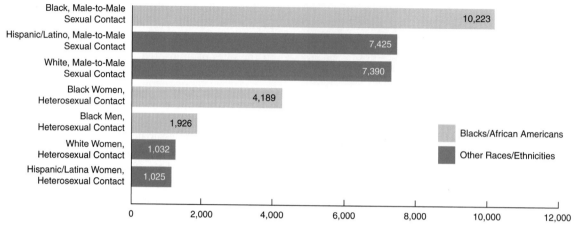

Fig. 4.4 HIV Diagnoses in the United States for the Most-Affected Subpopulations, 2016. (From Centers for Disease Control and Prevention, 2018, September 24. *HIV Among African Americans.* Retrieved from Centers for Disease Control and Prevention Website: https://www.cdc.gov/hiv/group/racialethnic/africanamericans/index.html.)

mortality rates for infants and adults. As part of the health care team, you should be aware of certain health conditions that adversely have an impact on racial and ethnic minorities. Human immunodeficiency virus (HIV), for instance, affects African Americans at higher rates than Whites (Fig. 4.4). According to the Centers for Disease Control and Prevention (CDC), nearly half of all new HIV diagnoses in 2016 were among African Americans, even though they make up only 12% of the U.S. population. Being African American in itself is not a risk factor for HIV, but a higher prevalence of the disease in African American communities combined with a tendency to choose sexual partners from within that community increases the risk of HIV transmission. Other risk factors include higher rates of other sexually transmitted diseases, limited access to quality health care, and lower income, putting African Americans at higher risk for HIV infection. In addition, because of stigma against those with HIV and lack of access to health care, approximately 1 in 6 African Americans living with HIV are unaware they even have the disease, making it more likely they will pass the disease on through unsafe sexual practices or sharing of needles (Centers for Disease Control and Prevention, 2018).

As another example, racial and ethnic minorities have higher rates of cardiovascular disease (CVD) and its risk factors, and experience worse health outcomes after a CVD diagnosis than whites. Age-adjusted deaths from CVD are approximately one third higher for African

Americans than for the overall U.S. population. High blood pressure is also more prevalent among African Americans, contributing to their increased risk of stroke (Graham, 2015). American Indians and Alaskan Natives are also disproportionately affected by heart disease. Approximately 15.4% of this population has been diagnosed with coronary artery disease, angina, heart attack, or another heart condition, whereas the rate among Blacks is 10.1%, and is 11.0% among Whites (Blackwell & Villaroel, 2018).

Diabetes is another disease that disproportionately affects racial and ethnic minorities. You may be surprised to learn that African Americans and Hispanics are 70% more likely to have a diabetes diagnosis compared with non-Hispanic White Americans; and Asian Americans, Native Hawaiian, and Pacific Islanders are approximately 20% more likely to have diabetes than non-Hispanic whites (Fig. 4.5). These minorities also have higher risks for complications related to diabetes, including limb amputation, blindness, and kidney failure (Centers for Disease Control and Prevention, 2017).

What can you, as a health care professional, do to alleviate some of the health disparities discussed above? Simple awareness of these types of disparities allows you to recognize risk factors and educate your patients. For example, you may have discussions with patients about safer sex practices, healthy food and lifestyle choices, and preventive health measures. Demonstrating how to check blood pressure or how to perform a glucose level

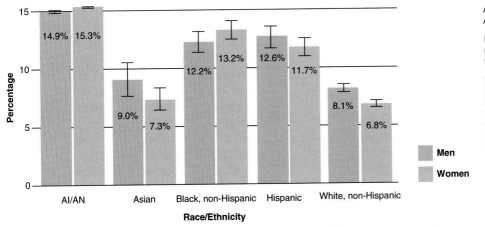

AI/AN = American Indian/Alaska Naitve.

Note: Error bars represent upper and lower bounds of the 95% confidence interval.

Data source: 2013–2015 National Health Interview Survey, except American Indian/Alaska Native data, which are from the 2015 Indian Health Service National Data Warehouse.

Fig. 4.5 Estimated age-adjusted prevalence of diagnosed diabetes by race/ethnicity and sex among adults aged ≥18 years, United States, 2013–2015. (Centers for Disease Control and Prevention. National Diabetes Statistics Report, 2017. Atlanta, GA: Centers for Disease Control and Prevention, US Department of Health and Human Services; 2017.)

check, and then allowing your patient to practice the procedure during a visit may provide your patients with the confidence they need to perform these procedures on their own. Ensuring your patient has the necessary home supplies, whether that means a supply of condoms, a portable blood pressure device, or a glucometer, could help the patient monitor his or her health at home. In busy clinics, information pamphlets tailored to different racial and ethnic groups can be a simple and effective means of providing important information. Education regarding prevention and early detection will likely lead to a reduction in the need for treatment-related visits and quite likely to improvement in the patient's quality of life.

Much work remains to be done if we are to eliminate racial and ethnic health disparities. But you have a unique opportunity to make a difference in your patients' lives through awareness, listening, and providing useful information and tools. So be attentive, be proactive, and be respectful.

Overcoming a Language Barrier

Increasing globalization means that we may be presented with patients whose primary language is not English. Some of these patients may have learned to speak or read English, some may have family members with them who speak English, and some may have little or no understanding of English. In these situations, it is important for health care professionals to have basic knowledge of the resources available in the health care center, and to advocate for use of those resources to benefit their patients. For example, when working with patients who do not speak English, or who have difficulty understanding English, particularly medical terms, you can advocate for your patient by calling for an interpreter. The interpreter can facilitate communications between you and your patient, interpreting what you and other health care professionals are communicating to the patient, and interpreting the patient's response back to you. Chapter 5 explores language barriers in detail.

✴ LEGAL EAGLE

Title VI of the Civil Rights Act of 1964 is a federal law that protects people from discrimination based on their race, color, or national origin. In health care, any facility or program that receives federal funds, such as Medicare, must provide the same service in the same way to everyone. Because the U.S. Supreme Court has ruled that discrimination against individuals who are not fluent in English is discrimination against national origin, providers must make sure they offer non-English speakers the same access to care as English speakers. They must provide language assistance at no cost, translate consent forms and other written materials, and post signs in alternate languages when other ethnic or cultural groups are prominent.

DIVERSITY IN SEX, GENDER, AND GENDER IDENTITY

In the not-so-distant past a chapter discussing diverse patient groups would not have included a section on sex and gender identity. We tended to think of male and female, and boy and girl, as terms that would encompass sex or genders. In essence, the words "sex" and "gender" were used almost interchangeably. More recently, however, gender is being viewed in a larger context. Terms such as *gender identity, gender expression, transgender, gender non-binary*, and *gender fluid* are being used by patients in identifying themselves. "Sex" and "gender" are now considered separate characteristics of personhood.

As health care professionals, we have a responsibility to provide care in a welcoming, inclusive manner to all of our patients, including those who do not conform to societal norms or our personal beliefs. In this section we will present some of the accepted terminology used with persons who identify outside of traditional gender norms. Keep in mind, however, that terminology continues to evolve, and you are certain to hear terms that are not addressed in this text. Being unfamiliar with proper terminology is not an excuse to treat your patients in a disrespectful manner. In general, do not be afraid to ask questions! It is a sign that you care about your patients and acknowledge their humanity.

Sex is a biological status, determined by a person's DNA, assigned at birth based on the appearance of external genitals to distinguish between males and females. In contrast, gender is influenced by an individual's life experiences, including one's perceptions of sexuality in addition to society's perceptions. Gender is the psychosocial condition of being male, female, or neither of those, whereas **sex** refers to the biological aspects of being male or female. Gender identity is the term used to describe how a person identifies their sex. Gender identity can be the same as the sex assigned at birth, or it can be different. Another term you may become familiar with is transgender. This is a term used for people whose gender identity or gender expression differs from what is typically associated with the sex they were assigned at birth. You may also hear the term cisgender, which describes a person whose gender identity aligns with the sex assigned at birth (i.e., a person who is not transgender).

Although the size of the transgender population is not well-known, it is estimated that about 1.4 million transgendered adults are living in the United States. This population may present with health care problems unique to their transgender status. They may also present with illnesses or health care issues that are unrelated to their being transgendered. Many transgender people are prescribed hormones by their health care professionals to align their bodies with their gender identity, and some people will also undergo surgery for this purpose; however, not all transgender people undergo these medical therapies and their transgender identity is not dependent on physical appearance nor on medical procedures.

Transition is a term used when a person is in the process of altering one's sex from his or her birth sex. There are various steps and therapies within the transition process, and the decisions to embark on any step or therapy is a very personal and emotional decision. Individuals may change their name or begin to dress differently. An individual may also seek medical interventions, such as hormone therapy or confirmation surgery. In the past we referred to a person undergoing a "sex change," but now refer to this as a person "in transition."

▓ SPOTLIGHT ON SUCCESS

Care for Transgender Patients
A recent study found that over half of all nurses surveyed expressed discomfort and lack of knowledge in caring for transgender patients (Carabez, Eliason, & Martinson, 2016). Taking the time and effort to learn about this marginalized group will give you the confidence and knowledge to serve these patients in a caring and professional manner.

While we tend to think of gender in *binary* terms (male or female), some people do not feel they fit neatly into either of those categories. Those who are nonbinary comprise a category of gender identities that are not exclusively masculine or feminine, such as identifying with both genders, neither gender, a third gender, or oscillating among genders. The term genderqueer is used to describe a non-binary gender identity that does not fit into either the male or female category. Genderqueer individuals may identify as both genders at once, neither man nor woman, or embody a third gender. Genderfluid is another term that has become more common. This term refers to a person who does not confine themselves to a single gender, fluctuating between presenting as masculine, feminine, or neither, or both.

This terminology may be new and confusing at first. Keep in mind that patients who do not conform to traditional gender identities will probably not expect you to be up to date on the latest terminology. But they will expect you to be respectful in your communication. One of the first steps in showing that you are making the effort to communicate effectively is to use the proper pronoun when caring for your patients. The words "they" and "their" can be used to describe someone who identifies as neither male nor female, as in the following sentence: "Each person should be able to express *their* gender is a way that feels comfortable to *them*." Table 4.1 lists gender neutral pronouns and examples of usage.

It is ok to ask questions and to clarify terms. A simple way of clarifying terms to ask the patient, "What are your pronouns?" By asking this question you are showing that you respect a person's self-identification and want to use the gender pronouns with which they identify. Alternatively, you can use

singular "they/them" pronouns if you do not know and have not asked about someone's pronouns. Either alternative may seem awkward at first, but making incorrect assumptions regarding someone's gender identity can be painful and embarrassing for both you and your patient.

COMMUNICATION GUIDELINES

Diversity in Sex, Gender, and Gender Identity
When communicating with others, the following guidelines can help:
- Ask, "What pronouns do you use?"
- Introduce yourself with your own pronouns, such as "My name is Ben and I use the pronouns he/him/his."
- Do not assume someone's pronouns based on their appearance.
- If someone doesn't share their pronouns with you, or doesn't want to share their pronouns, you can always use their name.
- It is not always possible to avoid mistakes, but a simple apology can go a long way. If you do make an error, you can say something like: "I apologize for using the wrong pronoun/name/terms. I did not mean to disrespect you."

TABLE 4.1 Gender Pronouns*

Nominative	Oblique	Possessive Determiner	Possessive Pronoun	Reflexive	Example
he	him	his	his	himself	He expresses himself.
she	her	her	hers	herself	She expresses herself.
they (singular)	them	their	theirs	themself	They express themselves.
ze (or zie) (pronounced "zee")	zir ("zere")	zir ("zere")	zirs ("zeres")	zirself ("zereself")	Ze expresses zirself.
ze ("zee")	hir ("here")	hir ("here")	hirs ("heres")	hirself ("hereself")	Ze expresses hirself.
sie ("zee")	sie ("zee")	hir ("here")	hirs ("heres")	hirself ("hereself")	Sie expresses hirself.
ey ("a")	em ("m")	eir ("ear")	eirs ("ears")	eirself ("earself")	Ey expresses eirself.
xe ("zee")	xem ("zem")	xyr ("zere")	xyrs ("zeres")	xemself ("zemself")	Xe expresses xemself.

*This is not a complete list of pronouns. Many others exist, but this should help you pronounce and conjugate non-binary forms.

WORDS AT WORK

Kylie was confused upon entering the room and seeing her patient sitting on the examination table. She held a chart with the name James Baker on the front, but the person she saw sitting there appeared to be female. Quickly realizing that her patient did not conform to the gender stereotypes she was accustomed to, she considered how best to address her patient.

"Hello, my name is Kylie, and I use she/her/hers. How shall I address you?"

The patient responded, "I go by Jamie."

Seeking further clarification, Kylie asked, "Hi Jamie, it's nice to meet you. What are your pronouns?"

"They, them, theirs." Jamie replied.

Jamie was more relaxed now that they realized Kylie was comfortable caring for persons who do not fit neatly into stereotypical gender roles.

Kylie avoided what could have been an embarrassing interaction for her and a hurtful experience for her patient by understanding gender diversity.

SEXUAL ORIENTATION

Sexual orientation is usually discussed in terms of three distinct categories: heterosexual, homosexual, and bisexual. In reality, sexual orientation ranges along a continuum, from exclusively attracted to someone of the opposite sex, to exclusively attracted to someone of the same sex. There are also people who feel no sexual attraction. The term for this is asexual. The term sexual orientation describes more than just the gender with which a person has sex; it encompasses who a person is attracted to romantically, emotionally, and sexually, and the sociocultural environment associated with this attraction. A person has a sexual orientation even if they have not had sex.

A person's sexual orientation may have no bearing on why that person is being seen for health care. A patient may think you are overstepping if you ask about sexual matters when the patient is being treated for the flu or a broken leg. When asking questions, be sure the questions are related to caring for the patient and that you are not asking simply because you are curious.

Gay, Lesbian, and Bisexual Patients

Gay and lesbian individuals are represented in every race, culture, religion, age group, and socioeconomic class. Depending on why a person is seeking health care, it may or may not be important to know a patient's sexual orientation; however, assuming all of your patients are heterosexual is disrespectful to those who fall outside of that traditional norm. Enhancing communication with your gay and lesbian patients will improve health outcomes and help ensure they will continue to seek care.

When health care professionals encounter gay, lesbian, or bisexual patients in their practice they can either create a welcoming atmosphere, or put up barriers owing to personal biases or lack of understanding. First impressions are important. A welcoming atmosphere can be offered even before a word is uttered. For example, step back and look around the patient areas of your facility. If all of your informational posters and flyers portray heterosexual couples and traditional families, gay and lesbian patients may feel excluded and marginalized. As a result, they may be less likely to disclose their sexual orientation. One way to convey a safe and supportive setting is by displaying a welcoming rainbow sign in a public area (Fig. 4.6). The pride flag is a succinct way to show that your workplace welcomes and affirms all types of patients.

Studies show that lesbian, gay, bisexual, and transgender youth have difficulty sharing their sexual orientation with their primary care provider (Heslin, Gore, King, & Fox, 2008), and lesbian women seek routine and preventive medical care at lower rates than the general population (Steele, Tinmouth, & Lu, 2006). Although attitudes are changing, gays and lesbians remain less likely to be cared for by culturally competent health care professionals. Negative attitudes of health care professionals, whether overt or perceived, may lead patients to delay or avoid health care. This can result in delayed or

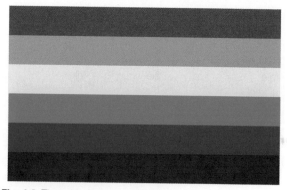

Fig. 4.6 The pride flag indicates support for diversity.

missed diagnoses, resulting in health outcomes that are less than optimal for your patient.

Healthy People 2020 described health disparities of gays and lesbians, including higher rates of smoking, alcohol, and other drug use, and higher rates of depression and anxiety (U.S. Department of Health and Human Services Office of Disease Prevention and Health Promotion, 2018). Heath care professionals may be better able to address these health disparities if they are aware of their patient's sexual orientation, and may be able to provide culturally competent written materials that may aid these patients in addressing these problems.

Meeting the needs of gay and lesbian patients can be accomplished simply by listening, asking the right questions, and making simple adjustments in how you practice. Remember to avoid assumptions. When admitting a new patient or taking a patient history, ask open-ended questions. If your patients state that they are married, then ask their spouse's name. Don't assume a woman is married to a man, or a man to a woman. Many gays and lesbians are in long-term relationships, but never marry. So when asking questions regarding social support networks, ask questions such as: "Are you married or in a relationship?" Questions like this are more likely to get the information you are trying to collect.

Certain diseases are more common in gay men or lesbians than in the general population. One example of this is HIV. Although HIV is found in all communities, the largest percentages of HIV infections are attributable to male-to-male sexual contact and gay males remain at the highest risk for contracting HIV. Knowing your patient's sexual orientation would be important if you are teaching prevention strategies to avoid HIV infection, or for teaching your patients living with HIV how to practice safer sex to avoid passing the virus on to a sexual partner. Although the physician or nurse may have the primary role in educating the patient, there will be times when this may be your role. You may have a patient who feels comfortable talking with you, and may ask you questions about something he has read or seen on the internet. You may have to decide when to seek guidance from other health care professionals, and when you have the background and knowledge to answer questions.

It is important to understand that not all men who have sex with men identify as gay. Simply because a man tells you he is heterosexual does not mean he has sex with women exclusively. A follow-up question about sexual activity would be important when communicating information about safe sex practices.

Current statistics indicate that lesbians are less likely to have health insurance and thus less likely to have mammograms, pap smears, and other routine health assessments (Gonzalez & Blewett, 2014). Communicating the importance of routine health care and providing information on free or discounted health resources available to your patients can be a way of keeping this marginalized population active in the health care system.

RELIGIOUS DIVERSITY

Religious traditions are often complex, incorporating teachings and rituals that are subject to interpretation by individuals and groups within the same tradition. Religious traditions can prove confusing if we are not familiar with them. It is not possible to predict how any one patient or family member's religious beliefs will interface with their understanding and choices of health care. When caring for patients, you will need to understand that religion often influences how patients react to illness, pain, and many health care decisions. Remaining nonjudgmental when a patient's religious beliefs are in conflict with your own is important in providing health care for diverse patient groups.

Some religious traditions have rules that directly affect medical decisions. Jehovah's Witnesses, for example, have a strict rule against receiving blood transfusions (Fig. 4.7). Muslims, along with some other religious traditions, consider suffering to be spiritually enriching and may refuse pain medications for this reason. Buddhists may also limit analgesics as they near the end of life over a concern for their consciousness during this time. In your role as a health care professional, you may witness how religion affects health care decisions. You are, however, more likely to be involved with nonmedical aspects of how religion affects your patient and how you care for them.

Some patients of the Buddhist, Hindu, and Muslim traditions have culturally based concerns regarding modesty. When hygiene therapies or procedures require disrobing or partial nudity, patients may request that a health care professional of the same sex provide that care. Your institution may have policies regarding how these personnel decisions are made.

Advance directive card carried by most Jehovah's Witnesses

Advance Directive to Refuse Specified Medical Treatment

1. I, _____ (print or type full name), born
_____ (date) complete this document to set forth my
treatment instructions in case of my incapacity. **The refusal of specified treatment(s) contained
herein continues to apply even if those medically responsible for my welfare and/or any other
persons believe that such treatments are necessary to sustain my life.**

2. I am one of Jehovah's Witnesses with firm religious convictions. With full realization of the implications
of this position I direct that **NO TRANSFUSIONS OF BLOOD or primary blood components (red cells,
white cells, plasma or platelets)** be administered to me in any circumstances, I also refuse to predonate
my blood for later infusion.

3. **Regarding minor fractions of blood** (for example: albumin, coagulation factors, immunoglobulins):
[Initial **one** of the three choices below.]

   (a) _____ I refuse all
   (b) _____ I accept all
   (c) _____ I want to quantify either (3a) or (3b) above and my treatment choices are as follows:
   _____

   _____

4. **Regarding autologous procedures** (involving my own blood, for example: haemodilution, heart bypass,
dialysis, intra-operative and post-operative blood salvage):
[Initial **one** of the three choices below.]

   (a) _____ I refuse all such procedures or therapies
   (b) _____ I am prepared to accept any such procedure
   (c) _____ I accept only the following procedures:
   _____

   _____

I am prepared to accept diagnostic procedures, such as blood samples for testing.

5. **Regarding other welfare instructions** (such as current medications, allergies, and medical problems):
_____

_____

_____

Fig. 4.7 Jehovah's Witnesses' beliefs prohibit them from receiving blood transfusions; many carry a durable power of attorney and advance directive to communicate their choice to health care providers in case they are unconscious. (From Lucy Yang, Zorica Jankovic. Orthotopic liver transplantation in Jehovah's Witnesses. *Current Anaesthesia & Critical Care.* 2008;19:34–41.)

Continued

6. I consent to my medical records and the details of my condition being shared with the Emergency Contact below and/or with member(s) of the Hospital Liaison Committee for Jehovah's Witnessess.

7. ______________________________ ______________________________
Signature Date

____
Address

8. **STATEMENT OF WITNESSES:** The person who signed this document did so in my presence. He or she appears to be of sound mind and free from duress, fraud, or undue influence. I am 18 years of age or older.

Signature of witness	Signature of witness
Name Occupation	Name Occupation
Address	Address
Telephone	Telephone
Mobile	Mobile

9. **EMERGENCY CONTACT:**

____
Name

____
Address

____
Telephone Mobile

10. **GENERAL PRACTITIONER CONTACT DETAILS:** A copy of this document is lodged with the Registered General Medical Practitioner whose details appear below.

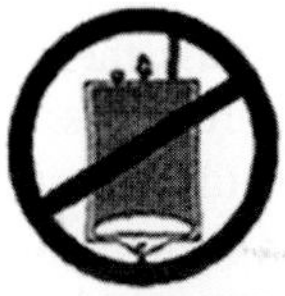

____
Name

____
Address

____
Telephone Number(s)

Page 2 of 2

NO BLOOD

(signed document inside)

Advance Decision to Refuse Specified Medical Treatment

Advance Decision to Refuse Specified Medical Treatment

(signed document inside)

NO BLOOD

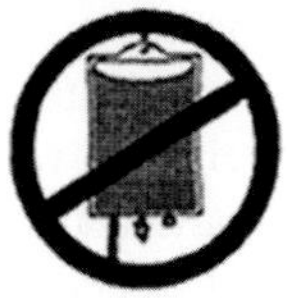

TABLE 4.2   Dietary Restrictions for Certain Religions

Religion	Restrictions
Hinduism	All meats are prohibited.
Islam	Pork and intoxicating beverages are prohibited.
Judaism	Pork, predatory fowl, shellfish, other water creatures (fish with scales are permissible), and blood by ingestion (e.g., blood sausage and raw meat) are prohibited. Foods should be kosher (meaning "properly preserved"). All animals must be ritually slaughtered by a shochet (i.e., quickly with the least pain possible) to be kosher. Mixing dairy and meat dishes at the same meal is prohibited.
Mormonism (Church of Jesus Christ of Latter-day Saints)	Alcohol, tobacco, and beverages containing caffeine (e.g., coffee, tea, colas, and select carbonated soft drinks) are prohibited.
Seventh-Day Adventism	Pork, certain seafood (including shellfish), and fermented beverages are prohibited. A vegetarian diet is encouraged.

From Nies M, McEwen M: *Community/Public Health Nursing*. St. Louis, 2019, Elsevier.

Many religions have dietary restrictions that may affect how you care for your patients, especially if you are working in an inpatient setting. Some religions require members to fast on certain days or certain times of the day. Some religions restrict certain foods altogether, or during times sacred or important to their religious tradition. Your patients may inform you of their dietary requirements or you can ask them. Table 4.2 lists dietary restrictions for certain religions.

Some religions require prayers at certain times of the day. Muslims, for example pray five times per day. Care should be taken to avoid disturbing your patient during these times whenever possible. Catholic patients may request daily communion, which can often be arranged through chaplain services at your institution or through a nearby parish. Jewish patients, especially those of the orthodox tradition, may strictly observe the rule not to work on the Sabbath (from sundown on Friday through sundown on Saturday). Under strict guidelines, this restricts turning on a light switch, pressing a call button, or raising and lowering their bed. Understanding these restrictions allows you to work with your patients to keep them safe and well-cared for during this time.

Not all patients adhere to religious traditions in the same manner or to the same extent. Therefore, you should encourage your patients and family members to express how their religious values may be relevant to their hospital stay, particularly in areas of personal needs, interaction with staff, and treatment decisions.

▶▶ TAKING THE CHAPTER TO WORK

Awareness of Spiritual Needs

Jane was caring for a patient recovering from knee surgery following an automobile accident. During morning rounds the nurse had told Jane that she wanted her to get the patient up and walking in the hallway so she could be discharged later that day. When Jane entered the room she told her patient, Mrs. Awan, that she was going to take her for a walk. Mrs. Awan, a Muslim, asked Jane if she could come back later because it was time for her morning prayer.

Jane dismissed Mrs. Awan's request. "I'll have you back really soon," she said, at the same time she was tightening a gait belt around the patient. "Right now it's more important that we get you up and moving so you can be discharged on time."

Mrs. Awan did not want to cause trouble or alienate the person caring for her, so she complied with Jane's orders; however, she felt disrespected, and disappointed that her religious requirements were ignored.

Jane did not mean to disrespect Mrs. Awan. In fact, she was not even aware she had done so. Jane did not realize the importance of praying at five specific times each day. Rather than talking to her patient about her religious needs, or asking if she could pray after her walk, Jane assumed the timing of prayers was unimportant. If she had taken a little extra time and asked Mrs. Awan why she needed to pray at that specific time, she could have learned a little about the Muslim faith and honored her patient's religious traditions by scheduling her care around Mrs. Awan's prayer schedule.

DIVERSITY IN AGE

We seldom consider age when we are thinking about diverse patient groups; however, age differences present another potential obstacle to effective communication. Obviously we communicate differently with children than with adults but we also communicate with small children differently than older children and we communicate with younger adults differently than with older adults. Take a few minutes now and notice how you are constantly adjusting your communication style based on your audience. In this next section we will discuss methods for communicating with different age groups.

Communicating With Children

Have you ever watched children at a playground or an amusement park? If so, you have undoubtedly noticed that children are not simply small versions of adults. You may also have noticed that, in most situations, children do not communicate in the same way as adults do, and that infants, toddlers, children, and adolescents all have unique methods and strategies for communication. Although the development of communication in children and young adults is fascinating, it also presents unique challenges for health care providers who care for children. Fortunately, several developmental theories can help us understand the intellectual capabilities of children at different ages. The CDC has published a chart depicting milestones for social/emotional, language/communication, cognitive/learning, and physical development of children from birth to 5 years of age. Swiss psychologist Jean Piaget (1896–1980) developed a commonly used theory of intellectual development based on the chronological age of a child. According to Piaget's theory, all children go through the same four developmental stages. Later research suggests that cultural context also plays a role in cognitive development. Accordingly, health care professionals should not be surprised when a child does not neatly fit within the development stage that corresponds with his or her chronological age. When caring for young patients, you may find it useful to consider the developmental stages below as general guidelines.

The Sensorimotor Stage

The **sensorimotor stage** lasts from birth to 2 years of age. In this stage children gain knowledge through their interactions with the environment. Physical growth and cognitive development occur quickly during this stage. Children

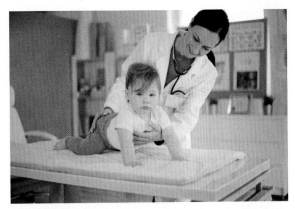

Fig. 4.8 A baby who crawls and does not yet speak is in the sensorimotor stage. (iStock.com/M_a_y_a.)

acquire physical skills, such as crawling and walking, and begin to acquire language skills (Fig. 4.8). Milestones of the sensorimotor stage include the following:

- Sucking and rooting (the ability to bring things to the mouth)
- Eye/hand (seeing an object and reaching for it)
- Discovering self-rewarding activities (thumb-sucking, playing with a favorite object)
- Anticipating ("I see the bottle. It must be for me.")
- Exploring ("If I pull this lamp cord, I wonder what will happen?")
- Verbal skills also develop during this stage as children learn to communicate and interact with caregivers.

Caring for patients in this developmental stage can be both challenging and rewarding. Patients of this age will not understand the limitations their illness or injury may place on them. They may experience your care as causing pain rather than helping them to heal; as a result, they develop a fear of health care professionals. Communicating with patients this young involves providing care in a gentle manner. Speaking in soft, soothing tones will help calm patients and their family members, if they are present. Providing care in this manner while parents or guardians are present also aids in building trust between patients, their familes, and you, the health care professional.

The Preoperational Stage

The **preoperational stage** includes ages 2 to age 7. This age is self-centered; these children believe the world revolves around them. They begin to learn from friends in their playgroup and at school and feel the need to blend with their peers. Milestones of this stage of development include:

- Engage in role playing, often pretending to a be mom, a dad, or a teacher
- Enjoy pretending, and engage in symbolic play
- Develop a memory, understand past and future
- Tend to be egocentric and struggle to see things from the perspective of others

While they are getting better with language and thinking, they still tend to think about things in very concrete terms. When communicating with patients at this stage, remember that it is not unusual for children to regress to earlier stages when ill or injured. Children may need more comforting than they would if healthy, and they may rely on you for comfort, especially when their parents or family members are unavailable. Basic explanations of what you are doing in providing care will help children of this age feel more comfortable during health care visits.

The Concrete Operational Stage

The concrete operational stage spans ages 7 to 11. With greater reasoning skills, children of this age understand that things and people change, that you might have a point of view different from theirs, and they can consider and accept differences of opinion. They understand abstract concepts and are beginning to exercise self-determination (autonomy). Peer groups are frequently more influential than family at this age. In addition, children in the concrete operational stage:

- Develop logical thinking skills, although thinking remains very concrete
- Begin using inductive logic, moving from specific information to a general principle

At this age children have a better understanding of your role as a health care professional. They will be able to follow basic instructions that are given to them. They will often want to know what you are doing and why you are performing certain tasks, so it is important to keep them in the loop (Fig. 4.9). Let them know what is happening, but do not overwhelm them.

The Formal Operational Stage

The formal operational stage includes ages 11 to 15. With deepening and developing levels of social skills, this age group recognizes its unique personality and begins to question authority for the full autonomy needed for adulthood.

- Begin to develop abstract thinking skills
- Can use reasoning skills to answer hypothetical problems

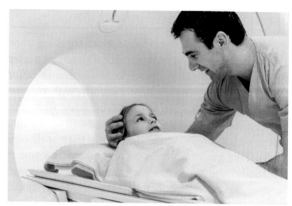

Fig. 4.9 Explaining a process and describing what you are doing will help younger patients feel more comfortable. (iStock.com/skynesher.)

- Consider ethical and moral issues from points of view other than their own
- Develop deductive reasoning skills, moving from the general principles to the specific instances

Children in the formal operational stage may be very interested and involved in their care (Fig. 4.10). They may explore their illness on the internet and attempt to act as experts on how they wish to be cared for. Communication should include partnering with your patient in developing a care plan. Getting buy-in from your patient will increase adherence to the care plan.

Each of these stages of development and comprehension will require different approaches for effective communication. Here are a few cues. Understanding the patient's developmental level and ability to comprehend before beginning an encounter will result in an

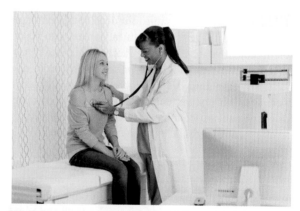

Fig. 4.10 The teenage patient in the formal operational stage is usually interested and involved in her care. (iStock.com/FatCamera.)

interaction that is less stressful and more productive for everyone. Try not to expect children to comprehend explanations or follow instructions beyond their level of understanding. Be patient. Remember that when children are ill, they may regress from their current level of development to an earlier level. For example, some children who are potty-trained may revert back to bedwetting or may have frequent accidents, requiring the use of diapers. Some children who had been testing their independence prior to an injury or illness may suddenly become more dependent on a parent or carer. Some children exhibit anger if their illness or injury prevents them from interacting with their friends or inhibits their ability to lead a "normal" life. These children may lash out or withdraw or they may alternate quickly from one behavior to another. Patience and understanding are important parts of communicating and caring for all patients, including children.

Remember that these developmental stages are a guide when communicating with children, regardless of their age or cultural background. Each child will develop at his or her own pace, and each will have unique characteristics that present during your communications with them. Your ability to adapt to each patient's communication style and needs is one of the most effective communication tools you possess.

▶ TAKING THE CHAPTER TO WORK

Understand the Adolescent's Need for Privacy

Jack was being seen in the clinic for his high school physical prior to starting his freshman year. Jack's mom was also in the room with them. Prior to the nurse practitioner performing the physical Emily was asking Jack some of the questions on the form.

- "Are you taking any medications?"
- "How many hours of sleep do you get each night?"
- "Are you sexually active?"

Emily could see Jack was embarrassed by the last question, but she recorded his "no" answer on the form. When the nurse practitioner began the physical she asked Jack's mother to leave the room. While performing the physical she discussed many health issues with Jack and asked him if he was sexually active. This time Jack said yes. The nurse practitioner inquired further about Jack's sexual activities and provided relevant education. This encounter taught Emily a valuable lesson that has guided many future encounters. Teenagers may be more honest and forthcoming if seen privately, rather than in the company of a parent. Emily now asks parents or guardians to wait outside when she works with teenage patients.

Communicating With Adults

We often group adults into a single category; however, just as we must consider the age and developmental milestones of a child when we are providing care, we must likewise consider the age and developmental decline of our adult patients. Younger adults and older adults may have very different life experiences and may interact within the health care system in very different ways. It is worth repeating that your ability to discern and adapt to each patient's communication style is a beneficial tool to the art of communication.

Communicating With Older Adults

In the United States, persons aged 65 and older are considered to be *older adults*. The Department of Health and Human Services, the Administration for Community Living, and the Administration on Aging (AoA) publish a yearly report called the Profile of Older Americans. This is a rich source of data, detailing the characteristics of this population and its expected future growth. This growing population numbered 49.2 million in 2016, and is projected to double to 98 million by 2060. The population of adults aged 85 and older is also projected to double from 6.4 million in 2016 to more than 14 million in 2040. Persons reaching age 65 can be expected to live about 20 additional years, with females having a slightly longer life expectancy than males. Racial and ethnic minorities comprise approximately 23% of this older population (AoA, Administration for Community Living, U.S. Department of Health and Human Services, 2018).

Generally, the need for health care increases as people age. In a 2017 survey, 45% of noninstitutionalized people aged 65 and older considered their health as excellent or very good, whereas 64% of younger adults reported excellent or very good health. Most older adults have at least one chronic health condition and many deal with multiple health problems. Older adults reported more overnight hospital stays and more health care visits than younger adults. Nearly 20% of older adults reported 10 or more health care visits in the past 12 months (Administration on Aging [AoA], 2018).

These numbers serve as a reminder that many of the patients we care for within the health care system will be older patients. Developing effective strategies to communicate successfully with older patients will result in better care, whether the patient is in an inpatient or outpatient setting.

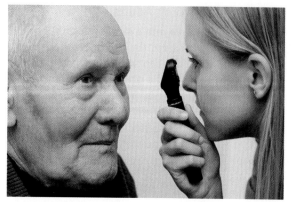

Fig. 4.11 Glaucoma is a common cause of vision deficits in older adults. (iStock.com/Barabas Atilla.)

Although language ability does not normally decline among older adults, some age-related changes can have an impact on communication. Hearing loss is common in older adults. By the time adults reach age 75, almost 50% experience significant hearing impairment, with men more likely to experience hearing problems than women. When speaking with a patient with a hearing deficit, position yourself in front of the patient, face to face and at eye level. Maintain eye contact, enunciate, speak clearly, and eliminate background noise whenever possible.

Vision deficits are also common with aging (Fig. 4.11). Reading small print and reading in dim light are common problems for older people. When providing written instructions to your older patients ensure that the type is large enough to be easily legible and avoid dark backgrounds because these can render written text more difficult to read. Chapter 5 discusses

communication through sensorineural deficits in more detail.

Older adults also experience comprehension difficulties that often result from a decline in working memory. Older adults often process information at a slower speed and thus have difficulty understanding complex sentences. When communicating with older adults, consider using concise sentences to convey information.

COMMUNICATION GUIDELINES

Older Adult Patients
Some additional cues to improve communications with older patients are:
- Address older patients by their surname and title, such as Mr. or Mrs. Smith, unless given permission by the patient to address them otherwise.
- Avoid the tendency to stereotype; treat each older patient as an individual.
- Avoid speaking in a patronizing manner. Never speak to older patients as if they were children.
- Face older adults when speaking with them and minimize background noise.
- Reinforce key points and consider visual aids to clarify important instructions.
- Seek clarification of instructions to verify comprehension.
- Consider older adult's living situation when planning discharge.
- Include caregivers when providing instructions, when appropriate.
- Express understanding and compassion to help the patient manage fear and unease with the health care system.

⏩ TAKING THE CHAPTER TO WORK

Working With Age-Related Sensory Deficits
Keith was helping to teach a class on art therapy for older adults. As each person entered the room Keith addressed them by their surname: "Good afternoon Mr. Carpenter," Nice to see you again Mrs. Clark," "How are you doing today Ms. Porter?"

Before explaining the art project Keith closed the door to the room to decrease outside noise and limit other distractions. He printed instructions in large block letters on the whiteboard at the front of the room and reinforced the steps with spoken instructions. Then, as the older adults

began their projects Keith approached several older adults individually to provide further instruction, as needed. He knew that some of the adults had vision problems and could not see what he had written, so he sought clarification that they understood the project. Keith interacted with the participants throughout the class. He was neither condescending nor patronizing, respecting each individual's circumstances. For many, this class was a highlight of their day. They enjoyed the camaraderie of the group and appreciated the respect shown to them by Keith.

CHECKING YOUR COMPREHENSION

Write a brief answer for each of the following assignments

1. How does the patient's perspective in the health care system differs from the perspective of the health care professional?
2. How do different cultural perspectives affect the delivery of health care?
3. Explain how health insurance affects health care for minority groups.
4. Explain the difference between sex and gender.
5. Give examples of ways that gender-nonconforming patients can be made to feel welcome.
6. List health disparities among gay, lesbian, and bisexual patients.
7. Describe three ways religious traditions might impact patient care.
8. List the stages of cognitive development according to Piaget.
9. What are some things that can impact your communication with older patients?

EXPANDING CRITICAL THINKING

1. Mrs. Rodriguez, an elderly female patient with breast cancer, confides in you that she is uncomfortable because her new nurse is male and she would feel better if she had a female nurse.
   What might be some reasons for this request and how would you respond?
2. Mr. Porter, an elderly African-American gentleman, returns to the clinic for a follow-up appointment for his hypertension. When getting his vital signs you notice that his blood pressure is high. He tells you he has not been taking his medications regularly. What further information would be important to gather from Mr. Porter?
3. A goal of Healthy People 2020 is to eliminate health disparities. What are some of the reasons health disparities exist?
4. Piaget describes four stages of intellectual development that all children pass through. You notice that many of your pediatric patients do not fit into the expected stage. Describe two possible explanations for this.
5. You notice when you are caring for Janet, a transgender patient, that some of the other staff consistently use the wrong gender pronouns when speaking with or about her. You can see this makes your patient uncomfortable, but she remains silent. How could you address this situation?

Communicating Through Barriers

Jaime Nguyen

CHAPTER OUTLINE

LEARNING OBJECTIVES

On successful completion of this chapter, you will be able to:

1. Discuss communication through language barriers and the use of interpreters.
2. Discuss communication and interaction with patients who have auditory and visual impairments.
3. Explain stress, the body's physiologic response to stress, common coping mechanisms, and actions health care professionals can take to help the stressed patient.

4. List best practices to address "challenging" patients and guidelines for responding to workplace violence.
5. List strategies to discuss sensitive topics with patients.
6. Discuss signs a patient may be a victim of intimate partner violence or abuse, and communication issues unique to these patients.

KEY TERMS

abuse general term for misuse or maltreatment, which may be emotional, physical, psychological, economic, and/or sexual trauma on another individual to satisfy a desire to control and have power over that individual

ad hoc interpreter use of an interpreter present during a clinical encounter, such as family members, friends, untrained members of the support staff, and even strangers found in waiting rooms

anacusis a type of auditory impairment where there is a total loss of hearing

bullying aggression among adolescents perpetrated by a person or persons against an individual, excluding a sibling or dating partner, which is based on a power imbalance

coping mechanism a person's strategy to manage stress

elder abuse abuse, neglect, or exploitation of people over the age of 60 years, which may include physical abuse, sexual abuse, emotional abuse, neglect, abandonment, and financial abuse

eustress good or positive stress with beneficial emotional and physical results

family violence a comprehensive term that addresses abuse throughout the life cycle and includes partner abuse, child abuse, and elder abuse

fight-or-flight response the body's physiologic reaction to a perceived threat consisting of the release of hormones that increase blood pressure and blood sugar and suppress the immune system to gain a boost of energy

intimate partner violence (IPV) an inclusive term that includes violence or abuse between two people, with or without marital status or sexual relationship, also referred to as domestic violence or spousal abuse

limited English proficiency (LEP) categorization of individuals that are not fluent in English or speak English "less than very well"

mandatory reporter a specific professional required to report suspected abuse, neglect, or violence to appropriate agencies

otosclerosis hardening of the structures of the ear which interferes with the transmission of sound from the structures of the ear to the cochlear nerve to the brain, resulting in a conductive hearing impairment

presbycusis a mixed auditory impairment common in older patients, literally meaning "old hearing"

remote interpreter service use of an interpreter where that person is not in-person, but instead provides services via phone or video

sensory barrier an impairment or disability of one or more senses: sight, hearing, smell, touch, taste, and spatial awareness

INTRODUCTION

As we have discussed, central to providing patient care is the ability to communicate effectively with patients, their families, and caregivers. In the health care setting, facts and ideas must be exchanged both between the health care provider and the health care team, as well as between the provider and the patient along with the family or caregivers. Talking, and asking and answering questions are essential parts of the relationship between the health care provider and the patient. Effective communication is critical to proper diagnosis, appropriate treatment, and ensuring patient adherence; mistakes can be harmful or even fatal. It is our duty as health care professionals to provide effective communication to all our patients and their families and caregivers.

Because of the nature of our work, many of our patients come to us with barriers in the way of communication. They may not speak the same language as we; they may suffer sensory impairments, such as poor eyesight or hearing; they may be victims of abuse or violence; they may be suffering under the weight of stress, anger, and anxiety, in general, or because of the stressfulness of their illness and the health care interaction. Although we interact with different people every day, many times communication fails because of these different types of barriers. Working with these patient populations requires special attention because of the consequences that may result in miscommunication, such as incomplete patient history, misdiagnosis, and inaccurate patient instruction.

Many patients will come to us with a combination of differences in languages, hearing and visual impairments, and behavioral and social problems. According to the American Community Survey (ACS), as of 2016 more than 40 million people or 12.8% of the population in the United States reportedly have some form of a disability, which includes visual and hearing impairments. About 36 of 1000 people have a hearing disability; 2.4% have a visual disability, meaning they are blind or have severe trouble seeing even with glasses. Approximately 9 of 100 people have difficulty understanding and speaking English. In addition, patients who are ill are under great stress, of course, and even those who are mildly or acutely ill are burdened by the possibility of illness.

These barriers have been recognized as the main reasons for poor clinical outcomes and quality of care, reduced patient satisfaction, and issues in patient safety.

Again, miscommunication in the health care setting can be life-threatening. By recognizing and understanding these barriers to communication can we better overcome them and focus on providing quality patient care.

In addition to establishing effective communication with our patients, a number of federal laws address disabilities and communication barriers in the health care setting. Thus, poor communication in health care can be serious and even fatal.

LANGUAGE BARRIERS

Although English is the primary language used in the United States, there are millions of Americans who speak more than 350 different languages. Many patients are only able to function adequately in a language other than English. According to the United

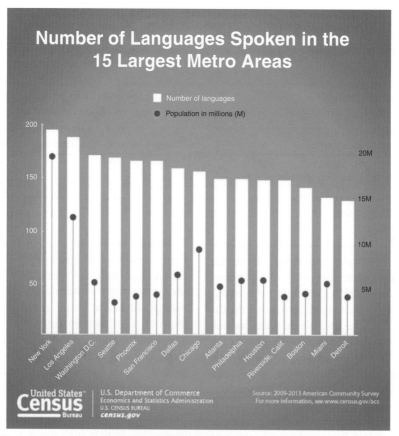

Fig. 5.1 Millions of people in the United States speak hundreds of languages. (From U.S. Census Bureau. [2015, November 3]. Census Bureau Reports at Least 350 Languages Spoken in U.S. Homes. Retrieved June 7, 2019, from U.S. Census Bureau Website: https://www.census.gov/newsroom/press-releases/2015/cb15-185.html.)

States Census Bureau, more than one-third of the population speaks a language other than English in the United States. In major metropolitan areas more than 100 different languages are spoken (Fig. 5.1). An estimated 8.5% of people over the age of 5 (or 25.4 million people) in the United States are reported as not fluent or speaking English "less than very well" and are considered to have limited English proficiency (LEP). Further, the largest group of people whose primary language is not English is composed of Spanish-speaking Hispanics and Latinos, comprising nearly 18% of the population in the United States. This population is expected to double to 29% by the year 2050 (U.S. Census Bureau, 2017). As of 2015, 37.4% of Hispanics over the age of 18 stated that they speak English "less than very well," although fluency in English is high and still increasing among younger Hispanics (Fig. 5.2). Additionally, speakers of some Asian languages, such as Chinese, Korean, and Vietnamese, are more likely to lack fluency in English (Ramakrishnan & Ahmad, 2014).

Language barriers can create challenges for patients to receive effective medical care. Studies show that language barriers between patients and health care professional can result in obstacles to patient care and negative clinical outcomes, including lower quality of health care and worse health outcomes. Patients with LEP are more likely to be misdiagnosed and not understand their diagnosis and treatment plans, which results in poor adherence to treatment and higher rates of adverse medication reactions and complications. They also have longer emergency care visits, higher readmission rates, receive fewer referrals to medical services, and have lower levels of patient satisfaction (Fernandez, et al., 2011).

What happens when the health care professional cannot accurately communicate medical information, such as a diagnosis or treatment plan, to patients? In interacting with patients, health care professionals may experience a loss of information, misinformation, and loss of control of getting information when there are language barriers. Language barriers can prevent health care professionals from obtaining an accurate patient history and limit their ability to fully communicate the risk and benefits of different procedures and treatment options. Patients with LEP may feel limited in their ability to fully express thoughts, understand instructions, and engage in self-management, and may experience challenges making health care decisions in collaboration with their health care provider.

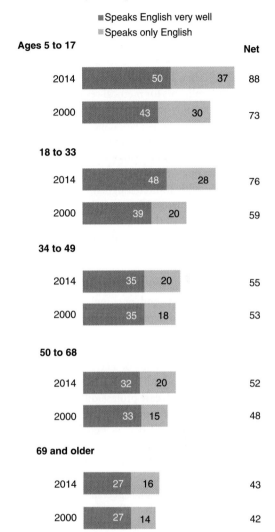

Fig. 5.2 The percentage of Hispanics who speak English proficiently is highest among younger speakers. (From Krogstad JM. (2016, April 20). Rise in English proficiency among U.S. Hispanics is driven by the young. Retrieved September 25, 2018, from Pew Research Center Website: http://www.pewresearch.org/fact-tank/2016/04/20/rise-in-english-proficiency-among-u-s-hispanics-is-driven-by-the-young/.)

Language barriers continue to exist because many health care professionals do not speak the primary language of their patients. For example, Spanish is the most common language spoken after English, but less than 5% of registered nurses and less than 8% of licensed practicing nurses reported being able to speak Spanish (Lo & Nguyen, 2018). In a 2013 study of non-English language skills among applicants for medical residency, more than four of five new physicians reported some proficiency in at least one non-English language. However, the survey revealed an overabundance of Hindi-speaking physicians and too few who spoke Spanish, Vietnamese, Korean, or Tagalog—four of the five top languages spoken by people with limited English. (Diamond, et al., 2014) Thus, the current demand for bilingual health professionals is one of the highest across all sectors, including registered nurses, medical assistants, pharmacists and pharmacy technicians, and medical billers and coders. The presence of bilingual or multilingual health care professionals means that communication will be more effective, timely, and personal, and ensures that everyone—the health care team, patient, and family—receives the same information.

Owing to time constraints, the health care professional may decide to use his or her own language skills when encountering a patient with LEP. In many situations, a bilingual health care professional using his or her own language skills is more efficient. Bilingual health care professionals would have a better understanding of the patient's diagnosis and treatment plan, would be more effective in explaining medical terms, and would be able to increase patient's confidence. However, it is not always possible or ideal, especially if the health care professional may have only rudimentary language skills, which may result in less than accurate interpretation and communication. In these situations, it is important for the health care provider to include an interpreter.

Using interpreters is not without its challenges, however. There may be a loss of accurate information through translation. The interpreter may also serve as a distraction during the patient encounter. Further, health care professionals may lose control in acquiring information when they communicate through interpreters. The health care professional may not be trained to use interpreters. Finally, there may be a lack of professionalism and training on the part of the interpreter in the health care setting.

★ LEGAL EAGLE

Miscommunication, especially when translating from one language to another, may have deadly consequences. Consider the case of Willie Ramirez. In 1980, 18-year-old Ramirez was brought to an emergency room in South Florida in a coma. When speaking with family, they described Ramirez as "intoxicado," which means *nauseated* in Spanish. However, the non–Spanish-speaking health care staff interpreted it literally as *intoxicated* and diagnosed Ramirez with a drug overdose. After several days in the hospital being worked up for a drug overdose with no improvements, Ramirez was reevaluated and discovered to have bleeding in his brain (intracerebellar hematoma) owing to a ruptured artery. But, by the time the correct diagnosis was made, Ramirez had suffered irreversible brain damage, which left him a quadriplegic. The family sued the South Florida hospital with a $71 million settlement.

(Foden-Vencil, 2014)

Legal Responsibility

The Civil Rights Act of 1964 requires that any health care provider or health care organization that participates in a federal program, such as receiving reimbursements for providing services to Medicare or Medicaid patients, must provide equal access to medical services. In 1998, the Office for Civil Rights of the Department of Health and Human Services issued a memorandum regarding the prohibition, under Title VI of the Civil Rights Act of 1964, against discrimination on the basis of national origin and this includes persons with limited English proficiency. This means health care providers must offer a qualified medical interpreter and provide translated written materials free of charge to the patient with a language barrier.

Use of an Interpreter

When a language barrier exists and no health professional is present with advanced and appropriate language skills, an interpreter should be used for assistance. Providing interpreted services for patients with LEP has been shown to have shorter emergency department stays, fewer follow-up appointments and returns to the emergency department, fewer laboratory tests and procedures, and lower overall medical costs (Bernstein, et al., 2002). Different forms of interpreter services may be used in the health care setting, with the most common being done in-person or remotely.

In-Person Interpreters

In-person interpretation, sometimes called face-to-face interpretation, in which the interpreter, patient, and health care professional are in the same room, is the most common method of providing interpretation. Owing to effort and time constraints required to locate a trained interpreter, health care professionals often will resort to using *ad hoc interpreters*, which may include family members or caregivers, friends, untrained members of the support staff, and even strangers found in waiting rooms who are able to speak the patient's language. Although many clinics and hospitals hire interpreters, many health care professionals often do not have time to wait 30 to 40 minutes for a trained interpreter to arrive. Family members, friends, and caregivers serving as *ad hoc* interpreters may also have the advantage of knowing the patient's history and can anticipate responses, which may save time and frustration.

Although convenient and cost effective, ad hoc interpreters are more likely than trained interpreters to commit errors that may result in adverse clinical consequences. *Ad hoc* interpreters have the potential for poor translation quality because the individual's competency is unknown. They are unlikely to have had training in medical terminology and may not adequately understand technical or medical information the health care professional gives. Further, there may also be issues with patient privacy and ethical considerations, especially when minor children are asked to interpret for their parents, or if abuse or domestic violence is suspected. *Ad hoc* interpreters may unintentionally omit parts of the conversation or omit parts intentionally out of embarrassment. Patients, too, may become embarrassed or more inhibited with a family member serving as interpreter.

Using *ad hoc* interpreters may not follow national standards for providing a qualified interpreter when providing health care. Thus, in most clinical situations, health care professionals should not use *ad hoc* interpreters unless the patient specifically requests to have a family member or friend interpret. However, they may need to be used in the case of an emergency involving an imminent threat to the safety or welfare of an individual or the public where there is no

---

BOX 5.1   EVALUATING THE AD HOC INTERPRETER

If a trained medical interpreter is unavailable, the following steps should be performed to evaluate the ad hoc interpreter:

- Ask the interpreter if he or she is comfortable in the situation and in interpreting.
- Assess the interpreter's level of English proficiency.
- Ask the interpreter to translate exactly what the patient says and not to edit or interpret.
- It may be beneficial to ask the interpreter to describe and translate basic body parts and functions.

Avoid using a minor unless it is an emergency situation and be cautious of any potential risks in confidentiality or conflicts of interest.

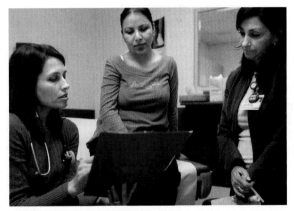

Fig. 5.3 A trained medical interpreter is culturally literate and understands medical terminology in both languages. (Jeanna Duerscherl/The Roanoke Times/Associated Press.)

interpreter available. If an *ad hoc* interpreter is used, it is important to assess the interpreter on his or her preparedness (Box 5.1).

Calling in a trained medical interpreter (Fig. 5.3) is still the safest way to address language barriers between patients and health care professionals effectively. Even on-site, bilingual health care professionals were much more likely to commit serious errors, such as neglecting to ask about drug allergies or mistranslating medication dosages, than were trained interpreters. Trained interpreters are associated with higher compliance and greater patient satisfaction and may be ideal for difficult conversations and procedural consent with patients.

COMMUNICATION GUIDELINES

Use of an Interpreter

Important points when using a trained interpreter are:

- Face both the interpreter and the patient so all parties will be able to read communication cues and body language. Patients need to see your face and may understand more English than they speak. If you are just facing the interpreter, the patient may not feel like he or she is an active participant in the conversation.
- Use short, clear sentences and avoid complex medical terms or jargon.
- Give patients time to form an answer. Some patients may mentally translate English into their own language, and then mentally translate their thoughts back into English for a response.
- To help establish rapport, learn several simple phrases in the most common languages your patient may speak. "Please," "Thank you," "Good day," and other greetings and pleasantries are easy to learn. Patients will appreciate your efforts to communicate and will be more responsive in return.
- Always document, in detail, the use of the medical interpreter or translator in the patient's medical record.

SPOTLIGHT ON SUCCESS

Become a Medical Interpreter

Being a medical interpreter is a very important and rewarding job. Do you have what it takes? Although there is no universal set of qualifications to be an interpreter, most states and health care organizations set the following criteria:

- Completion of general education, such as a high school diploma or equivalent, or an advanced degree
- Completion of an interpreter training program, interpreter certificate program from education institutions, or an advanced degree in interpreting
- Knowledge of medical terminology, including anatomic, technologic, and health system-related vocabulary
- Understanding and adherence to health care interpreting codes of ethics and standards of practice, such as the National Council on Interpreting in Health Care's National Code of Ethics and National Standards of Practice
- Continuing education undertaken by interpreters to maintain and improve skills
- Ability to anticipate and recognize misunderstandings that arise from the differing cultural assumptions and expectations of health care professionals and patients and to respond to such issues appropriately (refer to Chapter 4)

Remote Interpreter Services

One of the most effective ways for medical offices and other health care organizations to address the lack of on-site bilingual health care professionals is the use of remote interpreter services. Interpreter availability varies greatly by both language and location. A language that is rare in one area may be much more common in another, even within the same state. Even for the most common language spoken, such as Spanish, bilingual health care professionals may be scarce. It may also not be cost effective to hire and train a staff member or pay for a trained medical interpreter for dozens of possible languages that patients may speak. Thus, using a remote interpreter service may be an effective method of providing interpreter services that is both cost effective and close to resembling an in-person encounter. Examples of remote interpreter services include telephonic interpreters and video conferencing. Use of telephonic or video conferencing for interpretation can improve quality of care simply by increasing access to trained interpreters.

Telephonic interpreters would be effective for simple and short exchanges that do not require visual communication, such as providing patient education or a patient requesting a medication refill. The use of telephonic interpreters has significantly increased owing to its ease of use and that health care providers are able to access a larger number of different languages rapidly. A health care provider can easily access a telephonic interpreter by a cell phone at any point and at any location. Many hospitals have included a dual handset phone for remote simultaneous medical interpretations where the interpreter translates as he or she hears the dialogue.

Although telephonic interpreting is still one of the most prevalent methods of remote interpretation services, video remote interpretation (VRI) provides the quick access of telephonic interpretation, but also allows visual communication that more resembles an in-person interpretation. Not only can VRI be used for patients with LEP, but it may be used for patients who need American sign language (Fig. 5.4). Video conferencing allows for sharing a live, streaming video that can be used on an electronic tablet device or with any device using a wireless internet connection that can be used bedside or in the patient's room.

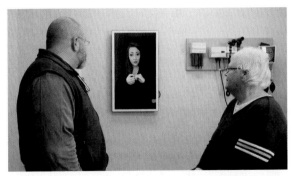

Fig. 5.4 A nurse and patient utilize a video remote interpreting (VRI) service to communicate. (Courtesy of Visual Communication Interpreting, Inc., Knoxville, Tennessee; videography by Wooden Films, Knoxville, Tennessee: woodenfilms.com.)

SENSORY BARRIERS

Communication requires many sensory interactions to be effective. An impairment in any of the systems involved in communication interrupts the flow of communication and leads to misunderstanding and frustration. Impairments in communication owing to a disability that affects one or more senses—sight, hearing, smell, touch, taste, and spatial awareness—are called **sensory barriers**. Sight and hearing losses are the most common sensory barriers that health care professionals will most likely face, although loss of other sensory functions are common in specific diseases.

Legal Requirements Addressing Communication Barriers

The Americans with Disabilities Act (ADA) of 1990 is legislation to protect civil rights and prohibits the discrimination against individuals with disabilities, applying to both state and federal agencies and requiring most businesses to provide accommodations for people with disabilities. The law mandates that all health care providers make accommodations for patients and their companions with disabilities, with § 36.303(c) specifically addressing effective communication: "A public accommodation shall furnish appropriate auxiliary aids and services where necessary to ensure effective communication…." Patients who have communication barriers or disabilities, such as vision, hearing, or speech, must be able to communicate with, receive information from, and convey information to, their health care providers. As a result, health care providers and organizations must provide auxiliary aids and services such as those listed in Box 5.2.

BOX 5.2 AUXILIARY AIDS AND SERVICES FOR PEOPLE WITH COMMUNICATION DISABILITIES

For people who are blind, have vision loss, or are deaf-blind, provide a qualified reader; information in large print, Braille, or electronically for use with a computer screen-reading program; or an audio recording of printed information. A "qualified" reader means someone who is able to read effectively, accurately, and impartially, using any necessary specialized vocabulary.

For people who are deaf, have hearing loss, or are deaf-blind, provide a qualified notetaker; a qualified sign language interpreter, oral interpreter, cued-speech interpreter, or tactile interpreter; real-time captioning; written materials; or printed patient information. A "qualified" interpreter means someone who is able to interpret effectively, accurately, and impartially, both receptively (i.e., understanding what the person with the disability is saying) and expressively (i.e., having the skill needed to convey information back to that person) using any necessary specialized vocabulary.

For people who have speech disabilities, provide a qualified speech-to-speech translator (a person trained to recognize unclear speech and repeat it clearly), especially if the person will be speaking at length, such as giving testimony in court, or just taking more time to communicate with someone who uses a communication board. (U.S. Department of Justice, Civil Rights Division, Disability Rights Section, 2014)

Visual Impairments

Visual impairments, also called *anopia* or *anopsia*, is a defect in vision or the visual field. It can range from complete or partial vision loss to a defect in visual acuity, such as farsightedness (*hyperopia*) and nearsightedness (*myopia*). Visually impaired patients may use aids, such as a white cane (support or probing cane) or a guide dog, but the impairment may not always be obvious. Undiagnosed patients or those unwilling to accept their impairment may display more subtle signs such as tripping, not being able to find the chair in which to sit, or having difficulty reading a patient form. Thus, it is important for health care professionals to be aware of these signs to promote a safe environment and a positive experience during the patient encounter.

Physical Environment

Accommodations must be made for patients with visual impairments, although what needs to be done will

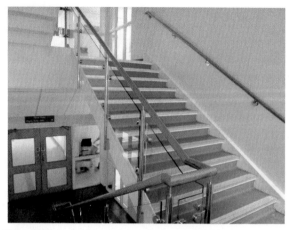

Fig. 5.5 The steps in this hospital are marked with yellow to increase contrast for people with visual impairments. (iStock.com/mtreasure.)

vary between patients and the severity of their impairments. Check the patient areas to ensure there is enough lighting, easy-to-read signage, and no obstacles, such as unmarked steps (Fig. 5.5), uneven floors, carpet, or obstructive furniture.

Patient Interaction

Some simple guidelines will help you put your visually impaired patients at ease.

- When approaching a door, let the patient know if it opens toward you or away, and if the door opens from the right or the left. Pass through the doorway first, allowing the patient to follow.
- Escort patients by having them take your arm, rather than taking theirs. This is more comfortable for patients and gives them a feeling of control. Do not pull or push the patient.
- Knock each time you enter the room and let patients know who you are. Tell them when you must leave the room.
- Ask the patient whether describing the space layout would help. For example, "the door is to your left" or "the sink is at your 3 o'clock."
- Explain each procedure and let patients know when you need to touch them. Remember that they cannot see that you have a thermometer in your hand or that you need to wrap the blood pressure cuff around their arm.
- If the patient is accompanied by a guide dog, the dog is legally permitted to go wherever the patient

goes. Do not distract the dog and do not handle or pet the dog unless the patient gives you permission.

> ## ▶▶ TAKING THE CHAPTER TO WORK
>
> ### Visual Impairment
>
> Elisa is working in an endocrinology clinic. Elisa starts every morning by reviewing her patient medical records. She notices that Mr. Ollie is scheduled for an appointment at 10 a.m. for insulin administration education. Elisa looks in the records and reads that Mr. Ollie has diabetes, cataracts, and retinopathy. He has also been having trouble seeing the numbers on the insulin syringe. Elisa finds the educational tools available for diabetic patients and obtains an insulin syringe magnifying glass. She also prints copies of insulin administration sheets in large print. When Mr. Ollie arrives for his appointment, the education session is completed in an organized and prompt manner because all of the needed materials were ready for him.

Auditory Impairments

Auditory impairments, or hearing losses, range from very slight, with the patient losing only a few sounds such as "s" or "th," to profound, with a total loss of hearing, called anacusis. Because many hearing losses are gradual, patients may not be aware they are missing or misunderstanding parts of a conversation and may wonder why they are having trouble communicating. In some cases, patients may refuse to admit they do not hear well, and trying to convince them may be more frustrating than productive. Patients who demonstrate any of the following may have a hearing impairment.

- Flat speech patterns with little inflection or variation in tone. We alter and vary our speech as we hear it, raising and lowering our pitch and tone for emphasis. Hearing-impaired patients may not change their speaking tones.
- Slurred or incomplete words. Patients may not be aware that they have not finished words or that the sounds were not distinct.
- Frequent requests that you repeat a statement. Questioning looks or puzzled expressions after you have spoken should tell you the patient did not understand.
- Apparent indifference to what you are saying. The patient may not know that you are speaking; we do not miss what we do not hear.
- A tendency to dominate the conversation. Patients may not be aware when you are speaking.

There are three main types of hearing impairment with degrees of loss within each.

- Conductive: This type of auditory loss is correctable and may be caused by a build-up of ear wax (cerumen) in the outer or middle ear or otosclerosis (hardening of the structures of the ear), which interferes with the transmission of sound through the structures of the ear to the cochlear nerve to the brain.
- Sensorineural: This deafness involves the cochlear nerve and sound transmission to the auditory (hearing) centers of the brain. If the hearing loss is profound, the patient may need a device called a cochlear implant that transmits sound past the cochlear nerve to the brain.
- Mixed deafness: This form of hearing loss is harder to diagnose and treat and may be a combination of both types—conductive and sensorineural—of impairment. The type of auditory impairment most common in older patients is called presbycusis (literally "old hearing").

Patient Interaction

Patients with hearing or auditory impairments may communicate in a variety of ways with health care professionals. Some patients speak and speech-read or lip-read; some use sign language or communicate by writing notes; and some bring someone with them to interpret. The following suggestions will accommodate your patient with auditory impairments.

- Before beginning the conversation, alert the patient to the topic. For example, you may tap her on the arm and say, "Mrs. Smith, this is how you should change your dressing." This will let her know she should be listening and gives her direction to the topic.
- Position yourself directly in front of the patient and face the patient while talking (Fig. 5.6). The

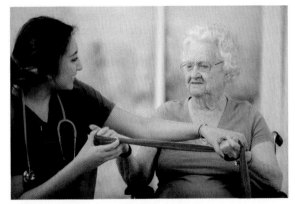

Fig. 5.6 Because this patient has difficulty hearing, the nurse makes sure to face the patient when explaining this exercise technique. (iStock.com/Pamela A. Moore.)

patient should be able to see your facial cues and expressions.

- Speak clearly and distinctly and avoid making exaggerated facial movements. If your patient relies on reading lips, distorting your face and mouth makes it very hard to distinguish the words.
- Speak with moderate force, but lower your normal speaking pitch. Many patients with auditory impairments may lose higher tones first, but still can hear low-pitched tones.
- As with other communication barriers, short words in short sentences are easier to interpret than complex words in lengthy sentences.
- Keep distractions to a minimum to cut down on confusion and to make your words easier to understand.
- If you must cover your mouth for treatment purposes, as in masking, write what the patient needs to know or have someone at the patient's side to interpret.
- If the patient cannot understand you, use magic slates, chalkboards, or note pads for writing.

▶▶ TAKING THE CHAPTER TO WORK

Auditory Impairment

Jack is a social worker at an adult inpatient behavioral health facility, where most of the patients spend anywhere from a week to a few months receiving treatment for mental health problems. One of Jack's new patients is Mr. Alexopoulos, a 50-year-old man whose life changed after a car accident 2 years ago. He sustained severe injuries after the accident including sensorineural hearing loss that caused tinnitus, the perception of a constant ringing in his ears. The tinnitus causes irritability and trouble concentrating and also makes sleeping very difficult.

Mr. Alexopoulos' great joy in life had been as a part-time musician, playing guitar at local bars nights and weekends, but his hearing impairment made this impossible. Mr. Alexopoulos could understand speech, but only if a person spoke directly at him and very loudly.

Although many of his bodily injuries healed, his hearing would never return. Mr. Alexopoulos became depressed and angry and, combined with the stressors of his impairment and poor sleep, his marriage fell apart. Six months ago his wife left, taking their teenage son with her. Mr. Alexopoulos' depression worsened. He is under Jack's care at the facility after threatening to kill himself.

The treatment for Mr. Alexopoulos' depression, suicidal ideation, and anger usually requires a mix of medication, counseling, and group therapy sessions. This required Jack and the staff to make adjustments to accommodate Mr. Alexopoulos' hearing impairment. They quickly found that the group therapy sessions would not work, because his inability to hear the other patients only heightened his anger and frustration. Because the staff had to shout to communicate with him, they were concerned that discussing his treatment might violate his privacy. They found it best to do most of the counseling in a separate room with the door closed; this way they could speak loudly without accidently disclosing his personal health information.

The nurses performed all the patient teaching in this separate room, making sure to sit face-to-face with their patient. The staff spoke loudly and clearly, using lower pitched voices to help Mr. Alexopoulos hear. For counseling, Jack brought in a whiteboard on an easel where they could write down key parts of his therapy for that day. Anytime the nurses performed medication teaching, they made sure to bring printouts and approached each piece of information slowly so that Mr. Alexopoulos could follow along.

Other smaller initiatives helped Mr. Alexopoulos feel more comfortable. For example, Jack turned on the closed captioning for the television in the day room. Other patients were asked to enunciate clearly and speak directly to Mr. Alexopoulos when communicating. The staff relied more heavily on physical group activities to help Mr. Alexopoulos build relationships with his peers. Jack and his colleagues found that with these adjustments they could accommodate the patient's impairment to communicate therapeutically.

PATIENTS AND STRESS

It is very difficult to communicate with patients overwhelmed by stress. Patients who are suffering from illness or the possibility of illness, regardless of what it is, are often under great stress. A part of our role in communicating with these patients is to recognize that stress is a side effect of illness, much like a fever or a rash. In some cases, stress may be the actual cause of the illness.

Although stress is usually undeniably a negative experience, some stresses are positive. This is called **eustress** (positive stress or good stress), such as pushing yourself to the limit for something you enjoy. Positive stress helps some people work more efficiently and perform better than they might without a certain degree of pressure. Some people may become more resourceful and creative, such as thinking of a better patient check-in process at a time when the clinic gets behind on patient appointments.

We all respond to stressful events differently; stressors for one person may not be a problem for another. For example, an action or event that stresses you (jumping out of an airplane) may be an enjoyable challenge to someone else. Responses also vary from day to day; stressors that overwhelm us today may be manageable tomorrow. For example, a fender-bender can be aggravating and costly but should not be devastating, unless we are already stressed because of an illness and feeling overwhelmed with having to manage another burden. Even minor, everyday irritations can add up and result in an overly stressful situation.

Mild stress can make us work more efficiently and think more clearly and challenges us to grow; however, severe or unrelieved stress can make us sick. If a stressor or stressful situation is not quickly resolved, the body's resources are exhausted, leaving no energy to cope with additional stressors. Unresolved stress may lead to physical signs and symptoms, such as the following.

- Headache, stiff neck, or tension in the back and shoulders
- Upset stomach, diarrhea or constipation, dry mouth and throat, difficulty swallowing
- Rapid heart rate and shortness of breath
- Anxiety that may lead to panic
- Exhaustion or lack of energy
- Disordered thoughts and poor concentration
- Loss of short-term memory
- Insomnia and nightmares

Chronic, psychological stress alters the immune function and can exacerbate the symptoms of many illnesses, both physically and psychologically. Evidence shows that stress can alter the health outcomes of patients with rheumatoid arthritis, multiple sclerosis, irritable bowel syndrome, and autoimmune diseases. This effect on the immune system caused by stress has also been linked to schizophrenia (Morey, Boggero, Scott, & Segerstrom, 2015). In most cases, a genetic predisposition must be present to cause a disease and disorder. But the presence of stress may overwhelm the immune system, resulting in patients being more susceptible to illnesses, especially those associated with the sympathetic response.

Review your anatomy and physiology or biology text to remember how the autonomic nervous system works to balance the response of its parasympathetic and sympathetic systems. As a matter of survival, the sympathetic branch of the nervous system controls the stress response when we sense a threat (Fig. 5.7). A perceived threat triggers our **fight-or-flight response**, a physiologic reaction intended to give the body energy to respond. For example, the heart beats faster to pump blood faster and the respiratory rate increases to increase the oxygen supply in the body, which will all help supply glucose to muscles to make them work more efficiently. Blood pressure rises to force blood into the tissues needed to fight or to run away. Pupils dilate to bring in every available visual image for processing. Digestion slows so that available energy is used for survival. Conversely, our parasympathetic system works to "rest and digest" or to calm and soothe the body when there is no crisis or threat, or when a crisis is over (Fig. 5.8), to conserve energy.

Many social factors also affect our ability to withstand a stressful situation. Think back to Maslow's pyramid discussed in Chapter 3. Are our hierarchical needs being met? Do we have a place to live and food to eat? Do we have the financial resources? Are we cared for, supported, and loved? All of these factors may affect our ability to manage stressors. Thus, to help keep our patients healthy, we must help them manage everyday stress, as well as any added stress from illnesses.

To manage our internal and external stress, we use various **coping mechanisms**—unconscious strategies to manage stressful events. Many different types of coping mechanisms exist that people may use depending on the situation. The most common coping mechanisms seen in health care are listed in Box 5.3. Coping mechanisms can be broadly categorized as either active or avoidant. An active coping mechanism acknowledges a source of stress and seeks to reduce or eliminate its effects. Avoidant coping mechanisms ignore a situation or problem, such as in denial. Short-term denial may help a patient delay facing a problem until he or she is ready and better able to adjust to the changes. However, denial may become harmful if it leads to a patient refusing treatment. For example, a patient may make no changes to his lifestyle, such as continuing to smoke and eat fatty foods, despite suffering a myocardial infarction (heart

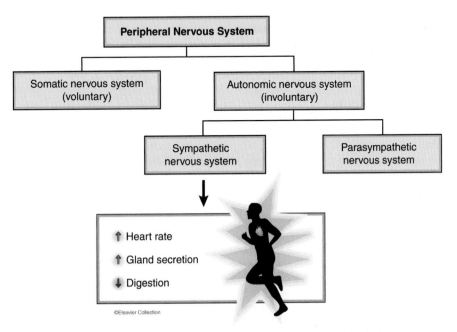

©Elsevier Collection

Fig. 5.7 The sympathetic nervous system reacts to stress with physiologic changes.

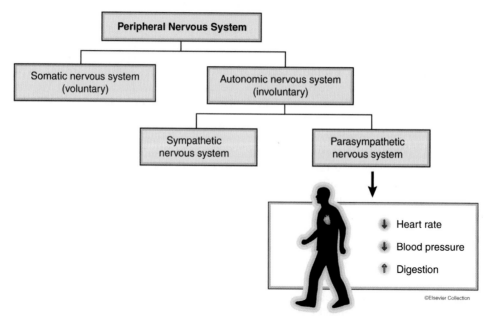

Fig. 5.8 The parasympathetic nervous system restores the body to homeostasis.

BOX 5.3 COPING MECHANISMS

The following methods of coping with stress are commonly seen in the health care setting:

Compensation: Developing strengths to overcome weaknesses. Patients with impaired vision may develop stronger hearing to compensate.

Displacement: Striking out at a substitute, usually someone or something unable to fight back, rather than the source of anger. Patients or caregivers may seem angry with you when they cannot direct their anger at the situation. For example, a caregiver may rage at you when the anger cannot be directed at the patient.

Fantasizing: Daydreaming as a means of escape. A patient may choose a fantasy, such as, "When I am well again, I will sell all of my belongings and travel around the world." This is not a bad strategy unless it interferes with adjustment.

Humor: Laughing at ourselves or at a situation. It may be hard to find humor in most medical situations, but some patients can genuinely laugh at themselves. Imagine the patient honestly laughing at herself in an unbecoming patient gown. Laughter helps relieve stress.

Projection: Attributing one's own unacceptable motives and characteristics to another person.

  A married man who feels attracted to a coworker might begin to suspect his own spouse is having an affair. A woman who is feeling guilty for drinking too often might harshly criticize another person for getting too drunk.

Rationalization: Justifying a behavior or situation by deceiving oneself into thinking it is acceptable. An example is the smoker who thinks, "I will have to die of something, I may as well enjoy myself."

Regression: Returning to an earlier developmental stage as an escape from stress. Patients may regress to tantrums, pouting, and other childish behaviors to get what they want or to avoid facing stressful decisions. Children frequently drop back to an earlier stage during illness or stress.

Repression: Involuntarily rejecting painful thoughts and realities from the conscious mind. Victims of child abuse and survivors of traumatic experiences sometimes protect themselves by storing the memories so deeply that it may take years of intensive psychotherapy to bring them back to a conscious level. Repressed memories and unacknowledged anger can lead to a number of mental or physical illnesses.

Suppression: Deliberately refusing to acknowledge something that causes mental pain or suffering. As opposed to regression, suppression is when patients consciously delay thinking painful thoughts or facing difficult decisions until they feel strong enough to face reality. This reaction, like denial, may be appropriate if it does not interfere with health care.

Undoing: Making amends; attempting to cancel out an unacceptable behavior by one that is more acceptable. Patients may think, "I was angry at her earlier, so I will be extra nice this time."

attack). If he continues to ignore his treatment plan and his physician's advice, this coping mechanism is no longer denial but is now termed maladaptive. Maladaptive coping strategies include such things as using alcohol and drugs to deal with a stressful situation, although substance use often adds to stressful situations.

Patient Interactions

The health care setting can be a frightening environment for patients. People around them are speaking in medical terms that may sound like a foreign language to them. Procedures are being performed that they may not understand. Even patients who present for nothing more serious than a follow-up visit or routine physical examination may be stressed and frightened as they wait, wondering if the twinge of pain they felt 2 weeks ago is something serious or not. Many other patients find even the idea of the hospital to be anxiety-provoking. As a result, health care professionals must develop methods to relieve patients' stress. First, we need to create a relaxing environment (Fig. 5.9). Second, lower the pitch of your voice and slow your speech patterns to alleviate the patient's anxiety. As with any exchange, sitting across from the patient, face-to-face, in a relaxed but professional manner inspires confidence and communicates compassion.

👤 COMMUNICATION GUIDELINES

Patients and Stress

To help patients successfully manage their stress, encourage them to try the following suggestions.

- Help them look at the situation objectively to see what they can change to make it more manageable.
- Help them adjust their priorities. What can wait versus what must be done now?
- List options and possible solutions in pro and con columns. Seeing the problem on paper may help put a problem into perspective.
- Encourage them to be realistic. Is it as bad as it seems? What can be done to make it better? Can the patient adjust or adapt if it does not improve?
- Help them to see that if what they are doing to resolve stress is not working, they should stop doing it and try something else. They should avoid digging themselves into a deeper hole of stress and depression.
- Be available if patients need help finding answers to their questions. Although no one has all of the answers, it is important to know where to look for answers and resources.

- Encourage patients to set limits and boundaries and say "No" when they need to. Does the patient need to serve on so many committees or take on everyone else's responsibilities?
- Encourage them to take breaks to rest their mind, such as listen to music, to spend time with family and friends, and to avoid depressing people or situations as much as possible.
- Help patients to laugh often and stay positive. Negativity increases stress.
- Discuss support groups available through community resources.
- Encourage patients to turn to their spiritual or religious leader for hope and encouragement if they are religious or spiritual.
- Let them be angry if they must and acknowledge that it is an understandable reaction. But help them look for acceptable outlets and move beyond anger.

These tips may help your patients manage their stresses. Remember, that even though the problem may still be there, the challenge is to meet the needs of the situation and to help patients manage psychological and physiologic stress.

Relaxation

Using techniques to relax may help alleviate the stress response; relieve short-term stress; and keep small, everyday aggravations from accumulating into large, more significant stressors. Several easy-to-perform relaxation techniques listed below may help to regulate vital signs and put patients in a frame of mind to listen and learn. As the body relaxes, vital signs return to normal, stress hormone levels drop, and every system involved in the stress response works toward balance. As you learn these techniques, teach them to your patients. Your patients can use these easy techniques as they wait for physical examinations or treatment procedures.

Stretching. Muscles tense during stress in preparation for a fight-or-flight response. Stretching the whole body with your hands over the your head is one of the easiest way to relieve muscle tension. This can be done sitting, but is more effective standing. Stretch through the shoulders, rib cage, hips, and legs. Work from the top of the head to the toes and then back again. Tighten every muscle group, then relax them. Many good stretching exercises are easy to do. Yoga stretching exercises are very good for relieving muscle tension and can fit into small timeframes for tension relief.

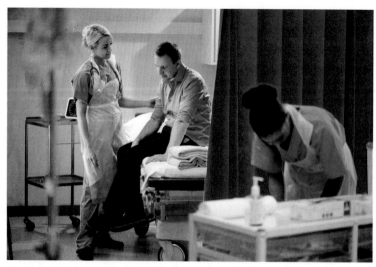

Fig. 5.9 Even in a hectic environment, such as the emergency department, you can relieve stress by limiting distractions and speaking slowly with a low pitch in your voice. (iStock.com/sturti.)

Patients can invest in either a good class or a good instruction book to learn proper technique.

Breathing Exercises. Learning to breathe correctly for tension relief helps to improve better exchange of oxygen and carbon dioxide. Focusing on your breaths may also take your mind off of stress. To optimize breathing, sit or stand with hands on your abdomen and your back straight for good posture (slumping interferes with respiration). Breathe deeply through the nose as the abdomen moves outward. Hold the breath for a few seconds and try to breathe in more deeply. Slowly exhale through pursed lips while pulling your abdomen inward toward the spine.

Visualization. With this technique, you would create a visual picture in your mind of a positive scenario, such as sitting on a sandy beach or getting a promotion. Concentrate on developing the pleasant image or creating a picture of a goal in your mind. This is a good method of stress relief or even more motivation, such as right before an examination.

Meditation. Similar to visualization, meditation is training the mind and body to relax and relieve stress. Setting aside as little as 5 or 10 minutes for meditation is a great stress reliever. Set a timer for the target period. Focus on a single point, such as a word or phrase, a thought or an image. Sometimes, it is even helpful in meditation to focus on breathing. Several yoga poses can be used to help in meditation. But simply sitting still and remaining quiet may help in clearing your mind to help you meditate. When the time has passed, take a deep breath, stretch, and go about the day in a better frame of mind. Meditation may help to lower blood pressure, improve circulation, lower heart rate, and reduce anxiety and stress.

Exercise. In addition to improving your overall health and well-being, exercise may help improve stress levels. Working through all the muscle groups relieves tension and releases endorphins, which are the body's natural mood elevators. Exercise may also help in improving your sleep, which may be affected by stress and anxiety. Fitting this time into your busy schedule is one of the most important variables in a healthy lifestyle and in managing stress.

"CHALLENGING" PATIENTS AND FAMILY MEMBERS

Almost every health care professional will encounter a patient or other person who is perceived as difficult or challenging. At times, patients and family members can become uncooperative, hostile, demanding, disruptive, and unpleasant. It is important to remember that there are a number of factors and influences on why patients present the way they do. For example, most patients are coming to the clinic or hospital to seek medical care and often are not feeling well, which may result in behavioral changes and feelings, such as frustration, anxiety, and anger. The type of disease and symptoms the patient has also plays a part in how the patient acts or feels. Patients with chronic diseases are also more likely to present with depression, and patients with chronic pain are more likely to be agitated, anxious, and depressed (National Center for Chronic Disease Prevention and Health Promotion, Division of Population Health, 2005).

Systematic and institutional issues may create difficult encounters. Limited resources, finances, and poor family support may contribute to negative interactions with the health care team. The health care provider may also contribute to a challenging patient encounter. For example, think of a patient who is not feeling well, and then waits an hour or more past the time of the appointment to see the provider (Fig. 5.10). If patients have to spend a substantial amount of time waiting to be seen, they may become frustrated and angry. They might feel disrespected of their time and may even be less receptive to the information the health care provider is offering. Further, how health care professionals interact and react to the "difficult" patient can make the situation worse. Health care professionals might find their body language is more defensive, they may listen less effectively and attentively, and they may be more likely to interrupt or talk over the patient.

Regardless of the reasons, these "challenging" patients and family members create challenging clinical encounters and result in poor patient satisfaction and health outcomes. These encounters and interactions may require more time and patience from the health care professional, which may cause the health care professional also to be stressed, frustrated, and anxious. This may result in a deterioration in the patient–health care professional relationship. Thus, it is important, first and foremost, to identify that you are encountering a "difficult" patient and a challenging patient. Only in this way, can we then move to addressing the patient's medical issues.

Do not take the anger personally. Staff members are also more likely to be the target of patients' anger and frustration because they often have more interaction with patients and may be seen as more approachable and "safer" to express dissatisfaction toward than the physician. Often, a patient who is angry or abusive may, in fact, be anxious and scared. Respect the patient's feelings and realize you may need to allow the patient to express his or her feelings even if it is venting.

If you find yourself with a "difficult" patient, the first thing you can do is confront the situation squarely. Communicate to the patient that there is an interaction problem. Being able to verbalize that there may be a communication or interaction issue allows both the patient and health care professional to have shared ownership in the process and to work toward a solution. It may help the patient see the health care provider as more of a "person" and create more trust between the two parties.

Also explore possible explanations for a patient's behavior—the angry patient's feelings may very well be justified. If an error was made, acknowledge and apologize if you, the health care provider, or the clinic is at fault. Then try to make amends. Do not continue to focus on who was at fault or what caused the disagreement.

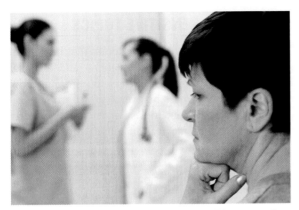

Fig. 5.10 The stress of illness combined with a sometimes frustrating medical system is burdensome to patients. (iStock. com/fotostorm.)

🔆 COMMUNICATION GUIDELINES

Angry or Upset Patients

The following suggestions will help you when communicating with an angry or upset patient or family member.

- Give calm, soft answers and responses. Avoid escalating the issue by arguing with the patient.
- Listen intently with attentive body language and closely observe body cues for either a decrease or increase in the patient's negative emotions and behaviors.
- Gently set limits and boundaries where appropriate, such as for profanity or verbal abuse.
- If the situation deteriorates further and the patient becomes aggressive and combative beyond your ability, call for the health care provider.
- Document the entire incident: what issue the patient was having, how the patient expressed it, and your actions to correct the situation.

Workplace Violence

There are times when the patient interaction may escalate to the point where it may be hazardous or dangerous for the health care professional. Violence or threats of violence against a worker in a workplace setting is called workplace violence. According to the National Institute for Occupational Safety and Health, workplace violence is the "violent acts, including physical assaults and threats of assault, directed toward persons at work or on duty." The violence may be a physical assault or threats or verbal violence, which includes threats, verbal abuse, hostility, and harassment. In some cases, verbal assaults may escalate to physical violence.

Health care professionals are at an increased risk of workplace violence. In fact, workplace violence is four times more likely to occur in a health care setting than another place of employment, with patients being the largest source of this violence. In 2013, 80% of serious violent incidents reported in health care settings were caused by interactions with patients (Fig. 5.11) (Occupational Health and Safety Administration, 2015). Many health care workers are at risk from violence caused by involuntary actions from patients, either while moving or subduing patients or from patients with mental disorders. Other violent situations may stem from disgruntled coworkers, visitors, or other people who come into the facility. Despite high numbers of incidents, it is important to note that violence and workplace bullying often go unreported owing to fear of retaliation.

There are signs that indicate a patient's emotional state is deteriorating and may become violent. Observe the patient for indications that his or her temper is rising. Look for changes in body language, including a tightened jaw, tense posture, clenched fists, raised voice, fidgeting, and any other significant change from his or her previous behavior. For example, a talkative person may suddenly become quiet, which may signal an upcoming emotional and violent outburst. It is difficult to always predict when and where violence can happen on the job. The best precaution a clinic or health care organization can make is to have a zero tolerance policy that covers anyone who may come into contact with personnel. Evaluation of potential hazards and employee training of how to handle a threat will help arm health care professionals with the tools to prevent workplace violence and to get out of a violent situation unharmed. Employees should be trained to recognize and manage escalating and volatile situations with patients, clients, and coworkers. Additional training in how to handle an active shooter situation is highly recommended.

Following are some important steps to take if you find yourself in a highly tense or dangerous encounter with a patient.

- Do not let the patient come between you and the door. Always have a clear path to an escape route.
- Move slowly and in full view to avoid any perceived threat to the patient.
- Use caution, but firmly tell the patient that his or her actions are unacceptable.
- Call for help from coworkers and the physician. If the situation is openly dangerous, a staff member must immediately call 911.
- When the crisis is over, document all that happened and how it was handled.

DISCUSSING SENSITIVE TOPICS

There are a number of sensitive topics that health care professionals must discuss with patients and, although they are deeply personal, barriers to communicating about these topics must be overcome to promote the patient's well-being. Examples are alcohol and drug use, sexual activity, medical diagnoses, and end-of-life issues. Often, the three factors that affect our ability to discuss sensitive topics with patients are:

1. The health care professional's anxiety in discussing the topic
2. The patient's anxiety in discussing the topic
3. Uncertainty about how to approach and ask about the topic

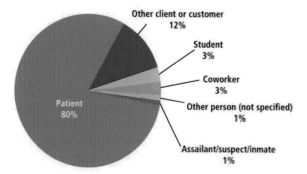

Fig. 5.11 Percentage of healthcare worker injuries resulting in days away from work, by source. (From Occupational Health and Safety Administration. [2013]. Workplace Violence in Healthcare. Retrieved September 27, 2018, from OSHA Website: https://www.osha.gov/Publications/OSHA3826.pdf.)

For both the health care professional and patients, discussing health and health behaviors may make them feel anxious, uncomfortable, and even embarrassed. Patients may feel judged and may worry about confidentiality. Thus, it is critical for the health care professional to assure patients that they are in a safe environment and that they can share personal and private information. However, it is important to remind patients that there are exceptions to confidentiality and that you may be required to report on information disclosed by the patient, such as child abuse, elder abuse, some sexually transmitted infections, and suicidal intentions. Patients should also be informed that they are not required to answer any questions that make them feel uncomfortable.

Health care professionals must be aware of their body language, tone, and how they ask about sensitive topics. When asking questions, it is best first to "normalize" a topic by using broad and general questions or statements. This helps to destigmatize the issue and limits any feelings of judgment from the patient. For example, you can begin by making the statement "Many people find it difficult to talk about their sexual concerns, so I find it important to ask all of our patients about it" or ask, "When was the last time you had sex?" A sensitive topic can also be approached by the health care professional asking permission: "Would it be okay if I asked you some questions about your relationship with your partner?" Avoid asking questions that suggest judgment or opinions, such as "How often do you get drunk?" or "Do you practice safe sex?" Instead, ask questions where patients can provide facts, such as "How often do you drink in a week?" or "How many sexual partners have you had in the last six months?"

To alleviate patient's anxiety and stress, carefully select your words and your line of questioning when asking about sensitive topics. For example, use close-ended questions, such as "How many drinks of alcohol do you have in an average week?" Close-ended questions will prevent ambiguous and unclear responses from the patient. Similar to close-ended questions, offering answer options will limit ambiguous answers. An example may be: "How often do you use condoms? Never, sometimes, most of the time, or always?" Asking specific questions increases the likelihood of receiving an accurate response compared with more general questions.

Questions about sexual health are often included during a patient's initial visit, preventative health, or well visits, or when there are signs of a sexually transmitted disease (STD). A sexual history can help the provider decide whether the patient is at risk for STDs and identify places on the body to test for certain STDs. You may find that a structured series of questions during the patient interview will help provide more details about the patient's sexual history.

► WORDS AT WORK

In the following dialogue, Shawna, a medical assistant at a free clinic, is asking Mr. Sims, a male patient, about his sexual history.

Shawna: It's important that I ask you some questions about your sexual health, which will help us better manage your overall health. Are you okay if I ask you some questions?

Mr. Sims: Okay.

Shawna: Just so you know, I ask these questions to all my patients, whether they are eighteen years old or eighty years old, men and women, married and single. You don't have to answer anything you don't feel comfortable with, but this information will be kept confidential, except for things that I am required to report, such as cases of abuse. Do you have any questions before we get started?

Mr. Sims: No, I understand.

Shawna: Are you currently sexually active?

Mr. Sims: Yes.

Shawna: In the last 6 months, how many sexual partners have you had?

Mr. Sims: Two or three, I think.

Shawna: With men, women, or both?

Mr. Sims: Well, both. I met this guy a while ago, but I don't exactly remember if it was in the last six months.

Shawna: That's okay. How many female sexual partners have you had in the past six months?

Mr. Sims: Two—my girlfriend and another woman right before we started dating.

Shawna: How many male sexual partners in the past twelve months?

Mr. Sims: Two.

Shawna: Do you use any kind of protection?

Mr. Sims: Sometimes. Not with my girlfriend—she's on the pill.

Shawna: Okay. Has your girlfriend had other sexual partners?

Mr. Sims: Yes.

Shawna: Have you ever had a conversation with her about STDs?

Mr. Sims: Yes, I know she's clean.	**Shawna**: Are you worried you might have an STD?
Shawna: Has she been tested for STDs?	**Mr. Sims**: Yes, a little.
Mr. Sims: Yes, they did it here a few months back.	**Shawna**: We can test you if you like. Would you like to be tested today?
Shawna: Okay. Do you use condoms with your male partners?	**Mr. Sims**: Okay.
Mr. Sims: Yes, I did.	**Shawna**: Is there anything you'd like to tell us about your sexual health or history?
Shawna: Have you ever had an STD?	
Mr. Sims: No, I don't think so. I've never been tested though.	

PATIENTS EXPERIENCING ABUSE

Health care professionals play a crucial role in identifying victims of abuse because they are in a position to ask patients about abuse, even if that is not the reason for the patient's medical visit. By directly asking about any incidences of abuse, there is an increased chance that victims of the abuse will disclose it to the health care professional and be able to receive medical treatment and assistance.

One of the more challenging topics health care professionals must discuss is family violence. Family violence is a comprehensive term that addresses abuse throughout the life cycle. Family violence includes partner abuse, child abuse, and elder abuse. Abuse is generally defined as a misuse or maltreatment. Regarding relationships, abuse can take many forms but include the following types and combinations thereof.

- Physical—pushing, hitting, shoving, punching, biting, choking, and physically trapping or impeding movement
- Verbal/emotional—criticizing, degrading, swearing, blaming, attacks that harm self-esteem
- Psychological—isolating you from your family and friends, controlling actions and decisions, stalking, invading privacy or space
- Sexual—forcing or demanding sex, forcing you to have unwanted sex with another person, forcing engagement into prostitution or pornography, refusing to use safe sex practices
- Economic—forbidding you from working, controlling access to money, exploiting your citizenship or lack of citizenship to work or to prevent you from working

Statutes in each state provide more specific details describing the behaviors that are considered grounds for abuse. Additionally, every state has mandatory reporting laws for abuse, specifically abuse against children and the elderly, whereas many states have requirements for reporting domestic violence.

Intimate Partner Violence

Although the terms domestic violence, spousal abuse, or partner abuse have been commonly used, intimate partner violence (IPV) is a more inclusive term to include relationships between two people, with or without marital status or sexual relationship. IPV describes physical, sexual, or psychological harm by a current or former partner or spouse and can occur between heterosexual or same-sex couples. According to the National Intimate Partner and Sexual Violence Survey conducted by the Centers for Disease Control (CDC), about one in three women and more than one in four men have experienced physical violence at the hands of an intimate partner. Additionally, more than 37% of women and 31% of men in the United States have experienced IPV, including sexual violence, physical violence, and/or stalking by an intimate partner in their lifetime, and nearly one in seven women (16.4%) has been sexually assaulted by an intimate partner in her lifetime (Smith, et al., 2017). However, these statistics are believed to be much higher owing to under reporting.

There are many forms of abuse in IPV, although two or more types of abuse are commonly present in the same relationship. Emotional abuse often occurs with or before physical or sexual abuse in the relationship. Abuse in IPV tends to occur in cycles, often escalating in severity over time, with the abuse not stopping without intervention. Some signs of IPV include the following.

- Repeated injuries or bruises
- Unusual marks, scars, or rashes
- Bite marks
- Swelling or pain anywhere on the body, including the genital area
- Venereal disease and genital abrasions or injuries
- Unexplained fractures
- Repeated accidental injuries
- Black eyes or wearing dark glasses
- Makeup worn to hide bruising

Many major medical associations and advocacy organizations have recommended universal screening for IPV by health care professionals in the hope of reducing its incidence and severity. Although the prevalence of screening for IPV differs across health care specialties, only 3% to 41% of health care providers reported routine screening for IPV (Strayton & Duncan, 2005). Further, 10% of health care providers had never screened a patient for partner abuse. The reasons for the low percentage of universal screening for IPV by health care providers were time constraints; lack of knowledge, education or training on the issue; and inadequate follow-up resources and support staff. Additionally, health care providers reported feeling uncomfortable discussing IPV, as well as fearing for their personal safety and misdiagnosing patients (Elliott, 2002).

When screening for IPV, it is important to ask questions when the patient is alone to determine whether the patient feels safe or fears for his or her safety (Fig. 5.12). Often, the abusive partner may insist on speaking for the patient and may be resistant to leaving the patient alone. The health care professional should observe the demeanor of the patient, such as acting apprehensive or fearful, or having an exaggerated concern for the partner. Prior to asking any questions about a patient's sexual history or experiences of abuse, many clinics will ask patients to complete a survey as a screening tool. Additionally, health care professionals should include questions about sexual history as a part of every new patient's intake. Not only will this provide important medical information, it will help to establish a patient's trust where he or she will then feel comfortable in confiding future concerns to the health care provider. The CDC provides a series of questions and screening tools and assessments for IPV and sexual violence: https://www.cdc.gov/violenceprevention/pdf/ipv/ipvandsvscreening.pdf.

🛈 COMMUNICATION GUIDELINES

Screening for Intimate Partner Violence

When screening a patient for IPV, the following steps should be taken.

- Always talk to patients alone and not within earshot of a partner or family member.
- Never use a family member or friend as an interpreter; use medically trained interpreters only.
- Do not expect a patient to disclose abuse immediately; it may require multiple visits before he or she feels comfortable or trustful enough to disclose abuse. However, be prepared if disclosure does happen.

If the patient does disclose abuse, thank the patient for sharing. Convey empathy for the patient who has experienced fear, anxiety, and shame. Let the patient know you will support him or her unconditionally without judgment. Ask the patient if he or she has any immediate safety concerns and discuss options. If no staff members are trained in IPV, refer the patient to an IPV service advocate for safety planning and additional support. It is important to follow up at the patient's next medical visit.

➡ WORDS AT WORK

An effective screening tool for intimate partner violence is the "SAFE" Questions:

"S" for Safe
Ask: "How safe do you feel in your relationship? Never, sometimes, most of the time, always?"

"A" for Afraid
Ask: "Do you ever feel afraid of a partner or family member? Now or in the past?"

"F" for Friends or Family
Ask: "Would you be able to tell your friends or family if you are hurt? Would they be able to help you?"

"E" for Emergency Plan
Ask: "Do you have a safe place to go in an emergency, such as if you ever felt your life was in danger?"

From Ashur M. Asking About Domestic Violence: *SAFE Questions*. JAMA.1993;269(18):2367.

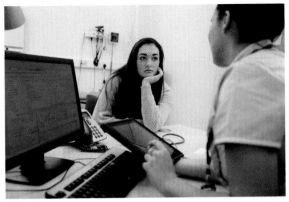

Fig. 5.12 The nurse uses a questionnaire to screen a patient for intimate partner violence (IPV).

Child Abuse

According to the CDC, there were more than 3.5 million reports of children being abused or neglected in the United States in 2016 (U.S. Department of Health & Human Services, Administration for Children and Families, Administration, 2018). Child abuse is a leading cause of death among children younger than 5 years of age. Every state has statutes that require specific professionals and persons to report suspected child abuse and neglect to appropriate agencies, called mandatory reporters. In fact, 48 states and the District of Columbia require that specific professions are designated as mandatory reporters of child abuse. The other two states—New Jersey and Wyoming—require that everyone reports incidences of child abuse, regardless of their profession. Although these mandatory reporters may vary by state, they often include the following.

- Social workers
- Teachers, principals, and other school personnel
- Physicians, nurses, and other health care professionals
- Counselors, therapists, and other mental health professionals
- Child care providers
- Medical examiners or coroners
- Law enforcement officers

Other states may require commercial film and photographic processors, animal control officers, and public and private college administrators to report child abuse. Additionally, many health care organizations and clinics have internal policies and procedures for handling reports of abuse, and these usually require the person who suspects abuse to notify the supervisor of the facility that abuse has been discovered or is suspected, which then needs to be reported to child protective services or other appropriate authorities. There are a number of signs of child abuse, such as

- Previously filed reports of physical or sexual abuse of the child
- Documented abuse of other family members
- Different stories between parents and child on how an accident happened; vague or poor explanations
- Stories of incidents and injuries that are suspicious
- Child brought in for a minor illness or complaint and serious injury is found

- Injuries blamed on other family members
- Repeated visits to the emergency department for injuries
- Discolorations/bruising on the buttocks, back, and abdomen; bruising on a child too young to walk or crawl
- Elbow, wrist, and shoulder dislocations
- Delays in the normal growth and development patterns
- Erratic school attendance
- Poor hygiene
- Malnutrition
- Obvious dental neglect
- Neglected well-baby procedures (e.g., immunizations)

🔲 COMMUNICATION GUIDELINES

Screening for Child Abuse

Child abuse is often identified during the patient intake. During the intake, questions should be open-ended. If the responses are unclear or suspicious, the questions should then be closed-ended, which requires simple and direct responses. Some questions that may be asked of children suspected of being abused are the following.

- "Have you ever been hurt by someone taking care of you? How did that happen?"
- "Have you ever been taken to the hospital/emergency room because you were hurt?"
- "Is anyone making you do anything that you feel uncomfortable about?"
- "What have you learned about "good touch/bad touch?" How did you learn that?"
- "What would you do if someone were trying to touch your private areas?"
- "What kind of things make you scared when you are at home?"
- "What is discipline like for you? Your brothers or sisters?"
- "Are there times when you feel bad about yourself? How does that happen?"

Child abuse may be difficult for health care professionals to identify and confirm because we often are dependent on parents or the child's caregiver for accurate information about the child's history and may not be critical or skeptical of the information provided, especially if the abuser is a parent or caregiver. The

BOX 5.4 TALKING WITH CHILDREN WHO REVEAL ABUSE

- Provide a private time and place to talk.
- Do not promise not to tell; tell them that you are required by law to report the abuse.
- Do not express shock or criticize their family.
- Use their vocabulary to discuss body parts.
- Avoid using any leading statements that can distort their report.
- Reassure them that they have done the right thing by telling.
- Tell them that the abuse is not their fault and that they are not bad or to blame.
- Determine their immediate need for safety.
- Let the child know what will happen when you report.

From Hockenberry MJ, Wilson D, Rodgers CC. *Wong's Essentials of Pediatric Nursing*, ed 10. St. Louis: Elsevier, 2017.

health care professional may also feel uncomfortable, intimidated, or threatened when asking parents or caregivers about concerns of abuse. These factors make it even more challenging to diagnose abuse. Guidelines for talking with children who reveal abuse are listed in Box 5.4. At the very least, the role of the health care provider is to identify children with suspicious injuries and report it to the child protection agency for investigation.

Elder Abuse

It is projected that 1 of 10 people over the age of 60 years has experienced some form of abuse, neglect, and exploitation, although this is likely an underestimate owing to under reporting (National Council on Aging, n.d.). The most common types of abuse among persons over the age of 60 are physical abuse, sexual abuse, emotional abuse, neglect, abandonment, and financial abuse. Elder abuse can also include inappropriate use of medications or physical restraints; force-feeding; failure to provide food, clothing, shelter, or other essentials, such as medical care or medications; and forging an older person's signature in order to steal money or possessions. Neglect, abandonment, and desertion can also include failing to pay nursing home or assisted-living facility costs if there is a legal responsibility to do so. Some signs of suspected elder abuse for health care professionals are

- Slap marks, most pressure marks, and certain types of burns or blisters (e.g., cigarette burns).

Explanations of the injury seems inconsistent with the pattern of the injury.

- Withdrawal from normal activities, unexplained change in alertness, or other unusual behavior may signal emotional abuse or neglect.
- Bruises around the breasts or genital area and unexplained sexually transmitted diseases can occur from sexual abuse.
- Sudden change in finances and accounts, altered wills and trusts, unusual bank withdrawals, checks written as "loans" or "gifts," and loss of property may suggest elder exploitation.
- Untreated bedsores, need for medical or dental care, unclean clothing, poor hygiene, overgrown hair and nails, and unusual weight loss.

A number of screening tools can be used by health care professionals to evaluate cases of suspected elder abuse, although there is no standard tool. Being proactive and having early identification of the abuse is key. In fact, it is recommended that every elderly patient is screened for any incidences of abuse. Studies have shown that patients, particularly women, favor routine screening of abuse as long as it is conducted in a safe environment by trained health care professionals (Perel-Levin, 2008).

Another method is to include broad questions and statements during the patient's intake or physical examination, which will help patients feel that they are not alone in their experiences. For example, a general question that could be asked to open the discussion may be "I don't know if you're experiencing this, but I find that I do have patients dealing with abusive relationships in their lives. Are you having any difficult relationships?" If the patient feels safe and trusts the health care provider, he or she may be comfortable in disclosing any abuse.

If the patient responds that there may be evidence of abuse or even hesitates when responding, it may be helpful to then ask more direct questions. Examples of direct questions may be

- "Do you feel safe at home?"
- "Are you afraid of anyone?"
- "Does anyone threaten or hurt you?"
- "Are you able to get out of the house and see your friends or other family members?"
- "Who takes care of your money and finances?"

• "What kind of help do you get at home when it comes to preparing your meals, shopping, or bathing?"

It is important to note that these questions should be asked only when the patient is alone with a health care professional. Any suspicions of elder abuse need to be documented and immediately reported to the health care provider.

Elderly patients may often be accompanied by a spouse, a family member, or caregiver. Almost 60% of elder abuse is perpetrated by a family member, with two-third being from adult children or a spouse (National Council on Aging, n.d.). Thus, it is important to closely monitor the family member's or caregiver's behavior and interaction during the patient visit. Some warning signs of suspicious behavior are

• Expressing a lack of concern or interest in the medical visit
• Closely monitoring the interaction between the patient and health care professionals
• Being overly protective and even answering questions for the patient
• Refusing to leave the room when asked
• Acting hostile and aggressive toward the medical team

In the case that the patient is unable to communicate or has dementia and is unable to disclose any abuse, the physical examination may need to be carefully evaluated for any suspicious and inconsistent findings.

⚹ LEGAL EAGLE

The Older Americans Act of 1987 (OAA) is federal legislation that protects adults older than the age 60 from abuse, neglect, abandonment, and exploitation. In addition to providing training, research, and community services, the OAA provides public education services and protection against elder abuse, neglect, and exploitation. In many states, elder abuse may be a criminal offense. Forty-eight states, the District of Columbia, and several territories require mandatory reporting of elder abuse, especially by health care professionals. A failure to report elder abuse may result in fines, imprisonment, and civil lawsuits for medical malpractice, depending on the state. In some states, reporting of the elder abuse must be made within five calendar days to the appropriate authorities.

👤 COMMUNICATION GUIDELINES

Talking About Abuse

When screening for family violence of any kind, it is often helpful to begin with broad statements or questions and then proceed with more direct questions. These broad statements will help normalize any problems and may reduce the patient's anxiety about discussing the problem.

Broad questions or statements include the following.

• "Because violence is common in so many relationships, we have been making it a practice to ask our patients about it."
• "Because difficult relationships can cause health problems, we are asking all of our patients the following question: Does anyone at home, such as a partner or family member, hurt, hit, or threaten you?"
• "Violence affects many families, which may result in emotional and physical problems for you and your children. We want to see if anything like that is going on in your family."

If you receive an affirmative answer or if you suspect abuse is happening with the patient, you may want to ask more direct questions.

"How are things at home?"

"How do you feel about the relationships in your life?"

"How does your husband/wife/partner treat you?"

"Every couple fights. What are your fights like? Do they ever get physical?"

"Do you feel you are in danger?"

"Are you afraid at home?"

Bullying

The term **bullying** refers to aggression among adolescents perpetrated on person or persons against an individual, excluding a sibling or dating partner, which is based on a power imbalance. Examples of power imbalances are physical characteristics, such as age or size; popularity with peers; socioeconomic class and being a part of majority or minority; being outnumbered; and the presence of weapons. According to the CDC, bullying is unwanted aggressive behavior(s) that is observed or perceived and is repeated multiple times or is highly likely to be repeated (U.S. Department of Health and Human Services, 2017). Bullying may inflict harm or distress on the targeted individual, which may include physical, psychological, social, or educational harm. Bullying may be physical violence like hitting or tripping; it may also be teasing, spreading rumors, or the threat of violence.

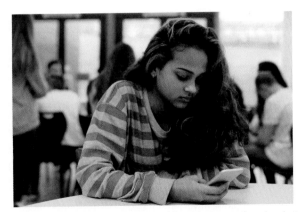

Fig. 5.13 Cyberbullying occurs with text messaging, in chat rooms, and on social media.

In 2015, 20% of 9th to 12th graders were bullied at school, whereas 16% were cyberbullied through chat rooms, text messages, and social media (Fig. 5.13). Most bullied children say that they are bullied because they are different or marginalized, such as having a disability or chronic disease, being overweight or underweight, being a member of a religious or ethnic minority, or identifying as a gender or sexual minority (Kann, et al., 2016) (McClowery, 2017). Boys and girls experience similar rates of bullying. Boys are more likely to experience physical bullying, whereas girls are more likely to experience verbal bulling, rumor-spreading, exclusion, and cyber-bulling. Healthy People 2020 includes an objective to reduce bullying among adolescents. According to the U.S. Department of Education (2010), possible consequences of bullying on individuals include

- Lowered academic achievement and aspirations
- Increased anxiety
- Loss of self-esteem and confidence
- Depression and posttraumatic stress
- Deterioration in physical health
- Self-harm and suicidal thinking
- Feelings of alienation
- Absenteeism

There may also be significant long-term effects of bullying. Adults who were bullied as children are more likely to suffer depression, anxiety, and substance use disorders (Lereya, Copeland, Costello, & Wolke, 2015).

Because 50% to 70% of victims do not report being abused to an adult, it is important for health care professionals to screen and counsel children for bulling because we are in a unique position. Signs a child might be a victim of bullying include the following.

- Behavioral or mood changes
- Unexplained injuries
- Frequent complaints of headaches, stomachaches, or feeling sick
- Changes in eating habits
- Difficulty sleeping or nightmares
- Declining grades, loss of interest in school, or not wanting to go to school
- Sudden loss of friends or avoidance of social situations (Abaza & Lu, 2017)

As a health care professional, pay careful attention when a child presents with a psychosomatic illness, and remember that being part of a marginalized group puts a child at a higher risk of being bullied.

COMMUNICATION GUIDELINES

Screening for Bullying

Screening for bullying can be as simple as asking the child, "Are you being bullied?" The child may be reluctant to verbalize the problem, however, so you may get better responses by offering a written survey with questions, such as

- "Do you feel safe at school?"
- "Do you have a group of friends at school?"
- "Has anyone ever hit you, tripped you, or spat on you?"
- "Have you been threatened by someone at school or online?"
- "How often have you been picked on or made fun of?"
- "Have any classmates started rumors about you?"
- "Has anyone posted anything about you online that is hurtful?"
- "Have you told anyone about any of these incidents?"

Early recognition of bullying is critical because, without intervention, it may lead to other behavioral problems. If you suspect a child is being bullied, counsel the patient's parents or caregiver on intervention strategies. Here again, effective communication is key. Parents must offer emotional support that promotes open communication and disclosure of any bullying incident. As the health care professional, you can help open the lines of communication by affirming to the parents and the child that the problem is unacceptable and that it has harmful consequences to the child's physical and mental health. The child must also be assured that he or she is not at fault, and that parents have a plan to address the child's safety. Parents should notify the school in writing, keep records of incidents, and refer to advocacy groups as needed (Abaza & Lu, 2017).

> ✳ **LEGAL EAGLE**
>
> Many states and local governments have taken action to protect children from bullying, cyberbullying, and any related behaviors and actions. A list of individual statistic antibullying laws and policies and their key components can be found at: https://www.stopbullying.gov/laws/key-components/index.html.
>
>   Although no federal laws specifically apply to bullying, there is federal legal protection in cases where the bullying is based on race, color, national origin, sex, disability, or religion. Additionally, schools, including colleges and universities, that receive federal funding must address discrimination based on these personal characteristics, per the following laws
>
> - Title VI of the Civil Rights Act of 1964 (referred to as Title VI) prohibits discrimination based on race, color, or national origin
> - Title IX of the Education Amendments of 1972 (referred to as Title IX) prohibits discrimination based on sex
> - Section 504 of the Rehabilitation Act of 1973 and Title II of the ADA (1990) prohibits discrimination based on disability
>
> School personnel and their employers may violate federal civil rights laws when the bullying and harassment creates a hostile environment and it is encouraged, tolerated, not adequately addressed, or ignored.

▌ CHECKING YOUR COMPREHENSION

1. What are the benefits of using a professional interpreter, as opposed to a family member?
2. What are the signs a person may have a vision problem he or she has not disclosed? What are the signs of a hearing problem?
3. Consider the last time you were faced with a stressful situation, such as trying to make an important deadline at work or having to pack up everything and move. Discuss how your body reacted during that situation. List three of your body's responses to the stress.
4. Thinking about the same stressful situation in Question 3, review the different coping mechanisms in Box 5.3. Which one did you use in the stressful situation? Discuss how it presented in the situation?
5. In your future health care profession, discuss what steps you would take in the case of an anxious or stressed patient? Or a violent patient?
6. Research the different community resources for intimate partner violence, such as counseling services and emergency shelters. How would you include these resources in a conversation where a patient discloses he or she is in an abusive relationship?
7. List five signs or behaviors that a patient experiencing elder abuse may exhibit.
8. List five signs or behaviors that a child experiencing abuse may exhibit.

▌ EXPANDING CRITICAL THINKING

1. A Spanish-speaking woman presents to the emergency department with vaginal bleeding. Her teenage son explains to the nurse that his mother has been acting tired and did not get out of bed all weekend. You will need to get more information from her and will have to ask her some sensitive questions about her sexual history. Her son has been doing a good job translating. What is the best course of action?
2. Consider a time when you were surrounded by people who were speaking a language that you did not understand. Discuss how you felt and what you did to communicate with these people.
3. Although Spanish is the most common language, other than English, spoken in the United States, only a small percentage of health care professionals speaks Spanish. What steps can you take to improve your language ability to communicate with a patient in your profession?
4. Lila is a nurse working in an emergency room. A couple comes in with their 13-year-old daughter, who complains of stomach pains and vaginal bleeding. Lila starts to ask questions about the daughter's symptoms and her medical history. But, every time she asks a question, one of the parents answers instead of the daughter. When Lila tries to direct a question to the daughter, she gives only one- or two-word responses before being interrupted by her parents. The daughter looks withdrawn and looks down almost the entire time. Lila suspects abuse and needs to get more information from the daughter. What should Lila do?

5. Kimberly, the medical office manager at a busy out-patient laboratory, is helping to check in a father with his 12-day-old baby. He explains that he has brought his infant son in for another heel stick to check his bilirubin levels. The pediatrician has been monitoring the baby for jaundice. The baby is crying now and the father looks distressed and exhausted. Kimberly suspects neither the baby nor his father have been getting much sleep. She begins to ask the father for the usual check-in information, such as the patient's name and birthday. When asked about insurance and if there are any changes in the insurance, the father loses his temper. "How could there be any changes in my insurance? I've been running back and forth between here and the doctor's office for the last week! And no one knows anything! And now you tell me that my insurance has changed!" As Kimberly tries to calm and explain the situation to him, the father grows increasingly loud and angry. What can Kimberly do to deescalate this situation and help this stressed and angry parent?

6. Jamie, the nurse at the family physician's office, is conducting the patient interview of Bryan, a 14-year-old boy in the office who is suffering from migraines. Bryan acts young for his age. He is bouncing in the chair and can't seem to sit still. He is wearing sweatpants and a t-shirt with a cartoon character on it. "We hate to miss another day of school," his mother says, "but we need to find out what's causing these headaches." His mother explains that Bryan was fine at church yesterday and at the church picnic afterward, spending all afternoon playing badminton with some of the younger children. But, after dinner, he began to complain of headaches. When it was time to get up for school this morning, the migraines were so bad that Bryan could not move. Bryan's mother states that this has been going on for several months since they transferred Bryan to a new school. Jamie wonders if the timing of Bryan's migraines is related to problems at school, and wonders if Bryan is being bullied. How should Jamie approach this subject with Bryan and his mother? What things can Jamie do to help them?

7. Sandra works as a nurse in a county health department that offers an STD and HIV-AIDS clinic. Devon comes in because he was contacted by the health department that he may have been exposed to an STD by a sexual partner. During the patient examination, Sandra takes blood and fluid samples for testing and prepares them for transportation to a testing laboratory. When she returns to the patient room, she overhears Devon talking to someone on the phone: "I'm still at the clinic. My girlfriend is waiting outside in the waiting room, but she doesn't know anything about you and why I need to be tested right now. Well, I'm not going to tell her about you and I'm just going to tell her this was all a mistake, nothing is wrong, and she doesn't need to be tested." Sandra wonders if Devon is cheating on his girlfriend with the person he is talking to on the phone. What should Sandra do in this situation?

8. Shannon is a medical assistant at a family medicine clinic. One of her patients this morning is Janice, who has been a patient at the clinic for several years. Janice is married and has three children at home. Her previous medical visits have been fairly routine, although her physical examination has noted frequent bruises and scratches on her body and a broken arm she said was caused by falls. Today, she is here for a follow-up medical visit and a refill of her prescriptions. Shannon calls Janice, who is sitting in the waiting room, back to the patient room and immediately notices bruises on her face, a swollen and cut lip, and a black eye. How should Shannon manage this patient visit? What would the discussion with Janice be like?

6

Communicating Through Illnesses and Disorders

Sharon Campton

LEARNING OBJECTIVES

Upon successful completion of this chapter, you will be able to:

1. Discuss the barriers to communicating with a patient who is ill.
2. Describe cancer, its various treatments, and considerations when interacting with cancer patients.
3. List and describe the common types of depression, its treatments, and considerations when interacting with depressed patients.
4. Define suicidal ideation and identify patients at risk for suicide.
5. Describe generalized anxiety disorder and considerations when interacting with anxious patients.
6. Explain the diagnostic criteria for substance use disorder (SUD) and recognize commonly abused substances.
7. Describe dementia and considerations when interacting with patients with dementia.
8. Discuss anorexia nervosa and bulimia nervosa and the unique challenges for communicating with patients who have eating disorders.
9. Discuss autism spectrum disorder and the unique challenges for communicating with patients with this disorder.
10. Define somatic symptom disorder and considerations when interacting with these patients.

KEY TERMS

activities of daily living (ADLs) self-care, such as bathing, preparing meals, cleaning, shopping, and other routines that require thought, planning, and physical motion

acute illness with a rapid onset and short duration

addiction physiologic and/or psychological dependence on a substance beyond voluntary control

advance directive legal document that provides guidance about the patient's desired treatments to sustain life when he or she becomes incapacitated

Alzheimer's disease progressive disease presenting with memory, thinking, and behavioral problems that become more severe over time

analgesic pain-relieving treatment

autism spectrum disorder a range of developmental conditions characterized by problems with social interactions, communication, and behavioral challenges.

anorexia nervosa eating disorder in which the individual fears gaining weight, has a disturbance in the view of his or her body, and restricts food intake to lose weight even weight is significantly low

benign noncancerous tumor that does not spread

biopsy removal of a living tissue sample for visual examination

bulimia nervosa eating disorder in which the individual compulsively eats large quantities of food (binge-eating) followed by compensating for the binge through purging (vomiting, use of laxatives, and/or exercise)

chronic slowly progressing illness that lasts longer than 3 months

cognitive behavioral therapy (CBT) intervention for treating mental disorders the solves problems by correcting distorted thinking and helping the patient develop new coping mechanisms

delirium tremens physical withdrawal from chronic high alcohol intake with symptoms of confusion, shaking, and hallucinations

dementia decline in mental ability caused by brain disease or injury sufficiently severe to interfere with daily life

Durable Power of Attorney (DPOA) type of advance directive that allows the patient to name another individual who legally makes health care decisions on the patient's behalf

informed consent patient's authorization to receive treatment following the provider's discussion of various treatment options and risks

dysthymia depressed mood lasting at least 2 years

generalized anxiety disorder a mental health disorder in which the patient suffers chronic, exaggerated worry or a sense of dread, sometimes without cause

malignant cancerous tumor

Maintenance condition of living with incurable cancer and managing the disease to allow for an acceptable quality of life

major depressive disorder mood disorder in which the patient suffers loss of interest, sadness, and a change in functioning, among other symptoms lasting a period of 2 weeks or more

metastasis spread of cancer to sites in the body beyond the cancer's origin

pathologist medical doctor who specializes in the causes and effects of diseases

Physician Order for Life Sustaining Treatment (POLST) portable document for a terminally ill patient containing physician orders for desired treatment in the event of an emergency

psychotropic substance that effects an individual's brain chemistry to produce a change in thinking, emotion, or behavior (literally, "turns the mind")

recovery state of abstaining from using a substance thereby improving health and well-being

relapse deteriorated condition after an improvement

remission complete or partial disappearance of the signs and symptoms of cancer in response to treatment

substance use disorder (SUD) disorder in which a patient has mental, social, and/or physiologic symptoms from continued use of a substance

suicidal ideation thoughts of causing one's own death

tolerance reduced effects following repeated use of a substance

withdrawal symptoms following cessation of substance use

❓ TEST YOUR COMMUNICATION IQ

1. A person with addiction can be considered cured after effective treatment.
2. Treatment of depression is highly successful for 80% or more of the people who seek treatment.
3. A cancer diagnosis is not the "death sentence" it once was.
4. If you suspect someone is contemplating committing suicide, asking him or her if (s)he's thinking of harming him or herself will only make him or her more likely to follow through.
5. Alzheimer's disease is a type of dementia.
6. Generalized anxiety disorder is a type of depression.
7. The rate of suicide is the highest in middle-aged men, predominantly white men.

Results

Statements 2, 3, 5, and 7 are true; the others are false. How did you do? Read the chapter to find more information on these topics.

INTRODUCTION

The nature of our health care service necessitates that most of our patients will not come to us in good health. Patients present in the health care system with varying degrees of pain, fatigue, discomfort, irritation, diminished function, and mental or emotional distress. To a certain extent, even the patient in good health who appears at the physician's office for a well-visit or annual physical examination may have a level of anxiety about having his or her body under scrutiny. But communication is especially challenging with those living with a disorder or who are severely ill. In general, patients must be prepared to face both physical and psychological pain as they heal, or must adjust to the fact that they may never fully recover. Some must realize that they cannot care for themselves and can no longer live independently. They may be required to endure treatments and procedures that frequently are painful and debilitating and may be long term. Their self-image, life role, and personal relationships may change to accommodate the effects of illness. All of these stressors are factors to consider during our interaction with all patients.

This chapter addresses some very specific illnesses and disorders that you are more likely to encounter in your work and the unique communication guidelines for them. Communicating with someone who is ill and/or has an identified disorder has its own unique challenges. In no way are the conditions included meant to be comprehensive; neither is the extent of the material about each condition. It is meant to give you some understanding of an illness or disorder because *understanding is always the first step in making any interaction more productive.* Our work is never to "fix" the patient or the patient's situation, but we can help the patient to clarify and understand better what he or she is experiencing by helping the patient say aloud and clarify his or her own thoughts and experiences. In this way, you actively demonstrate compassion.

You are encouraged to look into the following conditions in greater detail, to learn more about them and those that are not listed. The following are some especially reliable sources.

- The Centers for Disease Control and Prevention: one of the major operating components of the federal Department of Health and Human Services: https://www.cdc.gov
- The Mayo Clinic: a not-for-profit organization providing medical care, research, and education services: https://www.mayoclinic.org
- National Institute of Mental Health: the lead federal agency for research on mental disorders: https://www.nimh.nih.gov.
- The American Cancer Society: provides support to individuals battling cancer and funds research into treatments
- The Suicide Prevention Resource Center: offers articles and reports about suicide, as well as resources for education, screening, and treatment.
- The Substance Abuse and Mental Health Services Administration (SAMHSA): the federal agency whose mission is to reduce the impact of substance abuse and mental illness on America's communities: https://www.samhsa.gov.
- The Alzheimer's Association: enhances care, support, and research for those with Alzheimer's disease and dementia: https://www.alz.org.
- The National Eating Disorders Association (NEDA): staffs a support hotline, offers free and low-cost treatment resources, and advocates for public policy initiatives to prevent and heal eating disorders: https://www.nationaleatingdisorders.org.
- The Autism Society of America: offers information about autism spectrum disorders (ASDs), spearheads legislation, and helps people with autism live, learn, and work: http://www.autism-society.org.

INDIVIDUALS LIVING WITH ILLNESS

As you learn about and interact with patients who have illnesses and are diagnosed with a specific disorder, it is important to talk about these individuals as someone living with cancer, someone who is depressed, someone who is living with dementia, someone who has an eating disorder—not as the cancer patient, the depressive patient, the demented patient, the anorexic patient, for example. You are learning about many communication skills, but your ability to connect effectively with and support your patients is enhanced greatly by always thinking of, speaking about, and interacting with them as an individual who happens to have a disease, a condition, or a disorder; the individual is not the disease, condition or disorder.

Some illnesses present as acute, meaning that they have a rapid onset and are of short duration; other illnesses present as chronic, meaning that they develop gradually and extend over a long time (typically more than 3 months); some illnesses can present as both acute and chronic. A person who has pain for a short duration will communicate differently than someone who has endured pain for a long time.

Patients who are actively sick have difficulty listening to anything other than what is happening within their body. Pain, nausea, vertigo, and other symptoms of illness make it hard to communicate beyond the most basic information needed to relieve the most disturbing concerns. As discussed in Chapter 3, Educating Patients, individuals under great distress are not ready to exchange or retain information. Trying to communicate about topics other than relief at this time will increase their stress and may make the situation worse for them.

Even patients who are not acutely or actively ill have trouble may concentrating because of the psychological noise whirling around in their brains. Worrisome thoughts fill their minds, such as, "How will this affect my career, my marriage, my life?" "How can I pay for this?" "Will I be scarred, disabled, or sick for the rest of my life?" "Will I die from this?"

These circumstances make skillful communication all the more important. Patients need answers to questions they may be afraid to ask, such as, "Can I expect pain?" "Will I suffer?" "When will it become bearable, or will it always be unbearable?" "Will it ever end?" "Will I lose control of my bladder, my bowels, my mobility, and can I ever regain control?" Many questions tumble over in their minds and add to the confusion and depression associated with any illness.

Most patients do better with answers. When they know what lies ahead in 2 weeks, 2 months, or 2 years, patients can prepare for the next step in the progression of illness and also plan for the restoration of their health or the adaptations required to live with their illness or disorder. For the newly diagnosed patient, knowing what lies ahead can lead to the following:

- **Seeking knowledge.** When patients know the direction of the illness, some begin researching to know more about the disorder and how to handle it. With the help of family, social groups, and health care providers, many patients take control and work toward a reasonable level of wellness.
- **Seeking comfort.** Patients look for comfort and support from their social and spiritual groups and within the medical community. This love/belonging hierarchic need is never more important than during illness.
- **Learning self-care.** If the illness is extreme, patients need a strong ego and mental resources to adjust to the changes. Some changes can be devastating to the self-image, but knowing what to expect helps to prepare for self-care. Your role in this area of adjustment involves helping with procedures necessary for management of the illness.
- **Goal-setting.** Breaking the illness into small, manageable components makes the changes more acceptable. For example, "First, we will go over what to expect with the incision, then you can learn to change the dressing."
- **Planning alternative directions.** Life plans may be altered to fit the new self-image and physical limitations. Patients who realize this and make realistic adjustments fairly early in the illness usually respond better throughout the illness.

Patients with acute, short-term illnesses who are expected to recover fully and rather soon usually follow the provider's directions to encourage recovery. Knowing that the illness will be long and possibly painful or debilitating typically leads to difficult, if not poor, adjustment and, possibly, poor compliance. It is also somewhat easier to adapt with less stress to an illness that is not obvious to observers, even if it is long-term.

Tools for Communicating When the Patient Is Incapacitated

Ethically and legally, patients must authorize health care professionals to treat them before an intervention can be performed. With some exceptions made for emergencies, before any procedure or treatment the patient must be told of his diagnosis (if known), the options for treatment, any risks or side effects associated with the treatment, and the consequences of not intervening at all. Informed consent is given when a patient authorizes treatment following his or her understanding of this information. An informed consent form is signed by the patient and becomes part of the patient's health record, as discussed in Chapter 9.

Sometimes, illnesses or injuries can render the patient unable to communicate. Without the ability to understand her condition and the risks and side effects of treatment, or the faculties to convey her wishes to the physician, how can the health care team know what the patient desires for her care? For this reason, health care plans and providers recommend that adults have certain documents in place that identify the patient's wishes and provide guidance to their loved ones and medical providers.

An advance directive is a legal document that a person completes to provide guidance about his desires and the life-supporting interventions he deems acceptable when he is unable to communicate. This document may be called by different names that vary by state, but the terms advance directive, advance medical directive, living will, personal directive, medical directive, or advance decision all refer to the same legal instrument. Advance directives contain a section that outlines the specific medical interventions acceptable to the patient, the types of treatment the person desires to receive, and not receive. For example, the advance directive may state that if the physician determines a patient's condition to be incurable or irreversible, life-sustaining measures, such as mechanical ventilation, should be discontinued. Other situations commonly found on advance directives include whether to forgo food and water, instructions for the delivery of analgesic (pain-relieving) medications, and whether to revive the patient in the event that the heart or breathing stops. It is important to keep in mind that the advance directive is only applicable when the patient cannot speak for himself.

The durable power of attorney (DPOA) is one type of advance directive that allows the patient to name another individual who is delegated for making health care decisions on the patient's behalf. This person, sometimes called a *health care proxy* or *agent*, legally speaks on behalf of the patient to make medical decisions if the individual is incapable of making those decisions herself or himself. The person with this authority both ensures that the patient's directions are followed as described in the advance directive, and makes other decisions about the patient's care as they arise. Some states combine the DPOA and advance directive into a single document. Many health care providers make these documents available to their members; forms may be available online, but should be searched for the specific state in which a person lives. It is recommended that these documents be reviewed and updated regularly.

Five Wishes also is a unique legal advance directive written in everyday language. It also goes further than other advance directives by addressing medical, personal, emotional, and spiritual wishes. It is legally valid in most states; some require supplemental documents. Five Wishes also is available in Spanish and translations in other languages.

Physician Order for Life Sustaining Treatment (**POLST**) is a *medical order* directing emergency health care professionals (e.g., EMTs, firefighters, emergency room, and code responders) regarding specific treatments in the event of a medical crisis (Fig. 6.1). The POLST form is created to represent the conversation between the physician and patient about treatment options following diagnosis with a serious illness and those with advanced frailty near the end of life. It dictates whether or not to perform cardiopulmonary resuscitation or administer nutrition, and offers guidance on the level of treatment to be given (e.g., "comfort measures only"). Because the document contains a set of medical orders and is designed to stay with the patient, the POLST can communicate the patient's wishes to medical professionals in any setting. Often printed on a brightly colored single page, the POLST form is standardized to be found and read easily by professionals in emergency situations. This form does not replace an advance directive, but the two forms work together.

Communicating While Wearing Personal Protection Equipment

Some patients you will work with will have infectious diseases that can be transmitted through the air or by direct touch. Some patients may have such weakened immune systems that anyone who comes into contact with

SEND FORM WITH PERSON WHENEVER TRANSFERRED OR DISCHARGED
To follow these orders, an EMS provider must have an order from his/her medical command physician

pennsylvania
DEPARTMENT OF HEALTH

Pennsylvania
Orders for Life-Sustaining
Treatment (POLST)

Last Name

First/Middle Initial

Date of Birth

FIRST follow these orders, **THEN** contact physician, certified registered nurse practitioner or physician assistant. This is an Order Sheet based on the person's medical condition and wishes at the time the orders were issued. Everyone shall be treated with dignity and respect.

A
Check One

CARDIOPULMONARY RESUSCITATION (CPR): Person has no pulse and is not breathing.

☐ CPR/Attempt Resuscitation   ☐ DNR/Do Not Attempt Resuscitation (Allow Natural Death)
When not in cardiopulmonary arrest, follow orders in **B**, **C** and **D**.

B
Check One

MEDICAL INTERVENTIONS: Person has pulse and/or is breathing.

☐ **COMFORT MEASURES ONLY** Use medication by any route, positioning, wound care and other measures to relieve pain and suffering. Use oxygen, oral suction and manual treatment of airway obstruction as needed for comfort. *Do not transfer to hospital for life-sustaining treatment. Transfer if comfort needs cannot be met in current location.*

☐ **LIMITED ADDITIONAL INTERVENTIONS** Includes care described above. Use medical treatment, IV fluids and cardiac monitor as indicated. Do not use intubation, advanced airway interventions, or mechanical ventilation.

Transfer to hospital if indicated. Avoid intensive care if possible.

☐ **FULL TREATMENT** Includes care described above. Use intubation, advanced airway interventions, mechanical ventilation, and cardioversion as indicated.

Transfer to hospital if indicated. Includes intensive care.

Additional Orders _____ _____ _____

C
Check One

ANTIBIOTICS:

☐ No antibiotics. Use other measures to relieve symptoms.
☐ Determine use or limitation of antibiotics when infection occurs, with comfort as goal.
☐ Use antibiotics if life can be prolonged.

Additional Orders

D
Check One

ARTIFICIALLY ADMINISTERED HYDRATION / NUTRITION:
Always offer food and liquids by mouth if feasible

☐ No hydration and artificial nutrition by tube.
☐ Trial period of artificial hydration and nutrition by tube.
☐ Long-term artificial hydration and nutrition by tube.

Additional Orders

E
Check One

SUMMARY OF GOALS, MEDICAL CONDITION AND SIGNATURES:

Discussed with
☐ Patient
☐ Parent of Minor
☐ Health Care Agent
☐ Health Care Representative
☐ Court-Appointed Guardian
☐ Other:

Patient Goals/Medical Condition:

By signing this form, I acknowledge that this request regarding resuscitative measures is consistent with the known desires of, and in the best interest of, the individual who is the subject of the form.

Physician /PA/CRNP Printed Name:

Physician /PA/CRNP Phone Number

Physician/PA/CRNP Signature (Required):

DATE

Signature of Patient or Surrogate

Signature (required)

Name (print)

Relationship (write "self" if patient)

PaDOH version 10-14-10

1 of 2

Fig. 6.1 A POLST document is standardized and designed to be easy to read. It is often printed on brightly colored paper. (From the Pennsylvania Department of Health.)

SEND FORM WITH PERSON WHENEVER TRANSFERRED OR DISCHARGED

Other Contact Information

Surrogate	Relationship	Phone Number	
Health Care Professional Preparing Form	Preparer Title	Phone Number	Date Prepared

Directions for Healthcare Professionals

Any individual for whom a Pennsylvania Order for Life-Sustaining Treatment form is completed should ideally have an advance health care directive that provides instructions for the individual's health care and appoints an agent to make medical decisions whenever the patient is unable to make or communicate a healthcare decision. If the patient wants a DNR Order issued in section "A", the physician/PA/CRNP should discuss the issuance of an Out-of-Hospital DNR order, if the individual is eligible, to assure that an EMS provider can honor his/her wishes. Contact the Pennsylvania Department of Aging for information about sample forms for advance health care directives. Contact the Pennsylvania Department of Health, Bureau of EMS, for information about Out-of-Hospital Do-Not-Resuscitate orders, bracelets and necklaces. POLST forms may be obtained online from the Pennsylvania Department of Health.   www.health.state.pa.us

Completing POLST

Must be completed by a health care professional based on patient preferences and medical indications or decisions by the patient or a surrogate. This document refers to the person for whom the orders are issued as the "individual" or "patient" and refers to any other person authorized to make healthcare decisions for the patient covered by this document as the "surrogate."

At the time a POLST is completed, any current advance directive, if available, must be reviewed.

Must be signed by a physician/PA/CRNP and patient/surrogate to be valid. Verbal orders are acceptable with follow-up signature by physician/PA/CRNP in accordance with facility/community policy. A person designated by the patient or surrogate may document the patient's or surrogate's agreement. Use of original form is strongly encouraged. Photocopies and Faxes of signed POLST forms should be respected when necessary

Using POLST

If a person's condition changes and time permits, the patient or surrogate must be contacted to assure that the POLST is updated as appropriate.

If any section is not completed, then the healthcare provider should follow other appropriate methods to determine treatment.

An automated external defibrillator (AED) should not be used on a person who has chosen "Do Not Attempt Resuscitation"

Oral fluids and nutrition must always be offered if medically feasible.

When comfort cannot be achieved in the current setting, the person, including someone with "comfort measures only," should be transferred to a setting able to provide comfort (e.g., treatment of a hip fracture).

A person who chooses either "comfort measures only" or "limited additional interventions" may not require transfer or referral to a facility with a higher level of care.

An IV medication to enhance comfort may be appropriate for a person who has chosen "Comfort Measures Only."

Treatment of dehydration is a measure which may prolong life. A person who desires IV fluids should indicate "Limited Additional Interventions" or "Full Treatment.

A patient with or without capacity or the surrogate who gave consent to this order or who is otherwise specifically authorized to do so, can revoke consent to any part of this order providing for the withholding or withdrawal of life-sustaining treatment, at any time, and request alternative treatment.

Review

This form should be reviewed periodically (consider at least annually) and a new form completed if necessary when:
(1) The person is transferred from one care setting or care level to another, or
(2) There is a substantial change in the person's health status, or
(3) The person's treatment preferences change.

Revoking POLST

If the POLST becomes invalid or is replaced by an updated version, draw a line through sections A through E of the invalid POLST, write "VOID" in large letters across the form, and sign and date the form.

PaDOH version 10-14-10

2 of 2

Fig. 6.1, cont'd

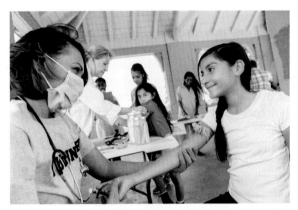

Fig. 6.2 When wearing a mask, remember to face the patient directly so he or she can see that you are talking and that you are also communicating with your eyes. (iStock.com/Steve Debenport.)

them needs to wear protective equipment to protect the patient from anything the person may transmit. Specific precautionary measures will be determined and made known to protect the health care professional and patient. Personal protection equipment (PPE) may include protective eyewear, face masks covering the nose and mouth, water-repellant gowns, gloves, hair coverings, and foot coverings (Fig. 6.2). Communication while wearing a face mask can be particularly challenging because it limits what others see of facial expressions and has an impact on the loudness of the voice. Remember to face the patient directly, so he or she can see that you are talking. Your eyes are still expressive, and it is possible to tell if you're smiling by your eyes, even when your mouth is covered.

CANCER

Cancer occurs when some of the body's cells grow abnormally and out of control, then crowd out normal, healthy cells, impacting how effectively the body works. Cancer can occur in skeletal structures (bone), blood, organs, and other tissues.

If a mass of abnormal cells is identified and its location is such that a small portion of the mass can be removed, it then is biopsied (studied microscopically to determine a diagnosis) by a pathologist, a medical doctor who specializes in the causes and effects of diseases. Not all abnormal cells are cancerous. If the abnormal tissue is benign, it means that the cells are not cancerous and will not spread to other areas of the body.

Sometimes benign masses affect a patient's ability to function and may need to be dealt with medically.

The other possible biopsy result is that the abnormal cells are malignant, which means the abnormal cells are cancerous. If that is the case, the patient is referred to an oncologist, who is a medical doctor specializing in the treatment of cancer.

Cell testing can usually determine the type of cancer, its source, and location(s), which determines the type of treatment to be done. Cancer is diagnosed in stages or staging, which indicates the degree of progression of the disease related to the size of the tumor, whether the cancer has spread to nearby lymph nodes and how many, and whether the cancer has metastasized (spread) to other parts of the body. These stages are represented by Roman numerals, I–IV; the lower the stage, the less the cancer has spread and the higher the number means a more serious cancer.

Treatment varies, depending on the type and stage of the cancer. Sometimes surgery to remove the affected tissue is involved; sometimes surgery is sufficient. Treatment may include *radiation therapy*, in which high-energy rays are directly targeted to a particular area of the body to kill cancer cells and shrink tumors. *Chemotherapy*, drugs administered to kill cancer cells, is another form of treatment. Hormone-origin cancers may be treated with *hormone therapy*. Some cancers respond well to *immunotherapy*. Depending on the type of cancer, treatment may include any combination of the above treatments. Each of these types of treatment have their own side effects, some permanent, some temporary; some relatively mild, some dangerous. Benefits and risks of each are reviewed with the patient, to help her or him determine the course of treatment. The patient's overall health and age also determine treatment; the patient's health insurance, or lack thereof, financial ability, proximity to care, and culture also may contribute to the type of treatment the patient seeks or is able to seek.

If there is complete or partial disappearance of the signs and symptoms of cancer in response to treatment, the patient may be determined to be in remission; however, a remission may not be a cure—there is the possibility of the cancer returning.

Maintenance is when people continue to live their lives with chronic cancer; they are not cured, but they continue to receive treatment that makes the cancer manageable and allows for an acceptable (to the patient) quality of life.

Patient Interaction

Cancer no longer is the death sentence that it was when diagnosed in earlier decades. Advanced research and treatment allow many people to survive cancer diagnoses for longer periods of time. However, hearing the word "cancer" still induces a tremendously impactful emotional reaction. There is a lot of waiting, especially in the unknown, that accompanies cancer—from the detection of a suspicious mass to awaiting biopsy/testing results, diagnosis, more specific diagnosis, treatment, further tests to determine effectiveness of treatment, side effects of treatment. And always present is the cloud of wondering whether the cancer will return or spread, even if remission or cure is determined, which is the overarching unknown.

It is not uncommon for the patient to come to terms with her or his cancer at a different pace and in different ways than those of loved ones. All of the waiting and unknowns that affect the patient also affect the patient's loved ones (a parent, partner, or child) often differently from one another, as well as from the patient herself or himself. Your professional, compassionate presence is critical to effective communication with cancer patients and their affected loved ones. You may be working with patients in a health care environment that is not related to cancer; cancer patients need to continue to be seen for care other than cancer that may or may not be impacted by their disease. Most cancer treatments weaken the patient's immune system, making them more susceptible to *opportunistic infections* (infections occur more frequently and may be more severe in those with a weakened immune system than in people with a stronger immune system) that need treatment independent of the cancer. Patients will be at varying phases of diagnosis, treatment, remission, and/or metastasis.

Sometimes loved ones, be they family or friends, react or respond to cancer diagnoses and treatment in unsupportive ways, such as withdrawing or denial. The American Cancer Society (ACS) provides extensive information, education, support for persons diagnosed with cancer, family and caregivers, and research on all types of cancers at www.cancer.org.

📇 COMMUNICATION GUIDELINES

Patients With Cancer

Your ability to appreciate the overall impact the disease has on the patient's life and identity physically, emotionally, and relationally and to accept the patient without judgment or pity helps the patient's ability to cope with the disease.

- Providing supportive material from resources, such as the ACS and regional cancer support groups, can be valuable for both patients and their loved ones.
- Do not attempt to be an expert or give advice on treatment decisions—just offer support.
- Do not call people "patients." Do not make the disease a part of their identity. Use patients names and rehumanize them after being poked and prodded in the medical setting.

▶ TAKING THE CHAPTER TO WORK

Cancer

Let's meet LaShanda, an assistant for a gastroenterologist. She is about to greet a new patient, Mr. Chung, age 74, who is to be examined for complications as a result of radiation treatment that he had received 2 years prior for prostate cancer; the cancer treatment has been successful thus far, but Mr. Chung continues to experience subsequent problems from radiation treatment to his bladder and now his intestines. LaShanda greets and introduces herself to the patient in the reception area and escorts him to a main area inside the treatment section. She takes his vital signs of temperature, blood pressure, respiration, and pulse then weighs the patient. LaShanda attempts to establish rapport, but notes that the patient remains very quiet, almost withdrawn even as she states the good news that his vital signs are all within limits. He is cooperative, but goes through the motions with minimal comment or interaction. When the patient is seated on the table in the examination room, LaShanda begins to enter his information in the computer.

"Mr. Chung, congratulations on 2 years of being cancer free!" LaShanda grins. "But I'm sorry that you are here because of some of the effects of your radiation treatment."

"You can call me Henry," he pauses, "Yeah, trade off one for the other…"

LaShanda turns away from the computer and faces the patient. "It sounds discouraging to have medical issues a couple of years after your cancer treatment has ended."

Mr. Chung looks down at his hands, folded in his lap. "Yeah, it is."

(Continued)

"We'll take good care of you, Henry," LaShanda assures him, "and do everything we can to make sure you get the best possible care."

Mr. Chung exhales a heavy sigh. "Oddly enough, I'm not so worried about my intestines. I mean, I'm not pleased about any of this, but I'm not worried about it—at least, not yet."

"You seem sad, though; are you discouraged?" The patient looks up at LaShanda, shrugs his shoulders and nods. "But it's not related to why you're here?"

Mr. Chung hesitates. He finally offers, "I'm afraid my cancer will come back."

"Oh, that's understandable," says LaShanda. "That's one of the frustrating aspects of the disease…"

"It sure is!" Mr. Chung's voice cracks a bit while he speaks. He sighs deeply again, only this time it appears he is about to cry. LaShanda notices a tear drop fall onto the patient's lap and slowly moves a little closer to him, but maintains respectful proxemics.

"I'm so sorry you're experiencing this. I imagine this is a scary time for you." LaShanda hands the patient a box of tissues.

Mr. Chung takes a tissue and wipes his eyes. "Thank you," he says softly. "Yeah, it *is* scary."

LaShanda says, "Have you spoken with your oncologist about your concerns, Henry?"

"Not yet… but I see her in 2 weeks. I suppose I can tell her then."

"That sounds like a good plan, Henry." LaShanda affirms. "I think she would want to know your concern."

Mr. Chung nods. "Yeah, okay; I'll do that. Thank you, LaShanda."

LaShanda replies, "You're welcome, Henry." She hands Mr. Chung a gown from the cabinet. "Now, please remove everything but your underwear and socks, and I'll let Dr. Gupta know you're ready."

LaShanda informs Dr. Gupta of her exchange with Mr. Chung and his fear of his cancer returning; this helps the physician to be specifically sensitive to the patient's concern and how she proceeds with her examination.

DEPRESSION

Depression is a mood disorder that affects the way a person feels, thinks, and acts. Depression can lead to a variety of physical and emotional problems that could have a negative impact on a person's ability to function at home or at work. You might hear a friend say "I'm depressed" in a casual manner to describe his gloomy mood, but clinical depression is a common and serious mental health disorder.

When diagnosing depression, health care professionals are careful to distinguish depression from normal feelings of sadness, as well as from the grief a person feels after a loss. According to the *Diagnostic and Statistical Manual of Mental Disorders (DSM-5)*, **major depressive disorder** is a 2-week period during which there is a change in functioning and either depressed mood or loss of interest or pleasure, and at least four other symptoms, such as problems with sleep, eating, fatigue or restlessness, concentration, guilt, or recurrent thoughts of death or suicide. Persistent depressive disorder, also called **dysthymia**, is a depressed mood that last for at least 2 years. Types of depressive disorders are listed in Box 6.1. Symptoms can range from mild to severe.

- Appetite changes, either eating less with weight loss or eating more with weight gain
- Sleep changes, either difficulty sleeping or sleeping too much (Fig. 6.3)
- Social interaction changes, ranging from isolation to excessive
- Feeling worthless or guilty
- Fatigue, loss of energy
- Loss of pleasure in things once enjoyed
- Loss of interest in daily activities and occupations
- Absenteeism from work or school
- Difficulty thinking clearly, concentrating, or making decisions
- Thoughts of self-harm or suicide

According to the Substance Abuse and Mental Health Services Administration

- 6.7% of U.S. adults have had a major depressive episode in the past year.
- Women are almost twice as likely as men to experience depression.
- Although depression can occur at any time in life, it typically appears during late adolescence and in the mid-twenties (Fig. 6.4).

BOX 6.1   SELECTED DEPRESSIVE DISORDERS

Major depressive disorder presents with a loss of interest or pleasure or a depressed mood in conjunction with altered sleep or eating habits, fatigue or restlessness, concentration, feelings of guilt, or recurrent thoughts of death or suicide. The patient with major depressive disorder displays impaired functioning and the depressive episodes are not attributable to another condition or a substance.

Persistent depressive disorder is a depressed mood that lasts for at least 2 years; it is also called dysthymia. Symptoms may become less severe at times, and the patient may have major depressive episodes at other times during the 2-year period.

Premenstrual dysphoric disorder is marked by sensitivity, irritability, anxiety, or depressed mood along with changes in sleep, eating, energy levels, and/or breast tenderness and "bloating" in the week before menstruation.

Peripartum depression is extreme sadness, anxiety, and exhaustion affecting women during pregnancy or after delivering the baby.

Seasonal affective disorder is a major depressive disorder "with seasonal pattern," (i.e., one that has an onset in the fall or winter), typically accompanied by social withdrawal, increased sleep, and weight gain. Symptoms remit in spring.

Bipolar disorder is not a depressive disorder, but the patient oscillates from "manic" or extremely high moods to low moods that meet the criteria for a major depressive episode. The disorder was formerly called *manic-depressive* disorder.

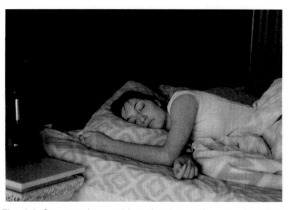

Fig. 6.3 Some patients with major depressive disorder struggle to get out of bed. (iStock.com/LENbIR.)

There are several theories about the potential causes of depression. Certain chemical imbalances in the brain would be a biochemical cause. Genetics can be a factor, because depression can run in families, crossing generations. Another theory is that depression can be a "learned emotion" by those living in depressed families. *Situational stressors*, such as the death of a loved one, loss of a job, end of a relationship, and a significant illness either as the patient or the caregiver, may result in depression. Personality can be a factor, as those who are generally pessimistic or who have low self-esteem may be susceptible to depression.

Exposure to violence, neglect, abuse, or poverty can lead to depression. Repressed memories or conflicts also can be a factor.

Treatment

Depression is among the most treatable mental disorders: 80% to 90% of people with depression eventually respond well to treatment (American Psychiatric Association, 2017). Antidepression medication often is prescribed to help modify the patient's brain chemistry. Unlike certain other psychotropic medications used in the treatment of a patient's mental state, antidepressants are *not* habit forming, allowing people to take them for long periods of time without adverse/serious side effects. Whereas the initial effects of antidepressants may be felt quickly by some, the typical amount of time for someone to feel the drug's full effect is 6 to 8 weeks.

Psychotherapy ("talk therapy") involves working with a licensed therapist who may help a person uncover incidents of loss and grief, abuse, repressed memories, dysfunctional coping, or relating skills that might result in depression. Psychotherapy may be used alone or in addition to the use of antidepressants. A wide variety of psychotherapeutic theories, methods, and approaches may be utilized. However, one approach can be particularly effective with many causes of depression: cognitive behavioral therapy (CBT) functions on the belief that "how you think affects the way you feel." This approach

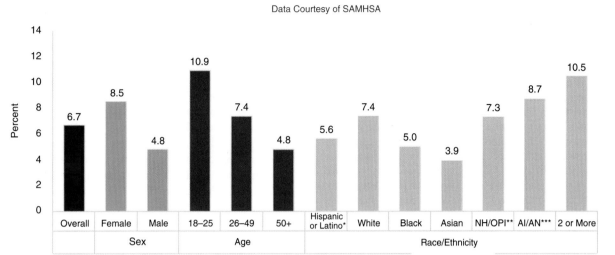

Fig. 6.4 Past year prevalence of major depressive episode among U.S. adults, 2016. *All other groups are non-Hispanic or non-Latino. **NH/OPI = Native Hawaiian/Other Pacific Islander. ***AI/AN = American Indian/Alaskan Native. (From National Institute of Mental Health. Major Depression. November 2017. Retrieved October 15, 2018, from National Institute of Mental Health: https://www.nimh.nih.gov/health/statistics/major-depression.shtml.)

allows people to identify "distorted thinking" that might be causing depression and finding new ways of thinking that will result in creative and healthy ways of thinking and feeling. CBT, unlike other forms of psychotherapy, focuses on the present and works best at solving problems.

Support groups can be another form of treatment. Sharing one's depressive struggles with other like-minded persons often lessens the isolation one often feels with depression.

Patient Interaction

In patient interactions, be aware of how the patient presents verbally and nonverbally. Look for sullenness, despair, desperation, hopelessness, and talk of having "the blahs" or "the blues." If the patient presents with any of these, ask the patient

- "How long have you been feeling this way? When did it begin?"
- "On a scale of 1 to 10, with 10 being the highest, how depressed would you say you currently are? What is the most depressed you have ever been?"
- "Is there anything that you've done or found helpful to find relief?"

- "Has it ever gotten to the point where you have thought of harming yourself?" (See Suicidal Ideation later in this chapter.)

🕴 COMMUNICATION GUIDELINES

Depression

Because of a persistent stigma toward mental health disorders, patients with major depressive disorders can be reluctant to seek treatment or to disclose the extent of their symptoms to health care professionals. Here, as elsewhere, approaching the patient in a respectful, compassionate, nonjudgmental manner will build trust and rapport.

- Practice active listening.
- Use open-ended questioning to elicit information from the patient. Depression may be the patient's problem, but it may not be the reason the patient came to the health care setting, e.g., "You said you haven't been sleeping well. Can you tell me more about that?").
- To encourage medication adherence, be patient and comprehensive when explaining the treatment plan. Some antidepressant therapies can take weeks or months before the patient begins to feel relief of symptoms.
- Accept the way the patient feels; refrain from offering advice.

An Opportunity to Help

Lynelle is a medical assistant for an internist. She is caring for a 52-year-old woman who comes into the office with very vague complaints. The patient states that she "has no energy," is having "trouble sleeping," and has to "force herself to eat" for nourishment. Lynelle looks at the medical record and sees that she has been a patient for 15 years and has no previous medical problems. As Lynelle takes the patient's blood pressure she notices that she appears despondent and withdrawn. The patient states that she "called in sick to work" again that day. Lynelle followed that response by asking the patient about work absenteeism. The patient states that "she doesn't care much about work or going out with her friends." The patient then explains that "her last child has gone off to college and that she is very lonely and sad." Lynelle communicates these observations and facts to the physician. The physician sees the patient and makes an initial diagnosis of depression. Lynelle's excellent communication and observation skills played an important role in helping this patient.

SUICIDAL IDEATION

Mental health directly affects the physical health of the body. Individuals with severe mental illnesses, such as schizophrenia, bipolar disorder, and major depressive disorder, suffer from nutritional and metabolic diseases, cardiovascular diseases, viral diseases, respiratory tract diseases, musculoskeletal diseases, sexual dysfunction, pregnancy complications, poor dental health, and some cancers at higher frequency than the general population (Hert, et al., 2011). Whereas some estimates translate these increased risks into a decreased life expectancy by 13 to 30 years (Hert, et al., 2011), at their worst, mental illnesses can lead to suicide. Studies have found that about 90% of people who die by suicide have a diagnosable mental disorder, with similar figures for those who attempt suicide (Nock, Hwang, Sampson, & Kessler, 2010). However, it is important to remember that other life events often contribute to suicide, such as those related to relationships, substance use, poor physical health, and financial, legal, employment, or housing stress. Often many factors combine to bring about suicide and suicide attempts.

The term suicidal ideation refers to a person's self-reported thoughts of killing himself or herself, which may range from having fleeting thoughts about what it would be like, to being preoccupied or fixated on suicide or death, to making a plan to commit suicide, to practicing a suicide

attempt. Most individuals with suicidal ideation never make a suicide attempt, and most attempts are unsuccessful (Fig. 6.5). However, suicidal ideation is a risk factor for suicide (Gliatto & Rai, 1999). In 2016, about 4% of those over the age of 18 reported having suicidal ideation, and this rate is more than double among those in the 18 to 25 age group (Fig. 6.6). According to the National Youth Risk Behavior Surveys, 17.2% of high school students seriously considered attempting suicide, and 13.6% made a suicide plan. Among sexual minority youth (SMY), including lesbian, gay, and bisexual high school students, reports of considering suicide are significantly higher, at 47.7%. Of sexual minority youth, 38% report making a plan to commit suicide in the past year (Centers for Disease Control and Prevention, National Center for HIV/AIDS, Viral Hepatitis, STD, and TB Prevention, Division of Adolescent and School Health, 2018).

The Centers for Disease Control and Prevention (CDC) Data & Statistics Fatal Injury Report (2017) provides the following statistics about suicide in the United States for 2016.

- The suicide rate increased by 19.5% from 2007 to 2016.
- The annual age-adjusted suicide rate is 13.42 per 100,000 individuals.
- Over 40,000 people die each year by suicide—on average, 123 suicides occur each day.
- It is the 10th leading cause of death.
- Men die by suicide 3.53 times more often than women, but women attempt suicide more frequently than men.
- The rate of suicide is highest in middle age, among white men in particular. White males accounted for 7 of 10 suicides.
- Firearms were used in 51% of all suicides.

Healthy People 2020, introduced in Chapter 4, is a collaboration among federal, state, and territorial governments and other organizations to identify causes of poor health, track trends, and set health promotion objectives to improve the well-being of all Americans. Mental health objectives in Healthy People 2020 target decreasing suicides, reducing teen suicide attempts, and reducing the number of adults and adolescents with major depressive episodes. To that end, the American Association of Suicidology (AAS) suggests health care professionals recognize warning signs suicidality, remembered in the mnemonic IS PATH WARM (Table 6.1). Box 6.2 lists risk factors for suicide, as well as protective factors that lessen a patient's risk for attempting suicide.

Past Year Suicidal Thoughts and Behaviors Among U.S. Adults (2016)

Data Courtesy of SAMHSA

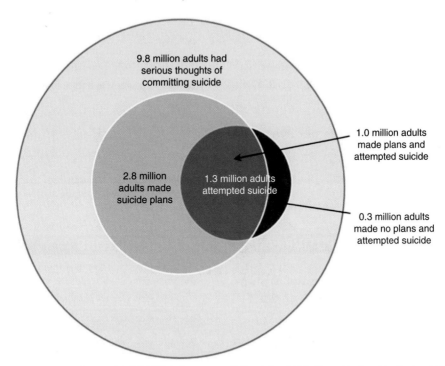

9.8 million adults had serious thoughts of committing suicide

2.8 million adults made suicide plans

1.3 million adults attempted suicide

1.0 million adults made plans and attempted suicide

0.3 million adults made no plans and attempted suicide

Fig. 6.5 Past year prevalence of suicidal ideation among U.S. adults, 2016. (From National Institute of Mental Health. Suicide. November 2017. Retrieved October 15, 2018, from National Institute of Mental Health: https://www.nimh.nih.gov/health/statistics/suicide.shtml.)

Past Year Prevalence of Suicidal Thoughts Among U.S. Adults (2016)

Data Courtesy of SAMHSA

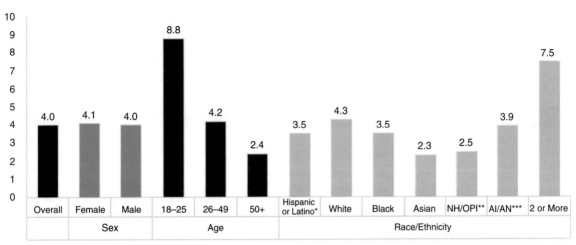

Fig. 6.6 Past year suicidal thoughts and behaviors among U.S. adults, 2016. *All other groups are non-Hispanic or non-Latino. **NH/OPI = Native Hawaiian/Other Pacific Islander. ***AI/AN = American Indian/Alaskan Native. (From National Institute of Mental Health. Suicide. November 2017. Retrieved October 15, 2018, from National Institute of Mental Health: https://www.nimh.nih.gov/health/statistics/suicide.shtml.)

TABLE 6.1 Suicide Warning Signs: "Is Path Warm"

Ideation	Does the patient report thoughts of suicide?
Substance abuse	Is the patient excessively using alcohol or drugs?
Purposelessness	Does the patient report feeling a lack or loss of purpose in life?
Anger	Does the patient exhibit or report feelings of rage. Does the patient speak of revenge?
Trapped	Does the patient say there is no way out of the current situation except to die?
Hopelessness	How does the patient view the future, him or herself, and others?
Withdrawal	Is the patient isolating him or herself from others?
Anxiety	Does the patient feel anxious, agitated, sleepless? Or does the patient sleep too much?
Recklessness	Does the patient engage in risky behaviors?
Mood changes	Does the patient report dramatic mood changes?

Modified from Juhnke, G.A., Granello, P.F., & Lebrón-Striker, M.A. (2007). *IS PATH WARM? A suicide assessment mnemonic for counselors (ACAPCD-03)*. Alexandria, VA: American Counseling Association.

BOX 6.2 SUICIDE: PROTECTIVE FACTORS AND RISK FACTORS

Protective Factors
- Effective clinical care for mental, physical, and substance abuse disorders
- Easy access to a variety of clinical interventions and support when seeking help
- Family and community support (connectedness)
- Support from ongoing medical and mental health care relationships
- Skills in problem solving, conflict resolution, and nonviolent ways of handling disputes
- Cultural and religious beliefs that discourage suicide and support instincts for self-preservation

Risk Factors
- Family history of suicide
- Family history of child maltreatment
- Previous suicide attempt(s)

- History of mental disorders, particularly clinical depression
- History of alcohol and substance abuse
- Feelings of hopelessness
- Impulsive or aggressive tendencies
- Cultural and religious beliefs (e.g., belief that suicide is noble resolution of a personal dilemma)
- Local epidemics of suicide
- Isolation, a feeling of being cut off from other people
- Barriers to accessing mental health treatment
- Loss (relational, social, work, or financial)
- Physical illness
- Easy access to lethal methods
- Unwillingness to seek help because of the stigma attached to mental health and substance abuse disorders or to suicidal thoughts

Adapted from Substance Abuse and Mental Health Services Administration, National Suicide Prevention Lifeline: *Risk factors for suicide*, n.d. http://www.suicidepreventionlifeline.org/learn/riskfactors.aspx. Accessed October 2018.

COMMUNICATION GUIDELINES

Suicidal Ideation
When interacting with patients, consider both warning signs and risk factors. If at any time you suspect a patient may be seeking to harm herself or himself, immediately discuss your concern with the physician. If the patient talks about feeling hopeless, despairing, incapable of going on in life, you can ask about the person's outlook
- "How does life seem to you?"

- "Have you ever felt that life was not worth living?"
- "Do you ever wish you could go to sleep and just not wake up?"

Do not be afraid or hesitant to ask directly about the presence of suicidal ideation. "Are you thinking about harming (or killing) yourself?" Studies show that asking at-risk individuals if they are suicidal does not increase suicides or suicidal thoughts; on the contrary, they may feel relieved

(Continued)

to be able to discuss their feelings. If the patient suggests he or she has suicidal ideation, you can ask questions to elicit details on the intensity of their thoughts.

- "How long have you had such thoughts? How often do you have them?"
- "Do you notice anything that causes these thoughts to occur?"
- "How close have you come to harming yourself?"
- "How likely do you think it is that you will act on these thoughts in the future?"

Listen carefully without judgment and learn what the individual is thinking and feeling. If the patient has suicidal ideations, ask if he or she has a plan for carrying this out; if so, what is it? Findings suggest acknowledging and talking about suicide may, in fact, reduce rather than increase suicidal thoughts. Do not attempt to moralize by telling a patient that it is wrong, or try to talk the person out of it; instead, immediately inform the provider. With your provider's guidance, you may also help the patient make a connection with a trusted individual, such as a family member, friend, spiritual advisor, or mental health professional. Also, you or someone else at the facility should attempt to stay connected with the patient. Having the appropriate person staying in touch after a crisis or after being discharged from care for an attempted suicide can make a difference. Studies show the number of suicide deaths goes down when someone follows up with the at-risk person. Box 6.3 contains information on resources to keep handy in the clinical setting.

WORDS AT WORK

In this scenario, note how the provider, Dalisay, uses open-ended questions to elicit more information from the patient, Darla.

Dalisay: "You say you've been having "dark thoughts" lately, Darla. Are you thinking of harming yourself?"

Darla: "Yeah, I've thought of it."

Dalisay: "What have you thought of?"

Darla: "I just can't deal with this anymore. I just want the whole thing to stop, I just want it to turn off."

Dalisay: "What do you mean by "it," Darla?"

Darla: "My thoughts, my life, the pain, ya know? All of it."

Dalisay: "Do you have a means of harming yourself?"

Darla: "I've been collecting pills. I always have a razor available, you know, for shaving my legs and pits."

Dalisay: OK, thank you for telling me. Have you ever attempted to harm yourself in the past?

Darla: "Well, once I made a cut on my wrist, just to see what it felt like. It creeped me out, so I bandaged it up right away. Never tried it again."

LEGAL EAGLE

Know the laws in your state about mandated reporting when a patient appears to be a threat to herself or someone else. At the very least, the health care worker must immediately report any observations directly to the physicians or provider. There are several established legal means for helping such patients.

BOX 6.3   RESOURCES FOR THE PATIENT WITH SUICIDAL IDEATION

- Keep the *National Suicide Prevention Lifeline's* number visibly posted in examination rooms and in your phone: 1-800-273-TALK (8255), open 24 hours/7 days a week; all calls are confidential.
- Keep updated resources available for your provider to give to patients, including
  - The nonemergency number for the local police department
  - The Crisis Text Line: Text HOME to 741741

GENERALIZED ANXIETY DISORDER

Our current culture fosters significant anxiety: global, national, and local events are shared immediately via numerous media sources. We are bombarded with disturbing events such as natural disasters, war and threats of war, terror attacks, mass killings, homicides, assault, political concerns, and climate changes, among many others, through written word, photos, and videos. Modern technology allows us to be available 24 hours, 7 days a week to family, friends, our work, which carries the expectation that we always will be available. We deal with daily life issues related to relationships, housing, finances, employment, health, insurance, and retirement.

All of these life issues can cause stress, which was addressed in Chapter 5. And, although a degree of stress in our lives is normal, stress can morph into distress. When worry and anxiety are experienced as ongoing and excessively disproportionate to the stress in our lives, it can interfere with our daily life and be an indication of generalized anxiety disorder.

Generalized anxiety disorder is the most common of several anxiety disorders. Symptoms can vary, but may include the following.

- Overthinking plans and solutions to all possible worst-case outcomes
- Being irritable
- Perceiving situations and events as threatening, even when they aren't
- Challenges in handling uncertainty
- Indecisiveness; fear of making the wrong decision
- Unable to let go of a worry, regardless of how large or small it is
- Inability to relax, feelings of restlessness, and feeling keyed up or on edge
- Difficulty concentrating; feeling your mind "goes blank"
- Losing perspective of the reality of a worry or concern

Environmental and genetic factors contribute to the risk of developing an anxiety disorder. These include a history of anxiety or other mental illness in biological relatives; childhood temperamental traits of inhibited behavior or shyness; early childhood or early adulthood exposure to negative and stressful life events or environments; certain health conditions, such as heart arrhythmias and thyroid problems; and caffeine, medications, or other substances. These factors can create or aggravate anxiety symptoms.

Stress from anxiety can have physical manifestations, including irritability, fatigue, sleep disturbances, nervousness, muscle aches and tension, intestinal problems, trembling, and sweating, which are all are common manifestations of a higher level of anxiety.

Depending on the type and severity of the anxiety disorder, treatment may include any combination of psychotherapy (in particular, cognitive behavioral therapy), medications, support groups, and stress management techniques.

🕯 COMMUNICATION GUIDELINES

Generalized Anxiety Disorder

When an anxious patient presents in the health care setting, your manner can help ease his stress and encourage the open communication necessary to diagnose and treat him.

- Be calm and approachable.
- Be patient and be prepared to spend extra time with an anxious individual.
- Normalize and accept the way the patient feels. Explain that anxiety is common and even appropriate.
- This patient may have a tendency to ramble. Summarize to keep the patient from talking too much and use reflective responses to get more of the information you need.

In the patient interview, try to elicit the following information about the history of the patient's symptoms.

- How long have you been feeling this way? When did this feeling begin?
- On a scale of 1 to 10, with 10 being the highest, how anxious would you say you currently are? What is the most anxious you have ever been?
- Is there anything that you've done or found helpful to find relief?
- Is there a family history of anxiety?

➤ WORDS AT WORK

In the exchange below, you can see how Lisa identifies intensity and duration information after summarizing and using a reflective response.

Lisa: "I'm sorry to hear that you're feeling so anxious, Pauline. Can you tell me how long you've been feeling this way?"

Pauline: "It's probably easier to tell you how long I haven't been feeling this way."

Lisa: "I'm so sorry. We see a lot of patients who are struggling just like you in this clinic. Is this a constant experience for you?"

Pauline: "Pretty much. Some days it's as soon as I get out of bed, as soon as that sort of fogginess of sleep clears up. It's as though I'm just waiting for something bad to happen, some kind of threat. Some bad news. Like the phone is going to ring, and—I don't know. Or my email notification on my phone—every time it goes off I'm just waiting for something bad."

Lisa: "That sounds terrible. You were saying that you've felt this way for a long time?"

Pauline: "I think—I don't know—I think I felt anxious in college, but it never seemed this bad, or this frequent. I was worried about grades and so on, exams, but I think it wasn't such a constant feeling. Then I went right to work out of school and that was an awful job. It's probably been that long, really, since then, I'd say."

Lisa: "Since you graduated college, so it's been about... 8 years?"

Pauline: "Yes, that sounds right. It seems like a long time."

Lisa: "On a scale of 1 to 10, with 10 being the most anxious, can you tell me where you would place your anxiety at this moment?"

Pauline: "I guess I'd say a 6. It's almost always around a 5 or 6."

Lisa: "OK, thank you. And what is the highest it's been?"

Pauline: "Wow, I guess close to 10, but that was when I had a lot going on at the same time."

Lisa: "OK, thank you. I appreciate you being specific. This is helpful, Pauline. We'll get the doctor in here and see if we can get you some help."

SUBSTANCE USE DISORDER AND ADDICTION

You are likely to work with patients affected by drugs, alcohol, and addiction at some point in your career. The growing epidemic of substance use in any form is a grave national and global concern; addiction has a profound impact on the individual, family dynamics, health care, and society in general. In this section, we are concerned with understanding the physical and mental health impact of substance use and addiction. Understanding is always the first step in making any interaction more productive.

Definitions and Terminology

In 2013, the American Psychological Association published its highly anticipated fifth edition of the *Diagnostic and Statistical Manual of Mental Disorders*, known as the DSM-5. Among many changes in language and conceptualization of mental disorders, the DSM-5 eliminates the old terminology of *substance abuse* and *substance dependence*. These terms were problematic because they were misleading. A person can abuse a substance to varying degrees and substance abuse occurs without dependence or addiction. Furthermore, a person can be

dependent on a substance without being addicted, as a patient might be dependent on blood thinners or insulin. Because of this, the DSM-5 reframes these pathologies as substance use disorders (SUDs), and places them in a range of severity. Diagnosis of SUD is made when two or more of the criteria below are seen within a period of 1 year. The criteria are in groupings of impaired control (numbers 1–4), social impairment (numbers 5–7), risky use (8–9), and pharmacological criteria (10–11).

1. The substance is taken for longer periods or in larger doses than intended.
2. There is a persistent desire or unsuccessful attempts to decrease the use of the substance.
3. Significant amount of time and energy is spent trying to get the substance or to recover from its effects.
4. A strong craving or desire to use the substance exists.
5. Recurrent substance use is resulting in a failure to complete obligations at work, school, or home.
6. Substance use continues despite experiencing social or interpersonal consequences.
7. Limiting social and/or recreational activities to use of the substance
8. Recurrent substance use in physically dangerous situations, like driving.
9. Continued substance use when the individual knows it is causing physical and/or psychological harm
10. The development of tolerance, reduced effects following repeated use of the substance
11. Experiencing withdrawal symptoms following cessation of substance use

Two or three criteria suggest a diagnosis of moderate substance use disorder. Four or more places someone at the level of severe substance use disorder.

In this way, the medical community draws a distinction between using a substance and overusing a substance to the extent that it harms a person's health and well-being or the health and well-being of others. Many people can use substances for their intended purposes, such as taking a drug for a prescribed treatment or having wine with dinner. Further, it is possible for a person to use or even overuse a substance without being addicted.

Addiction is when the person has a mental obsession to control the use of the substance *and* a physical allergy to the use of the substance. Addiction is defined as physiologic and/or psychological dependence on a substance and/or behavior beyond voluntary control. *Physiological addiction* affects body chemistry at such a deep level and to such an extent that withdrawing the substance produces a reaction at the cellular level, sometimes causing severe physical complications, such as delirium tremens (DTs), an uncontrolled shaking with confusion and hallucinations, in chronic alcoholics. Many persons who develop a physiologic addiction may be biologically susceptible to certain substances, such as alcohol or nicotine. They seem to metabolize the chemicals differently than others who use, but do not abuse, potentially addicting chemicals. The susceptibly addictive person may be addicted after brief exposure to a substance that others can use occasionally without developing an addiction.

If addiction does not involve a biologically based need, but fills a psychological need, the substance may be used as an escape from stress or to alter an unpleasant reality and may be made more intense by the person's personality/temperament, culture, and/or a combination of factors. Many studies suggest that addictive personalities usually have a low frustration threshold and poor self-esteem and need the support of the substance as a coping mechanism. People who are *psychologically addicted* may be so attached to this form of stress relief that they subconsciously increase stress levels as an excuse to fall back into the behavior. For example, the smoker or alcoholic who is trying to stop, but starts a fight with a spouse as an excuse to say, "See, you made me start smoking (or drinking) again when I was trying so hard to stop." (Both alcohol and nicotine may be physiologically addicting as well.) Addictive personalities may not be physiologically addicted and usually do not suffer the same physical symptoms on withdrawal as someone who is addicted at the cellular level. These persons need to develop coping skills rather than resorting to chemical substances as a defense mechanism. Psychological addiction, also called *habituation*, becomes a habit and is seen in people who function better in social situations with a cigarette and drink in hand to overcome awkwardness, but may not need the substances at other times.

Patients affected by commonly abused substances should be under the supervision of trained health care specialists. Problems of this significance require careful assessment and management and are not likely to be within your scope of practice. Potential or at-risk patients deal with stress that may lead to abuse or addiction; they need productive, healthy, coping mechanisms; substance abuse in addition to a stressful situation mul-tiplies the problem; the stress is still there but is made worse by adding addiction. If and when instructed to do so by your employer, it is caring to provide patients with educational resources and support groups.

SPOTLIGHT ON SUCCESS

Substance Use Disorder in the Workplace

Medications are so readily available and stress levels are so high in health care that it may not be just patients whose substance abuse causes concern. Health care professionals are at high risk for addiction. It is not your place to verify, confront, or make accusations. Report your concerns to a supervisor or human resources department. Not only may your co-worker's life be in jeopardy, but the lives of patients may be at risk, as well.

Recognizing Substances

Every substance discussed below can be dangerous to the substance user and to the public at large. The U.S. Drug Enforcement Administration classifies drugs into five schedules of varying potential for misuse and addictive qualities (Table 6.2). Be aware of the most common drugs in your area and some of their common street names (Table 6.3); also be alert for signs of abuse in your high-risk patients. Of the following, alcohol and nicotine are not illegal and are readily available; however, many of the other substances listed below potentially can result in "drug-seeking behaviors" or clusters of patients asking for specific medications that have a high potential for abuse and an equally high street value.

Many substances also have adverse and potentially deadly effects during pregnancy. Infants born to addicted mothers usually are addicted to the same substances they received from their mothers *in utero* and will go through all of the horrors of drug withdrawal during the neonatal period. For example, fetal alcohol syndrome is well documented; for certain metabolisms, even a small amount of maternal alcohol intake may result in fetal damage. Even secondhand smoke has been shown to affect the fetus, resulting in fragile, low–birth-weight infants. Patients who are pregnant and abuse any of the following substances must be referred for counseling, not just for their own safety, but to protect the health of the fetus.

Following is a brief overview of only *some* of the most commonly abused substances with the highest risk of addiction.

TABLE 6.2 Drug Schedules from U.S. Drug Enforcement Administration

Schedule	Definition	Examples
Schedule I	No currently accepted medical use and a high potential for abuse	Heroin, lysergic acid diethylamide (LSD), marijuana (cannabis), 3,4-methylenedioxymethamphetamine (ecstasy), methaqualone, and peyote
Schedule II	High potential for abuse, with use potentially leading to severe psychological or physical dependence	Combination products with <15 mg of hydrocodone per dosage unit (Vicodin), cocaine, fentanyl, methamphetamine, methadone, hydromorphone (Dilaudid), meperidine (Demerol), oxycodone (OxyContin), fentanyl, Dexedrine, Adderall, and Ritalin
Schedule III	Moderate to low potential for physical and psychological dependence	Products containing <90 mg of codeine per dosage unit (Tylenol with codeine), ketamine, anabolic steroids, testosterone
Schedule IV	Low potential for abuse and low risk of dependence	Xanax, Soma, Darvon, Darvocet, Valium, Ativan, Talwin, Ambien, Tramadol
Schedule V	Lower potential for abuse; generally used for antidiarrheal, antitussive, and analgesic purposes	Cough preparations with <200 mg of codeine or per 100 mL (Robitussin AC), Lomotil, Motofen, Lyrica, Parepectolin

From United States Drug Enforcement Administration. (n.d.). *Drug Scheduling: Drug Schedules*. Retrieved October 17, 2018, from United States Drug Enforcement Administration Web site: https://www.dea.gov/drug-scheduling.

TABLE 6.3 Substance Names and Slang Terminology

Drug Class/ Generic (Trade) Names	Slang Terms
Benzodiazepine	Benzos; bennies
Clonazepam (Klonopin)	Benzos; K; K-Pin; Pin; Super Valium; Tranks
Alprazolam (Xanax)	Bars; Benzos; Bicycle Handle Bars; Bicycle Parts; Bricks; Footballs; Handlebars; Hulk; L7; Ladders; Palitroque; Planks; School Bus; Sticks; Upjohns; White Boys; White Girls; Xanies; Yellow Boys; Zanbars; Zannies; Z-Bars
Flunitrazepam (Rohypnol)	542; Circles; Date Rape Drug; Forget Pill; La Rocha; Lunch Money; Mexican Valium; Mind Eraser; Pingus; R2; Reynolds; Roach; Roapies; Rochas; Roofies; Rope; Rophies; Ro-Shay; Trip-and-Fall; Wolfies
Barbiturates Phenobarbital, amobarbital (Amytal), pentobarbital (Nembutal), and secobarbital (Seconal)	Barbs; Tooties; Dolls; Nembies; Goofballs; Downers; Wallbangers. *Street name is often based on the color of the pills or capsule*: Bluebirds; Blue Heaven; Blue Devil; Yellows; Yellow Jackets; Purple Hearts; Reds; Red Birds; Pinks; Pink Ladies
Stimulants	Uppers
Amphetamine	Acelerador; Amy; Amps; Bam; B-Bombs; Beans; Bennies; Benz; Black and Whites; Black Beauties; Black Birds; Black Bombers; Black Mollies; Blacks; Blue Boys; Bombita; Brain Ticklers; Brownies; Bumblebees; Cartwheels; Chalk; Chicken Powder; Chochos; Chocolates; Christina; Chunk; Co-Pilot; Coast-to-Coasts; Crisscross; Cross Roads; Cross Tops; Crosses; Debs; Dexies; Diablos; Diamonds; Diet Pills; Dolls; Dominoes;

(Continued)

TABLE 6.3 **Substance Names and Slang Terminology—cont'd**

Drug Class/ Generic (Trade) Names	Slang Terms
	Double Cross; Drivers; Dulces; Fives; Flour; Footballs; French Blues; Geeked Up; Goofballs; Greenies; Head Drugs; Hearts; Horse Heads; In-Betweens; Jelly Babies; Jelly Beans; Jolly Beans; Jugs; LA Turnaround; Leapers; Lid Poppers; Lightening; Little Bombs; Marathons; Mini Beans; Mini Bennies; Morning Shot; Nuggets; Oranges; Pastas; Pastillas; Peaches; Pep Pills; Pepper; Pingas; Pink Hearts; Pixies; Pollutants; Purple Hearts; Rhythm; Rippers; Road Dope; Roses; Rueda; Snaps; Snow Pallets; Sparkle Plenty; Sparklers; Speed; Splash; Sweeties; Sweets; Tens; Thrusters; TR-6s; Truck Drivers; Turnabouts; Uppers; Wake Ups; West Coast Turnarounds; Wheels; Whiffle Dust; White Crosses; Whites; Zoomers
Adderall	A-Train; Abby; Addy; Amps; Christmas Trees; Co-Pilots; Lid Poppers; Smart Pills; Smarties; Study Buddies; Study Skittles; Truck Drivers; Zing
Cocaine	7; 62; 77; 777; 921; A-1; Adidas; All-American Drug; Ancla; Angel Powder; Angie; Animals; Apache; Apodo; Arriba; Audi; Aunt Nora; Azucar; Baby Powder; Barrato; Basuco; Bazooka (cocaine paste mixed with marijuana); Beach; Belushi (cocaine mixed with heroin); Bernice; Bernie's Flakes; Bernie's Gold Dust; Big Bird; Big Bloke; Big C; Big Flake; Big Rush; Billie Hoke; Bird; Birdie Powder; Blanca Nieves; Blanco; Blast; Blizzard; Blonde; Blocks; Blow; BMW; Board; Bobo; Bolitas; Bolivian Marching Powder; Bombita (cocaine mixed with heroin); Booger Sugar; Bose; Bouncing Powder; Brisa; Bump; C-Dust; Caballo; Caca; Cadillac; California Pancakes; Calves; Canelon; Candy; Car; Carney; Carrie Nation; Cars; Case; Cebolla; Cecil; Cement; Charlie; Chevy; Cheyenne; Chica; Chicanitas; Chinos; Chiva; Cielo; Clear Kind; Clear Tires; Coca; Coca-Cola; Cocazo; Coconut; Coke; Cola; Colorado; Comida; Comida Dulce; Connie; Cookie; Cosa; Coso; Cosos; Crow; Crusty Treats; Cuadro; Death Valley; Designer Jeans; Devil's Dandruff; Diamonds; Diente; Dienton; Diesel; Diosa Blanca; Dona Blanca; Double Bubble; Double Letters; Dove; Dream; Dulces; Duracell; Durazno; Duro; Dust; Escama; Escorpino; Falopa; Fef1; Fichas; Fiesta; Fire (cocaine base); Fish (liquid cocaine); Fish Scale; Flake; Flea Market Jeans; Florida Snow; Flour; Food; Foolish Powder; Fox; Freeze; Friskie Powder; Frula; Funtime; Gabacho; Galaxy; Gallos; Gato; Gift of the Sun; Gin; Girl; Girlfriend; Glad Stuff; Gold Dust; Green Gold; Gringa; Gringito; Grout; Guerillo; Gueros; Guitar; H1; Hai Hit; Hamburger; Happy Dust; Happy Powder; Happy Trails; Heaven; Heaven Dust; Heavy One; Hen; Henry VIII; HH; HHJ; High Heat; HMH; Hooter; Hundai; Hunter; Ice Cream; Icing; Inca Message; Izzy; Jam; Jaime Blanco; Jaula; Jeep; Jelly; John Deere; Joy Flakes; Joy Powder; Juguetes; Jump Rope; Junk; K13; King's Habit; Kordell; La Familia; Lady; Lady Snow; Late Night; Lavada; Leaf; Libreta; Line; Loaf; Love Affair; LV; Maca Flour; Madera; Mama Coca; Mandango; Manita; Maradona; Marbol; Material; Mayback (62 g); Mayo; Melcocha; Media Lata; Mercedes; Milk; Milonga; Mojo; Mona Lisa; Monte; Morro; Mosquitos; Movie Star Drug; Muchacha; Muebles; Mujer; Napkin; Nieve; Niña; Normal; Nose Candy; Nose Powder; Old Lady; Oyster Stew; Paint; Paloma; Paleta; Palomos; Pantalones; Papas; Paradise; Paradise White; Parrot; Pearl; Pedrito; Perico; Personal; Peruvian; Peruvian Flake; Peruvian Lady; Pescado; Peta; Pez; Pichicata; Pillow; Pimp; Pingas; Pingos; Pintura Blanca; Poli; Pollo; Polvo; Powder; Powder Diamonds; Puma; Puritain; Quadros; Queso Blanco; Racehorse Charlie; Rambo; Refresco; Refrescas; Regular Kind; Regular Work; Reindeer Dust; Richie; Rims; Rocky Mountain; Rolex; Rolex HH; Rooster; Scale; Schmeck; Schoolboy; Scorpion; Scottie; Seed; Serpico; Sierra; Shirt; Ski Equipment; Sleigh Ride; Sneeze; Sniff; Snow; Snow Bird; Snow Cone; Snow White; Snowball; Snowflake; Society High; Soda; Soditas; Soft; Space (cocaine mixed with PCP); Special; Speedball (cocaine mixed with heroin); Stardust; Star Spangled Powder; Studio Fuel; Suave; Sugar; Superman; Sweet Stuff; Tabique; Tablas; Talco; Talquito; Tamales; Taxi; Tecate; Teenager; Teeth; Tequila; Thunder; Tire; Tonto; Toot; Tortes; Tortuga; Toyota; T-Shirts; Tubo; Tucibi (pink variety); Turkey; Tutti-Frutti; Vaquita; Wash; Wet; Whack (cocaine mixed with PCP); White; White Bitch; White Cross; White Dove; White Girl; White Goat; White Horse; White Lady; White Mercedes Benz; White Mosquito; White Paint; White Powder; White Rock; White Root; White Shirt; White T; White Wall Tires; Whitey; Whiz Bang; Wings; Wooly; Work; Yayo; Yeyo; Yoda; Zapato; Zip

TABLE 6.3 Substance Names and Slang Terminology—cont'd

Drug Class/ Generic (Trade) Names	Slang Terms
Crack Cocaine	51s; 151s; 501s; Apple Jack; Baby T; Base; Baseball; Bazooka; Beam Me Up; Beautiful Boulders; Beemer; Bill Blass; Bings; BJ; Black Rock; Blowcaine; Blowout; Blue; Bobo; Bolo; Bomb; Bone Crusher; Bone; BooBoo; Boulder; Boy; Breakfast of Champions; Bubble Gum; Bullion; Bump; Candy; Caps; Casper the Ghost; Caviar; CD; Cheap Basing; Chewies; Chingy; Clicker; Climax; Cloud; Cloud Nine; Cookies; CRC; Crib; Crunch and Munch; Devil; Devil Smoke; Dice; Dime Special; Dirty Basing; Dirty Fentanyl (crack cocaine mixed with fentanyl); Double Yoke; Durin; Eastside Player; Egg; Eye Opener; Famous Dimes; Fat Bags; Fifty-One; Fish Scales; Freebase; French Fries; Garbage Rock; Geek; Glo; Gold; Golf Ball; Gravel; Great White Hope; Grit; Groceries; Hail; Hamburger Helper; Hard; Hotcakes; Hubba; Ice; Ice Cubes; Issues; Jelly Beans; Johnson; Kangaroo; Kokoma; Kryptonite; Love; Mixed Jive; Moon Rock; Nickle; Nuggets; One-Fifty-One; Paste; Pebbles; Pee Wee; Piedras; Pile; Pony; Primo; Quarters; Raw; Ready Rock; Red Caps; RIP (Rest in Peace); Roca; Rock; Rock Attack; Rocks of Hell; Rocky III; Rooster; Rox; Roxanne; Roz; Schoolcraft; Scotty; Scramble; Scruples; Seven-Up; Sherms; Sight Ball; Slab; Sleet; Smoke; Speed Boat; Square Time Bomb; Stone; Sugar Block; Takeover (crack cocaine mixed with fentanyl); Teeth; Tension; Tissue; Top Gun; Troop; Ultimate; Up; Uzi; Wave; White Ball; White Ghost; White Sugar; White Tornado; Wrecking Crew; Yahoo; Yale; Yimyom
Methamphetamine	Accordion; Amp; Aqua; Arroz; Assembled (crystal meth); Batu; Begok; Biker's Coffee; Blue; Blue Bell Ice Cream; Beers; Bottles; Bucio; Bud Light; Bump; Cajitas; Chalk; Chandelier; Chavalone; Chicken; Chicken Feed; Chicken Powder; Chris; Christine; Christy; Clear; Clothing Cleaner; Cold; Cold One; Colorado Rockies; Crank; Cream; Cri-Cri; Crink; Crisco; Crissy; Christy; Crypto; Crystal; Cuadro; Day; Diamond; Dunk; El Gata Diablo; Evil Sister; Eye Glasses; Fire; Fizz; Flowers; Foco; Food; Frio; Fruit; Gak; Garbage; G-Funk; Gifts; Girls; Glass; Go-Fast; Go-Go; Goofball (methamphetamine mixed with heroin); Groceries; Hard Ones; Hare; Hawaiian Salt; Hielo; Hiropon; Hot Ice; Hubbers; Ice; Ice Cream; Ice Water; Icehead; Jale; Jug of Water; L.A. Glass; L.A. Ice; Lemons; Lemon Drop; Light; Light Beige; Livianas; Madera; Mamph; Meth; Methlies Quick; Mexican Crack; Mexican Crank; Miss Girl; Montura; Motor; Muchacha; Nails; One Pot; No-Doze; Paint; Pantalones; Patudas; Peanut Butter Crank; Piñata; Pointy Ones; Pollito; Popsicle; Purple; Raspado; Rims; Rocket Fuel; Salt; Shabu; Shards; Shatter; Shaved Ice; Shiny Girl; Small Girl; Soap Dope; Soft Ones; Speed; Speed Dog; Spicy Kind; Spin; Stove Top; Stuff; Super Ice; Table; Tina; Tires; Trash; Truck; Tupperware; Tweak; Unassembled (powder meth); Uppers; Ventanas; Vidrio; Walking Zombie; Water; Wazz; White; Whizz; Windows; Witches Teeth; Yaba; Yellow Barn; Yellow Cake; Yellow Kind; Zip
Methylphenidate (Ritalin)	Diet Coke; Jif; Johnny; Kibbles and Bits; Kiddie Cocaine; Kiddie Coke; MPH; Pineapple; Poor Man's Cocaine; R-Ball; R-Pop; Rids; Rittys; Skippy; Skittles; Smarties; Study Buddies; Truck Drivers; Vitamin R
Synthetic Cathinones (Bath Salts)	Bath Blow; Bath Salts; Bliss; Bloom; Blow; Blue Silk; Bubbles; Cloud 9; Cosmic Beast; Drone; Energy-1; Explosion; Flakka (Alpha-PVP); Gravel (Alpha-PVP); Insect Repellent; Ivory Wave; Jewelry Cleaner; Lunar Wave; M-Cat; Meow-Meow; Ocean Burst; Phone Screen Cleaner; Plant Feeder; Plant Food; Pure Ivory; Purple Wave; Recharge; Red Dove; Salting; Scarface; Snow Leopard; Stardust; Vanilla Sky; White Dove; White Knight; White Lightening; White Magic; Wicked X; Zoom

(Continued)

TABLE 6.3   Substance Names and Slang Terminology—cont'd

Drug Class/ Generic (Trade) Names	Slang Terms
Hallucinogens	
LSD	Aceite; Acelide; Acid; Acido; Alice; Angels in a Sky; Animal; Avandaro; Backbreaker (LSD mixed with strychnine); Barrel; Bart Simpson; Battery Acid; Beast; Big D; Black Acid (LSD mixed with PCP); Black Star; Black Sunshine; Black Tabs; Blanco de España; Blotter Acid; Blotter Cube; Blue Acid; Blue Barrel; Blue Chair; Blue Cheer; Blue Heaven; Blue Microdots; Blue Mist; Blue Moon; Blue Sky; Blue Star; Blue Tabs; Bomba; Brown Bomber; Brown Dots; California Sunshine; Cherry Dome; Chief; Chinese Dragons; Cid; Coffee; Colorines; Conductor; Contact Lens; Crackers; Crystal Tea; Cubo; Cupcakes; Dental Floss; Dinosaurs; Divina; Domes; Dots; Double Dome; El Cid; Electric Kool Aid; Elefante Blanco; Ellis Day; Fields; Flash; Flat Blues; Ghost; Golden Dragon; Golf Balls; Goofy; Gota; Grape Parfait; Green Wedge; Grey Shields; Hats; Hawaiian Sunshine; Hawk; Haze; Headlights; Heavenly Blue; Hits; Instant Zen; Jesus Christ Acid; Kaleidoscope; Leary; Lens; Lentejuela; Lime Acid; Live, Spit and Die; Lluvia de Estrellas; Looney Tunes; Lucy; Maje; Mellow Yellow; Mica; Microdot; Micropunto Azul (white tablet with drop of blue LSD); Micropunto Morado (white tablet with drop of purple LSD); Mighty Quinn; Mind Detergent; Mother of God; Mureler; Nave; Newspapers; Orange Barrels; Orange Cubes; Orange Haze; Orange Micros; Orange Wedges; Owsley; Paper Acid; Pearly Gates; Pellets; Phoenix; Pink Blotters; Pink Panthers; Pink Robots; Pink Wedges; Pink Witches; Pizza; Pop; Potato; Pure Love; Purple Barrels; Purple Haze; Purple Hearts; Purple Flats; Recycle; Royal Blues; Russian Sickles; Sacrament; Sandoz; Smears; Square Dancing Tickets; Sugar Cubes; Sugar Lumps; Sunshine; Superman; Tabs; Tacatosa; Tail Lights; Teddy Bears; Ticket; Uncle Sid; Valley Dolls; Vodka Acid; Wedding Bells; Wedge; White Dust; White Fluff; White Lightening; White Owsley; Window Glass; Window Pane; Yellow Dimples; Yellow Sunshine; Zen
MDMA (Ecstasy)	Adam; Baby Slits; Beans; Blue Kisses; Blue Superman; Bombs; Booty Juice (dissolved in liquid); Candy; Chocolate Chips; Clarity; Dancing Shoes; Decadence; Disco Biscuits; Doctor; Domex (ecstasy mixed with PCP); Drop; E; E-Bomb; Essence; Eve; Go; Goog; Green Apple; Happy Pill; Hug; Hug Drug; Kleenex; Love Doctor; Love Drug; Love Flip (taken with mescaline); Love Potion #9; Love Trip (ecstasy mixed with mescaline); Lover's Speed; Malcolm X; Molly; Moon Rock; Peace; Pingaz; Pingers; Rolls; Rolling; Running; Scooby Snacks; Skittle; Smacks; Slits; Smarties; Speed for Lovers; Sweets; Tacha; Thizz; Vitamin E; Vowels; White Mercedes; X; XTC; Yokes
Mescaline/Peyote	Big Chief; Black Button; Blue Caps; Britton; Buttons; Cactus; Green Button; Half Moon; Hikori; Hikuli; Hyatari; Love Flip (taken with Ecstasy); Media Luna; Mescal; Mescapade; Mezcakuba; Microdot; Moon; Nubs; San Pedro; Seni; Shaman; Topi; Tops

TABLE 6.3   Substance Names and Slang Terminology—cont'd

Drug Class/ Generic (Trade) Names	Slang Terms
PCP (Phencyclidine)	Ace; Alien Sex Fiend (PCP mixed with heroin); Amoeba; Angel; Angel Dust; Angel Hair; Angel Mist; Angel Poke; Animal Tranquilizer; Ashy Larry; Aurora Borealis; Bionic (PCP mixed with marijuana); Black Acid (PCP mixed with LSD); Black Whack; Blue Madman; Blue Star; Boat; Busy Bee; Butt Naked; Cadillac; Cliffhanger; Columbo; Cozmos; Crazy Coke; Crazy Eddie; Cucuy; Cyclones; Detroit Pink; Dipper; Domex (PCP mixed with MDMA); Dummy Dust; Dust; Dust Joint; Dust of Angels; Elephant; Elephant Tranquilizer; Embalming Fluid; Energizer; Fake STP; Flakes; Goon; Gorilla Tab; Gorilla Biscuits; Green Leaves; Green Tea; Heaven and Hell; Hog; Horse Tracks; Horse Tranquilizers; Jet Fuel; Juice; Kaps; K-Blast; Killer; Kools; Leaky Leak; Lemon 714; Lethal Weapon; Love Boat; Mad Dog; Mad Man; Magic Dust; Mean Green; Mint Leaf; Mint Weed; Mist; Monkey Dust; Monkey Tranquilizer; New Acid; New Magic; Orange Crystal; Ozone; Paz; Peace Pill; Peep; Peter Pan; Pig Killer; Puffy; Purple Rain; Red Devil; Rocket Fuel; Rupture; Scuffle; Sheets; Sherms; Shermstick; Space (PCP mixed with cocaine); Spores; Stardust; STP; Super Grass; Super Kools; Super Weed; Surfer; Synthetic Cocaine; Taking a Cruise; T-Buzz; Tic Tac; Tish; Trank; Venom; Wack (PCP mixed with cocaine); Water; Wet (marijuana dipped in PCP); White Horizon; Wobble Weed; Wolf; Worm; Yellow Fever; Zombie; Zoom (PCP mixed with marijuana)
Psilocybin Mushrooms	Alice; Blue Meanies; Boomers; Buttons; Caps; Champiñones; Cubes; God's Flesh; Hongos; Lazers; Liberties; Liberty Caps; Little Smoke; Magic; Mushies; Musk; Pizza Toppings; Psilly Billy; Purple Passion; Shrooms; Silly Putty; Simple Simon; Stemmies; Tweezes
Opioids	
Fentanyl	Apache; Birria (fentanyl mixed with heroin); Blonde; Blue Diamond; Blue Dolphin; Blues; Butter; China Girl; China Town; China White; Chinese; Chinese Buffet; Chinese Food; Crazy; Crazy One; Dance Fever; Dragon; Dragon's Breath; F; Food; Freddy; Fuf (furanyl fentanyl); Facebook (fentanyl mixed with heroin in pill form); Fent; Fenty; Fire; Friend; Girl; Goodfella; Great Bear; Gray Stuff; He-Man; Heineken; Huerfanito; Humid; Jackpot; King Ivory; Lollipop; Murder 8; Nal; Nil; Nyl; Opes; Pharmacy; Poison; Shoes; Snowflake; Tango and Cash; TNT; Toe Tag Dope; White Girl; White Ladies
Heroin	Abajo; A-Bomb (heroin mixed with marijuana); Achivia; Adormidera; Amarilla; Anestesia de Caballo (heroin mixed with the horse anesthetic xylazine); Antifreeze; Apodo; Arpon; Aunt Hazel; Avocado; Azucar; Bad Seed; Baja Corte (diluted heroin); Ballot; Basketball; Basura; Beast; Beyonce; Big Bag; Big H; Big Harry; Bird; Birdie Powder; Birria; Birria Blanca; Black; Black Bitch; Black Goat; Black Olives; Black Paint; Black Pearl; Black Sheep; Black Shirt; Black Tar; Blanco; Blue; Blow Dope; Blue Hero; Bombita (heroin mixed with cocaine); Bombs Away; Bonita; Boy; Bozo; Brea Negra; Brick Gum; Brown; Brown Crystal; Brown Rhine; Brown Sugar; Bubble Gum; Burrito; Butter; Caballo; Caballo Negro; Caca; Café; Cajeta; Capital H; Cardio (white heroin); Carga; Caro; Cement; Certificada (pure heroin); Chapopote; Charlie; Charlie Horse; Chavo; Cheese; Chicle; Chiclosa; China; China Blanca (white heroin); China Cat; China White; Chinese Buffet (white heroin); Chinese Food; Chinese Red; Chip; Chiva; Chiva Blanca; Chiva Loca (heroin mixed with fentanyl); Chiva Negra; Chivones; Chocolate; Chocolate Balls; Chocolate Shake; Choko; Chorizo; Churro Negro; Chutazo; Coco; Coffee; Cohete; Comida; Crown Crap; Curley Hair; Dark; Dark Girl; Dark Kind; Dead on Arrival (DOA); Diesel; Dirt; Dog Food; Doggie; Doojee; Dope; Dorado; Down; Downtown; Dragon; Dreck; Dynamite; Dyno; El Diablo; Engines; Enrique Grande; Esquina; Esquinilla; Fairy Dust; Flea Powder; Food (white heroin); Foolish Powder; Galloping Horse; Gamot; Gato; George Smack; Girl; Globo (balloon of heroin); Goat; Golden Girl; Good and Plenty; Good H; Goofball (heroin mixed with methamphetamine); Goma; Gorda; Gras; Grasin; Gravy; Gum; H; H-Caps; Hairy; Hard Candy; Hard One; Harry; Hats; Hazel; Heaven Dust; Heavy; Helen; Helicopter; Hell Dust; Henry; Hercules; Hero; Him; Hombre; Horse; Hot Dope; Huera; Hummers; Jojee; Joy Flakes; Joy

TABLE 6.3	Substance Names and Slang Terminology—cont'd
Drug Class/ Generic (Trade) Names	**Slang Terms**
	Powder; Junk; Kabayo; Karachi; Karate; King's Tickets; La Tierra; Lemonade; Lenta; Lifesaver; Manteca; Marias; Marrion; Mayo; Mazpan; Meal; Menthol; Mexican Brown; Mexican Food (black tar heroin); Mexican
	Horse; Mexican Mud; Mexican Treat; Modelo Negra; Mojo; Mole; Mongega; Morena; Morenita; Mortal Combat; Motors; Mud; Mujer; Murcielago; Muzzle; Nanoo; Negra; Negra Tomasa; Negrita; Nice and Easy; Night; Noise; Obama; Old Steve; Pants; Patty; Peg; P-Funk; Piezas; Plata; Poison; Polvo; Polvo de Alegria; Polvo de Estrellas; Polvo Feliz; Poppy; Powder; Prostituta Negra; Puppy; Pure; Rambo; Raw (uncut heroin); Red Chicken; Red Eagle; Reindeer Dust; Roofing Tar; Ruby; Sack; Salt; Sand; Scag; Scat; Schmeck; Scramble (uncut heroin); Sheep; Shirts; Shoes; Skag; Skunk; Slime; Smack; Smeck; Snickers; Soda; Speedball (heroin mixed with cocaine); Spider Blue; Sticky Kind; Stufa; Sugar; Sweet Jesus; Tan; Tar; Tecata; Thunder; Tires; Tomasa; Tootsie Roll; Tragic Magic; Trees; Turtle; Vidrio; Weights; Whiskey; White; White Boy; White Girl
	White Junk; White Lady; White Nurse; White Shirt; White Stuff; Wings; Witch; Witch Hazel; Zapapote
Oxycodone (OxyContin)	30s; 40s; 512s; Beans; Blues; Buttons; Cotton; Greens; Hillbilly Heroin; Kickers; Killers; Muchachas; Mujeres; OC; Oxy; Oxy 80s; Roxy; Roxy Shorts; Whites
Percocet	512s; Bananas; Blue; Blue Dynamite; Blueberries; Buttons; Ercs; Greenies; Hillbilly Heroin; Kickers; M-30s; Paulas; Percs; Rims; Tires; Wheels
Suboxone	Boxes, Bupes; Oranges; Sobos; Stop Signs; Stops; Subs
Hydrocodone (Norco, Vicodin)	357s; Bananas; Dones, Dro; Droco; Fluff; Hydros; Idiot Pills; Lemonade; Lorries; Scratch; Tabs; Triple V (Vicodin taken with Valium and Vodka); Veeks; Vics; Vikes; Watsons
Marijuana/Cannabis	420; A-Bomb (marijuana mixed with heroin); Acapulco Gold; Acapulco Red; Ace; African Black; African Bush; Airplane; Alfalfa; Alfombra; Alice B Toklas; All-Star; Almohada; Angola; Animal Cookies (hydroponic); Arizona; Ashes; Aunt Mary; AZ; Baby; Bale; Bambalachacha; Barbara Jean; Bareta; Bash; Bazooka (marijuana mixed with cocaine paste); BC Budd; Bernie; Bhang; Big Pillows; Biggy; Bionic (marijuana mixed with PCP); Black Bart; Black Gold; Black Maria; Blondie; Blue Cheese; Blue Crush; Blue Dream; Blue Jeans; Blue Sage; Blueberry; Bobo Bush; Boo; Boom; Branches; Broccoli; Bud; Budda; Burritos Verdes; Bush; Cabbage
	Café; Cajita; Cali; Camara; Canadian Black; Catnip; Cheeba; Chernobyl; Cheese; Chicago Black; Chicago Green; Chippie; Chistosa; Christmas Tree; Chronic; Churro; Cigars; Citrol; Cola; Colorado Cocktail; Cookie (hydroponic); Cotorritos; Crazy Weed; Creeper Bud; Crippy; Crying Weed; Culican; Dank; Devils's Lettuce; Dew; Diesel; Dimba; Dinkie Dow; Diosa Verde; Dirt Grass; Ditch Weed; Dizz; Djamba; Dody; Dojo; Domestic
	Donna Juana; Doobie; Downtown Brown; Drag Weed; Dro (hydroponic); Droski (hydroponic); Dry High; Elefante Pata; Endo; Escoba; Fattie; Fine Stuff; Fire; Flower; Flower Tops; Fluffy; Fuzzy Lady; Gallina; Gallito;

TABLE 6.3 Substance Names and Slang Terminology—cont'd

Drug Class/ Generic (Trade) Names	Slang Terms
	Garden; Garifa; Gauge; Gangster; Ganja; Gash; Gato; Ghana; Gigi (hydroponic); Giggle Smoke; Giggle Weed; Girl Scout Cookies (hydroponic); Gloria; Gold; Gold Leaf; Gold Star; Gong; Good Giggles; Gorilla; Gorilla Glue; Grand Daddy Purp; Grass; Grasshopper; Green; Green Crack; Green-Eyed Girl; Green Eyes; Green Goblin; Green Goddess; Green Mercedes Benz; Green Paint; Green Skunk; Greenhouse; Grenuda; Greta; Guardada; Gummy Bears; Gunga; Hairy Ones; Hash; Hawaiian; Hay; Hemp; Herb; Hierba; Holy Grail; Homegrown; Hooch; Hoja; Humo; Hydro; Indian Boy; Indian Hay; Jamaican Gold; Jamaican Red; Jane; Jive; Jolly Green; Jon-Jem; Joy Smoke; Juan Valdez; Juanita; Jungle Juice; Kaff; Kali; Kaya; KB; Kentucky Blue; KGB; Khalifa; Kiff; Killa; Kilter; King Louie; Kona Gold; Kumba; Kush; Laughing Grass; Laughing Weed; Leaf; Lechuga; Lemon-Lime; Leña; Liamba; Lime Pillows; Little Green Friends; Little Smoke; Llesca; Loaf; Lobo; Loco Weed; Loud; Love Nuggets; Love Weed; Lucas; M.J.; Machinery; Macoña; Mafafa; Magic Smoke; Manhattan Silver; Manteca; Maracachafa; Maria; Marimba; Mariquita; Mary Ann; Mary Jane; Mary Jones; Mary Warner; Mary Weaver; Matchbox; Matraca; Maui Wowie; Meg; Method; Mersh; Mexican Brown; Mexicali Haze; Mexican Green; Mexican Red; MMJ; Mochie (hydroponic); Moña; Monte; Moocah; Mootie; Mora; Morisqueta; Mostaza; Mota; Mother; Mowing the Lawn; Muggie; My Brother; Narizona; Northern Lights; Nug; O-Boy; OG; O.J.; Owl; Paja; Palm; Paloma; Palomita; Panama Cut; Panama Gold; Panama Red; Pakalolo; Parsley; Pasto; Pasture; Peliroja; Pelosa; Phoenix; Pine; Pink Panther; Pintura; Plant; Platinum Cookies (hydroponic); Platinum Jack; Pocket Rocket; Popcorn; Porro; Pot; Pretendo; Prop 215; Puff; Purple Haze; Purple OG; Queen Ann's Lace; Red Hair; Ragweed; Railroad Weed; Rainy Day Woman; Rasta Weed; Red Cross; Red Dirt; Reefer; Reggie Repollo; Righteous Bush; Root; Rope; Rosa Maria; Salt and Pepper; Santa Marta; Sasafras; Sativa; Shoes; Sinsemilla; Shmagma; Shora; Shrimp; Shwag; Skunk; Skywalker (hydroponic); Smoke; Smoochy Woochy Poochy; Smoke Canada; Sour OG; Spliff; Stems; Sticky; Stink Weed; Sugar Weed; Sweet Lucy; Tahoe (hydroponic); Tangy OG; Terp; Terpenes; Tex-Mex; Texas Tea; Tigitty; Tila; Tims; Top Shelf; Tosca; Train Wreck; Trees; Trinity OG; Tweeds; Valle; Wake and Bake; Weed; Weed Tea; Wet (marijuana dipped in PCP); Wheat; White-Haired Lady; Wooz; Yellow Submarine; Yen Pop; Yerba; Yesca; Young Girls; Zacate; Zacatecas Zambi; Zip; Zoom (marijuana mixed with PCP)
Synthetic Cannabinoids	4-20; Abyss; Ace of Spades; AK-47; Amnesia; Atomic Blast; Big Bang; Black Magic Smoke; Black Mamba; Blaze; Bliss; Blue Cheese; Bombay Blue; Brain Freeze; Buzz Haze; Cherry Bomb; Chill; Chrome; Clockwork Orange; Cloud 10; Cowboy Kush; Crystal Skull; Dead Man; Devil's Venom; Dr. Feel Good; Dragon Eye; Earth Blend; Exodus; Extreme; Fake Bake; Fire; Fruit Candy Flavors; Funky Buddha; Funky Monkey; Garden Salad; Genie; G-Force; GI Joe; Green Dream; Green Peace; Hammer Head; Helix; Hipster; Hysteria; Ice Dragon; Joker; Juicy Leaf; Jungle Juice; Just Chill; K2; Kaos; Karma; Kong; Krazy Kandy; Kryp2nite; Kush; Layer Cake; Limitless; Mad Hatter; Mile High; Mystique; Ninja; Odyssey; OMG; Pandora's Box; Phoenix; Pineapple Express; Posh; Potpourri; Pow; Rapture; Red Magic; Rewind; Scooby Snax; Sexy; Sky High; Snake Bite; Solar Flare; Spice; Spike Diamond; Storm; Sweet Leaf; Synthetic Marijuana; Terraband; Time Traveler; Top Gear; Train Wreck; Ultimate; Viper; Voodoo Child; Wazabi; Wicked; Wizard; Xtreme; Yucatan; Yucatan Fire; Zero Gravity; Zohai; Zombie

Adapted from United States Drug Enforcement Administration. (2018). Slang Terms and Code Words: A Reference for Law Enforcement Personnel. DEA Intelligence Report, Houston Division. Retrieved October 18, 2018, from https://ndews.umd.edu/sites/ndews.umd.edu/files/dea-drug-slang-terms-and-code-words-july2018.pdf.

Alcohol

Alcohol is one of the most socially acceptable and most frequently misused drugs in our society. Alcohol depresses the central nervous system, causing relaxation, loss of coordination, slurred speech, and double vision. In large amounts, alcohol depresses respiration and heart rate and may cause the individual to lose consciousness (Fig. 6.7). Withdrawal may result in delirium tremens (DTs), a painful, dangerous physiologic response to the absence of alcohol in the blood stream. There are no medical applications for ingested alcohol except to delay withdrawal in situations in which DTs would be dangerous to the patient, such as during surgery and recovery. All states recognize blood alcohol content of greater than 0.08% as the legal definition of intoxication. Death

by alcohol poisoning may result with blood alcohol levels over 0.40%. Prolonged misuse of alcohol may lead to alcohol use disorder, malnutrition, cirrhosis of the liver, and death. Alcohol use disorder can have devastating effects on the life of the alcoholic and his or her family, because life functioning is likely to be impaired.

Sedative-Hypnotics and Anxiolytics

Sedatives-hypnotic drugs are taken to produce a calming effect and induce sleep. These are sometimes called depressants. The term *anxiolytic* refers to drugs that treat anxiety. Often, all of these actions occur from the same substance.

Benzodiazepine. Benzodiazepine is a tranquilizer drug, prescription use only, for quieting the central nervous system, most particularly the sympathetic nervous system responsible for the "flight or fight" response to stress. The names of its generic forms and derivatives have the pharmacologic suffix "-pam." Drugs in this class include Valium, Ativan, Xanax, and Klonopin, among many other trade names. Benzodiazepine is given to control anxiety, panic, insomnia, agitation, and DTs, and to relax patients prior to surgery or certain procedures. With prolonged use and abuse, this drug can become habit forming and may cause confusion, slurred speech, seizures, drowsiness, and a decrease in heart rate and respirations. The addiction is hard to break, with a strong rebound effect, which means a return to symptoms that frequently are stronger than the initial reasons for treatment. Withdrawal may result in seizures and true psychosis.

Barbiturates. Barbiturates depress the central nervous system. Used therapeutically as prescription drugs, they reduce anxiety in certain stress disorders, prevent seizures, relieve insomnia, and aid in pain relief. Several forms are highly addictive. Patients who are not physically addicted frequently are so dependent on the effects of this class of drugs that they cannot function normally after withdrawal. Because the effects of these drugs are depressive, abusers may appear drowsy and lethargic, their speech may be slurred, and their heart rate and blood pressure are usually low. Overdose may lead to respiratory depression, coma, and death. Commonly prescribed in the 1960s and 1970s, they have fallen out of favor in medicine following the development of benzodiazepines.

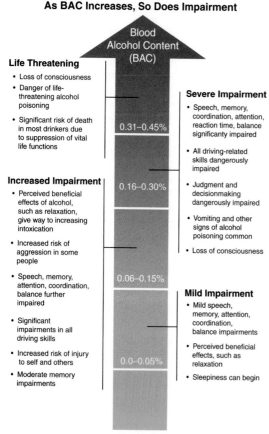

Fig. 6.7 Percent of alcohol in the blood had increasingly pathologic effects. (From Aware Awake Alive. [n.d.]. Blood Alcohol Concentration & Calculator. Retrieved October 15, 2018, from Blood Alcohol Concentration & Calculator Website: http://awareawakealive.org/educate/blood-alcohol-content.)

Hallucinogens

Hallucinogens excite the central nervous system, causing hallucinations, mood changes, and delusions. These drugs elevate all vital signs, including body temperature. LSD, PCP, mescaline, and peyote are illegal psychologically addicting hallucinogens. Abuse may result in memory loss, seizures, coma, cardiopulmonary collapse, and death. Abusers may experience hallucinations for up to a year after withdrawal. Because reality and pain perception are so altered, abusers may injure themselves or others while under the influence. Signs of abuse vary with the hallucinogen, but most include agitation and loss of reality. Current studies are being done on potential medical benefits of mircrodosing some drugs in strictly controlled psychiatric venues.

MDMA (Ecstasy). The synthetic drug 3,4-methylenedioxymethamphetamine (MDMA), often called *ecstasy* or *molly*, is included here as a hallucinogen, but in fact its hallucinogenic effects are mild and it shares chemical similarities with stimulants. It acts on the neurotransmitters serotonin, dopamine, and noradrenaline in parts of the brain to alter mood and perception, producing feelings of increased energy, pleasure, self-confidence, inner peace, an altered sense of time, and strong emotional attachment to others. The effects typically last 3 to 4 hours. MDMA is illegal in most countries; in the United States it is listed as a Schedule I drug with no medical use, despite its promise as an aid in psychotherapy. Often used recreationally at parties and raves, the drug is usually pressed in a tablet with a colorful design and taken orally. It may also be in powder form and snorted. In the short term, adverse effects of MDMA are dehydration, nausea, muscle cramping, loss of appetite, erectile dysfunction, involuntary teeth clenching, blurred vision, chills, sweating, insomnia, rapid heartbeat, and hypertension. The substance is addictive and can cause memory problems and paranoia. In the week after a person uses MDMA, he or she can suffer insomnia, anxiety, loss of appetite, irritability, decreased libido, and depression. Long-term effects are not known.

An added health risk is that a recreational user cannot know if the tablet, capsule, or powder sold as MDMA is pure. It may contain *adulterants*, other drugs instead of or in addition to MDMA. Testing on the product seized by law enforcement yielded the presence of adulterants such as cocaine, ketamine, methamphetamine, over-the-counter cough medicine, or synthetic cathinones (bath salts).

Stimulants

Stimulants include prescription amphetamine (e.g., Ritalin, Adderall) and its derivatives. These excite the central nervous system to produce wakefulness and euphoria. Stimulants are used medically to treat narcolepsy, short-term fatigue, certain respiratory conditions, attention-deficit/hyperactivity disorder, and depression. Signs include those associated with stimulation, such as agitation and increased heart rate and respirations. The many adverse effects include paranoia, hallucinations, and suicidal tendencies.

Methamphetamine. Methamphetamine or "meth" is an illegal stimulant made into a white or blue crystal and usually smoked in a glass pipe. It is highly addictive, producing energy, motivation, and feelings of confidence. Over time, methamphetamine use causes memory loss, anxiety, aggression, and damage to the cardiovascular system that may result in stroke or coma. In the long term users can display psychotic behavior; some report feeling covered with bugs and they may develop sores from picking at their skin. The chronic user can have "meth mouth," a condition of cracked and decayed teeth.

Once the user comes down from the initial high, subsequent highs become more difficult to achieve. "Tweaking" is a slang term for the intense cravings and despair felt by the user when he or she can no longer achieve a high. Often a tweaker has not slept for days or even weeks, becoming irritable, paranoid, and even developing psychotic symptoms such as delusions (false beliefs) and hallucinations (imagined auditory or visual perceptions). Many users seek treatment during the desperation of the tweaking phase, presenting to emergency departments and other health care settings. The long-term insomnia ends in a crash during which the user will be hungry, thirsty, and fatigued for several weeks.

Cocaine and Crack. Cocaine and crack cocaine are derived from the leaves of the coca plant, but can be synthetically reproduced in laboratories. Both have strong stimulant effects on the central nervous system. As a recreational drug, cocaine is ingested, rubbed on the mucous membranes, sniffed into the nose, or injected. Its euphoric effects last only about 30 minutes, meaning that the user needs frequent doses to maintain a "high." It is quickly and severely addicting, with multiple possible side effects that include hypertension, cardiac arrhythmias, seizures, respiratory arrest, paranoia, and death. The crack form of cocaine is smoked, enters the cardiovascular system quickly, and can lead to cardiopulmonary collapse and death.

Synthetic Canthinone (Bath Salts). Cathinone is a substance derived from the khat plant, native to East Africa and the Arabian Peninsula, where people chew the leaves

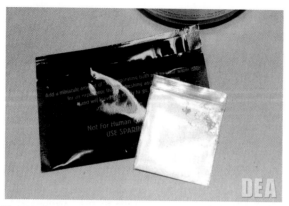

Fig. 6.8 Synthetic cathinone, commonly known as bath salts, comes in the form of a fine white powder, usually in a foil pouch. (Courtesy of the U.S. Drug Enforcement Administration.)

for its stimulant effects. Synthetic cathinone is far more potent. The drug comes in the form of a fine white powder, usually in a foil pouch (Fig. 6.8). It was so named because of originally being disguised as "bath salts" to use when soaking in a bathtub, these substances might also be sold as "plant food," "phone screen cleaner," or "jewelry cleaner." To evade law enforcement authorities, the package is usually labeled "not for human consumption," and sold openly online and at smoke shops and head shops.

Bath salts are swallowed, snorted, injected, or inserted into the rectum or vagina. The intended effects on the user are euphoria, excitement, increased sex drive, and hallucinations. Negative effects reported from users of bath salts are heart palpitations, headaches, nausea, panic attacks, violent responses to vivid and disturbing hallucinations, and paranoid delusions. Because they are amphetamine derivatives they pose special risks to the cardiovascular system, including hypertension, tachycardia, hyperthermia, diaphoresis, seizures, arrhythmias, and respiratory distress, which can lead to a heart attack, stroke, coma, or death (Slomski, 2012). An added complication is that routine urine toxicology screening in emergency departments is not available and the results from sending samples to a laboratory for testing take several days.

Marijuana/Cannabis

Marijuana is manufactured from the dried tops of the cannabis, or hemp, plant. The product can be smoked or ingested. It produces euphoria and alters judgment, cognition, and sensory perception. Medically, there are specific properties that studies show to be effective for certain symptoms. Tetrahydrocannabinol (THC) is a chemical in marijuana that increases appetite, reduces nausea, and decreases pain and inflammation; it can be particularly effective to treat chemotherapy side effects in patients with cancer. Another plant chemical is cannabidiol (CBD), which does not create any "high" and also helps reduce pain and inflammation and is particularly effective in controlling certain types of pediatric epilepsy. Medical marijuana may be in edible, cream, and oil formats and is lawful and strictly regulated in some states. Some states have legalized over-the-counter sales of recreational marijuana, again strictly regulated; be sure to know your state and municipal laws. Even low doses may alter certain perceptions, depressing some, such as concentration and complex interpretations, and increasing or altering others, such as touch, taste, and smell. If mental illness is present in any form, the mind-altering chemicals increase the incidence of paranoia and schizophrenia. Signs of marijuana use include conjunctivitis, hunger, and either agitation or lethargy.

Synthetic Cannabinoids (K2/Spice). Synthetic cannabinoids, sometimes found under the names K2 or Spice, are artificial chemicals that bind to the same receptors in the brain as THC. These chemicals are sprayed onto dried plant material and sold in small pouches. The user smokes the plant material, much like marijuana. Because synthetic cannabinoids are unregulated and sold openly online, at "head shops," gas stations, and the like, some users may mistakenly think they are safe. In reality, some synthetic cannabinoids produce much stronger effects than marijuana. The effects of various synthetic cannabinoid products are unpredictable; some can elicit an elevated mood and relaxation, whereas others can send the user to the emergency room with psychotic symptoms, vomiting, tachycardia, violent behavior, and suicidal ideations.

Opioids

Opioids are substances that act on opioid receptors in the brain to relieve pain in the user. The term *opioid* is often misused by laypeople and the media. "Opioid" refers to *any* synthetic, semisynthetic, or naturally occurring drug that acts on opioid receptors in the brain. In contrast, an *opiate* is a drug derived from the opium poppy; an opiate is a type of opioid.

Opioids can alter sensory perception and produce euphoria. Medically, they are prescribed to treat pain, suppress the cough reflex, constrict pupils, and decrease gastrointestinal motility in cases of nausea and vomiting.

Included in the prescription opioid group are codeine, morphine, fentanyl, meperidine (Demerol), oxycodone (OxyContin), tramadol (Ultram), and hydrocodone (Vicodin). Heroin is a nonprescription street drug.

Fentanyl. Fentanyl is a synthetic opioid that is particularly dangerous because it is cheap and easy to manufacture, easily sent across borders by mail in small packages, and is hundreds of times more potent than heroin. Irresponsible drug manufacturers cut illicitly manufactured fentanyl (IMF) into heroin as a cost-cutting measure, whereas on the street, unsuspecting users overdose not knowing the product has been laced. A fatal dose of IMF is very small (Fig. 6.9) and therefore its proliferation contributes to the increasing number of often fatal overdoses (Fig. 6.10).

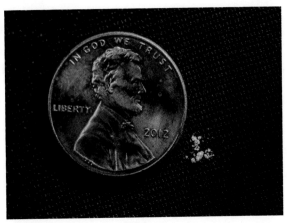

Fig. 6.9 Two milligrams of fentanyl is a fatal dose for most people. (Courtesy of the U.S. Drug Enforcement Administration.)

► WORDS AT WORK

Questions about substance abuse are often included in the initial patient intake about lifestyle. However, you may find that a structured series of questions during the patient interview will help provide more details about the patient's substance use. In the following dialogue, a medical assistant at a sexual health clinic, Kiara, is asking about a patient's drug use.

Kiara: "As a part of your routine health screening, I'd like to ask you some questions about your drug use. Will that be okay?"

Patient: "That's fine."

Kiara: "When was the last time you used any kind of drug? That includes drugs that have been prescribed to you or to someone else and drugs that were not prescribed?"

Patient: "A while ago."

Kiara: Okay. "Have you used in the 6 months, 1 month, or within the last week?"

Patient: "I've done something in the last week."

Kiara: "How many different types of drugs have you used in the last week?"

Patient: "I don't remember, maybe three."

Kiara: "Okay. Were any of these drugs prescribed to you or someone else? Or did you get them or buy them from someone else?"

Patient: "I got them from someone else."

Kiara: "I'm just going to ask you what they were to make sure we don't prescribe you something that may interact with them. Was it marijuana?"

Patient: "No."

Kiara: "Was it a pain medication such as oxycodone or methadone?"

Patient: "Yes."

Kiara: "How did you take it—by mouth, snorting it, or injecting it?"

Nicotine/Tobacco

Tobacco. Tobacco use is the single largest preventable cause of disease and death in the United States. Smoking tobacco causes cancer, heart disease, stroke, lung diseases, diabetes, and chronic obstructive pulmonary disease, which includes emphysema and chronic bronchitis. It increases risks for problems with the immune system and causes erectile dysfunction in males. Smokers are far more likely than nonsmokers to develop cardiovascular disease and cancers of the lungs, mouth, throat, stomach, and bladder (U.S. Department of Health and Human Services, 2014). On average, smokers die 10 years younger than nonsmokers (Jha, et al., 2013).

Nicotine. Nicotine, a stimulant, is the physiologically addictive substance in tobacco. Nicotine is highly addictive whether it is smoked or chewed. When a user attempts cessation, he suffers physiologic withdrawal that includes insomnia, anxiety, and agitation. Nicotine has been proven to harm adolescent brain development, continuing into the early 20s (Goriouinova & Mansvelder, 2012). Breaking nicotine addiction is extremely difficult and many smokers cannot do it alone. Social support groups can be very effective. Several new drugs have shown promise in breaking the addiction. They are available as patches, oral medications, and prescription gum.

Vaping. E-cigarettes, electronic nicotine delivery systems have become a very popular device in recent years for those who already smoke cigarettes, as well as an enticement to those who have not. Commonly called vaping, the device heats a liquid, often containing nicotine, which produces a vapor inhaled by the user. The safety of vaping is unknown. There may be harmful

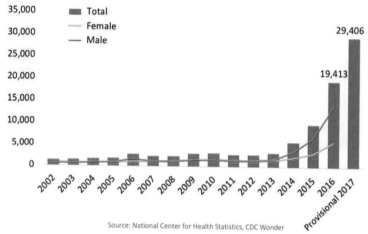

Fig. 6.10 The number of fatal overdoses from fentanyl has increased six-fold since 2013. (From National Institute on Drug Abuse. Overdose Death Rates. November 2017. Retrieved October 15, 2018, from National Institute on Drug Abuse Website: https://www.drugabuse.gov/related-topics/trends-statistics/overdose-death-rates.)

chemicals that are inhaled into the lungs. Even as research continues, the CDC considers them unsafe for youth, young adults, pregnant women, and people who do not smoke regular cigarettes. Since 2016, the U.S. Food and Drug Administration deemed e-cigarette devices and e-liquids to be tobacco products, giving the federal government authority to regulate the marketing, labeling, and manufacture of devices and liquids.

Product marketing is particularly targeted to the younger demographic, boasting a variety of flavors and that they are a safer alternative to regular cigarettes; e-cigarettes are the most commonly used tobacco product among youth as an alternative to smoking cigarettes.

Treatment

Many treatment options are available to people who desire to overcome their addiction. However, because of the very nature of addiction, people often **relapse** and use the substance again, making the success rate often quite low, with many individuals going through treatment programs more than once. When an addicted person is in treatment, she or he is considered to be in **recovery**, a state of abstaining from using the substance to improve health and well-being. One is never *cured* of addiction, but rather one is in recovery for the rest of his or her life.

COMMUNICATION GUIDELINES

Substance Use Disorder
- Withhold judgment. Never moralize with addictive patients to shame them or make them feel guilty; they know it is wrong, but are powerless to stop. They need help, not lectures. As always, talk with the provider first about the patient and document your concerns.
- Help patients realize they can ask for help for anxiety, depression, or loneliness. With proper support, they are less likely to abuse potentially addicting substances.

- Know the local names and forms of the drugs you may encounter (see Table 6.3) Almost all drugs are widely used, but some are more common in certain populations and geographic locations than others, and the names and forms may change frequently. If a patient mentions a slang term for a street drug with which you are unfamiliar, just ask. Say, "You know, I never heard of that. Does it go by other names?" Patients may even appreciate the chance to tell you about their experience. You can ask, "Tell me a little bit more about this. Why do you think it is popular here?"

- Learn to recognize the signs and symptoms of chronic abuse and overdose for all of the substances of abuse. With the variety and availability of destructive drugs, you may be the patient's first and best resource for assistance.
- Educate patients to talk candidly with physicians regarding potentially addicting medications. Patients who we know or suspect to be at risk for addiction may be offered other less potentially addictive medication choices by their providers.
- Be alert to drug-seeking behaviors, such as patients who ask for specific controlled substances before trying other means to relieve symptoms and those who seek prescription pain medications late in the day on

Fridays. Patients who self-diagnose and self-prescribe may be at risk.

- Be mindful of clusters of patients asking for the same controlled substances. Many addictive drugs have significant street value.
- Keep current supportive resource materials updated and available for the provider to refer, such as in-patient and out-patient treatment programs, 12-Step programs, and other support group and treatment options.
- *Seek immediate help if you are frightened by drug-related psychosis and/or behavior in a patient.* Patients in drug-induced paranoia or other states will not listen to reason. Refer to Chapter 5 for ways to protect yourself from workplace violence. Do not put yourself in danger.

▶ TAKING THE CHAPTER TO WORK

Drug-Seeking Behavior

Let's meet Maria, who assists a general practitioner, Dr. Gibbons. It is 4:30 p.m. on a Friday, and the office closes at 5:00 p.m. A new patient, Mrs. Heely, was seen for the first and only time by the doctor 2 weeks ago, complaining of severe back pain. Dr. Gibbons examined the patient and referred her to an orthopaedist and prescribed a short-term dose of the painkiller hydrocodone (an opioid). Mrs. Heely has called the office and asked to speak with Dr. Gibbons. As the doctor is with a patient, the receptionist puts the call through to Maria. Maria pulls up the patient's chart on the computer as she answers the call.

Maria: "Hello, Mrs. Heely, this is Maria, Dr. Gibbons' assistant. He's currently with a patient, so may I help you?"

Mrs. Heely: "Oh, hi, Maria. Look, I'm still in a lot of pain; my back is killing me. I know it's late and you probably can't squeeze me in today, but…"

Maria: "I'm sorry to hear that you're still experiencing so much pain, Mrs. Heely. Are you able to go to urgent care?"

Mrs. Heely: "Yeah, OK. I may be able to do that… But if I can't get there until tomorrow at the earliest, can Dr. Gibbons renew my pain medication prescription? I'm out of it and I won't be able to see the orthopaedist he referred me to for another couple of weeks. I just need some more to see me through until then."

Maria: "Did the medication help your pain?"

Mrs. Heely: "Oh yeah, it really made a difference for me to just move around and do simple things. But I don't have any left and I'm scared about how bad the pain will get; I'm feeling it more intensely, already."

Maria: "I'll speak with Dr. Gibbons and will get back to you, Mrs. Heely, but I strongly urge you to get to urgent care today or tomorrow if your pain is so bad. Is there someone who can take you? You shouldn't drive if you have any of the medication still in your system."

Mrs. Heely: "I don't know… I don't think so. My son is working late today and I don't know his plans for tomorrow. The medication will help see me through the weekend, though."

Maria: "I'm so sorry you're experiencing so much pain, Mrs. Heely. I'll check with the doctor and get back to you as soon as I can. Is the number you're calling from the best one to call you back on?"

Mrs. Heely: "Yeah. Call that one."

Maria: "OK, thank you; I will. In the meantime, I hope you can find a friend or Uber or Lyft or some other options to get yourself to urgent care."

Mrs. Heely: "Yeah, OK. OK. Yes, please let me know, even if he can just give me enough to get me through the weekend, OK? That would be great."

Maria: "Is there anything else I can help you with at this time?"

Mrs. Heely: "No, that's it. Thank you, Maria."

Maria: "You're welcome Mrs. Heely."

DEMENTIA

Dementia is a general term for a decline in mental ability severe enough to interfere with daily life. When brain cells are damaged, their ability to communicate with each other is disrupted. The location in the brain of these damaged cells determines what brain functions are affected. Dementia is not a disease, but rather a symptom that appears in many forms in many diseases and other conditions. Alzheimer's disease is the most common type of dementia, accounting for 60% to 80% of cases. Vascular dementia, occurring after a stroke, is the next most common type. The term "senile" or "senile dementia" is no longer a correct term to use, because it presumes that serious mental decline is a normal part of aging, which is not true.

Dementia can be from brain injuries as a result of brain trauma (e.g., an accident), degenerative changes (such as frontotemporal dementia or Alzheimer's disease), stroke, diseases (e.g., Parkinson's and Huntington's), genetic conditions (e.g., Down syndrome), and from many other causes. Many dementias get progressively worse over time; however, some are treatable and reversible, such as with thyroid conditions or chemical imbalances, nutritional deficiencies, depression, medication side effects, excess use of alcohol, among others.

Symptoms of dementia may include

- Memory loss, usually noted by a partner or someone else
- Difficulty with language/finding the right words
- Inability to focus and pay attention
- Difficulty reasoning and using judgment
- Challenges in motor functions and coordination
- Diminished visual perception
- Confusion and disorientation

Psychological changes may include the following: personality changes, anxiety, depression, agitation, paranoia, inappropriate behavior, and hallucinations. Although dementia is not a normal part of aging, the risk of dementia increases with age. People with mild cognitive impairment that does not negatively impact daily function are at higher risk of getting dementia. People with the genetic developmental disorder of Down syndrome are particularly susceptible to getting early onset Alzheimer's disease. Family history of dementia also places one at greater risk, but this is not conclusive.

Alzheimer's disease accounts for the vast majority of dementia cases. It is a progressive disease that causes problems with memory, thinking, and behavior. It has distinctive, predictable symptoms and progression. The disease progresses through three stages: mild (early stage), moderate (middle stage), and severe (late stage). Each stage has its own particular symptoms and related behaviors. In the early stages the patient experiences mild memory loss, but after a period of years, the late-stage Alzheimer's patients lose the ability to carry on a conversation and respond to their environment. There is no cure.

If you will work in a long-term care setting, such as a hospital or live-in skilled nursing facility, you will be trained on particular caregiving for those with dementia, especially those with progressive dementia that interferes with **activities of daily living (ADLs)**, the routines that require thought, planning, and physical motion, such as toileting, brushing teeth, eating nutritionally, and otherwise living independently.

Patients who have dementia as a result of brain trauma often have other cognitive and motor skill limitations. They may look their actual age, but have the mental cognition of someone much younger. You will provide the best communication and care if you find out from the person's caregiver what level of development the patient understands and adjust your vocabulary accordingly.

Patient Interaction

Studies provide new understanding about dementia and help improve how we communicate with and care for patients with dementia. Researchers have found that working with and caring for patients with dementia is best when it is *person-centered care*, rather than *task-centered care*. Person-centered care focuses on putting the needs of the person first, whereas traditional care models were based on tasks, processes, and schedules to be performed that fit the needs of the organization. A task-centered model says to the patient with dementia, "We need you to get out of bed, get a shower, and get dressed in 30 minutes before going to breakfast." A person-centered model considers that the experience of each of these patients with dementia is unique and puts first and foremost the idea of love and care for the individual. Decisions about how provide care are made in a way that sustains a patient's identity, comfort, attachment, inclusion, and occupation. It strives to keep that patient involved both in her care and in her life. In terms of daily activities, this may mean some things happen more slowly or not at all. Health care professionals who embrace person-centered care focus less on "what is done" and more on "how it is done" (Kitwood, 1997).

When the patient has a cognitive communication barrier, assume that all that patient's behavior is communication. As she becomes less capable of verbalizing what her needs and wants are, she will try to communicate her needs and wants through nonverbal means. What you experience as belligerent behavior may be the patient's frustration on being forced to do something she does not want to do.

Severely cognitively impaired patients usually are accompanied by a caregiver to whom you will direct most of your interview or instruction. You should consult with caregivers accompanying patients for their experiences with the patient's behavior and their methods for effective communication (Fig. 6.11). However, do not exclude the patient. As with any other impairment or challenge, patients need to feel as involved as possible and may make small, limited decisions. Because disabilities vary so widely, some level of interaction may be possible.

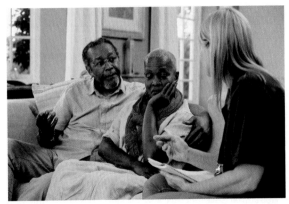

Fig. 6.11 A home health aide speaks with a patient who has dementia and her spouse. Consulting with caregivers can provide excellent information about the communication strategies that work for the patient. (iStock.com/Monkeybusinessimages.)

COMMUNICATION GUIDELINES

Dementia

The following suggestions work in many situations involving cognitively impaired patients.

- Do not assume all patients with dementia present similarly; you will need to adjust your vocabulary and interactions according to the level of the patient's cognitive ability.
- Some patients may have little-to-no short-term memory, but they can remember specific details from 40 or more years ago. Engaging the patient in life review of happy memories helps to build rapport.
- Interact in an environment as free of distractions as possible; noisy, busy areas make focus and attention even more challenging.
- Approach the patient slowly from the front; do not come up suddenly from behind or beside the patient without the patient being able to see you.
- Look directly at the patient and engage his attention before beginning. Touching the patient may bring his or her attention to you. Holding his or her hand and talking directly to him or her may help keep his or her attention focused on you and your words.
- Offer your hand, palm up; the patient may put his or her hand in yours or choose not to.
- Address the patient at his or her eye level.
- Assume that the situation is new each time; reintroduce yourself.
- Use the patient's name at the beginning of speaking to them so they know that you are talking to them.

- Address both the patient and the caregiver; do not talk about the patient in the third person.
- Lower the pitch of your voice and do not talk in a singsong, child-like voice. Patients may pay more attention if you speak in soft, low-pitched tones. Never shout; they may be easily frightened.
- Use the Rule of Fives: sentences no longer than five words, words no longer than five letters.
- Use short, concise sentences; say less and say it slowly.
- Use realistic, clear language with no euphemisms.
- It is appropriate to use pictures and drawings to communicate.
- Give small, limited choices, such as, "Would you rather I take your temperature first, or weigh you first?" Small choices give patients a degree of control and increase self-esteem.
- Closed-ended questions are appropriate in this situation, as are yes/no questions. Open-ended questions may be confusing.
- Never correct patients and never argue. It does not matter whether they are right or wrong. Trying to convince the cognitively impaired patient is frustrating for both of you. Agree and continue with your tasks.
- Praise the patient for cooperation. Respond positively to efforts to contribute.
- Be patient and allow time for the patient to respond.

▶▶ TAKING THE CHAPTER TO WORK

Patient-Centered Care

Let's meet Carlos, a home health aide at a memory care facility. He is to help Mr. Rosenthal get dressed to go to breakfast. Mr. Rosenthal is a 91-year-old widower who has been living at the facility for 2 years. He has dementia as the result of a stroke, limited motor ability on his left side, is hard of hearing and uses hearing aids, and has minimal speech capability. The patient is known to be unpredictably resistant with aides who need to assist him with his ADLs, so Carlos is unsure what mood he will find Mr. Rosenthal in this day. Carlos assists Mr. Rosenthal several days a week and knows he often responds well to light humor.

Carlos knocks on Mr. Rosenthal's door, which is partway open, and calls the patient's name. Carlos notes that the patient is in his pajamas in his wheelchair, watching a closed-captioned nature channel on TV; he is seated with his side to the door and appears not to have heard or seen Carlos. Carlos carefully and slowly approaches the patient, so as not to startle him, until he is in the patient's line of vision, without blocking the TV. Carlos drops to one knee just in front of and to the side of Mr. Rosenthal's wheelchair. He notes the patient's hearing aids on the side table.

Carlos speaks more loudly this time. "Good morning, Mr. Rosenthal. It's Carlos." Carlos puts his hand on his chest to indicate he's talking about himself. Mr. Rosenthal looks suddenly at Carlos, without recognition.

Remembering his patient's hearing loss, Carlos speaks even louder. "I'm Carlos, Mr. Rosenthal. I visit you many mornings." Carlos places his hand, palm up, toward the patient's right hand, without touching the patient. "You show me pictures of your dog, Penny." He points to a framed picture of the younger-looking patient laughing with a small black dog on his lap sitting on the side table next to the hearing aids.

Mr. Rosenthal opens his eyes wide, looking from Carlos to the photograph and back to Carlos. A smile of comprehension crosses the patient's face and he smiles and places his right hand in Carlos' outstretched hand. Carlos smiles in return and places his other hand on top of the patient's hand. "I'm glad you remember me, Mr. Rosenthal. I'm here to help you get dressed to go to breakfast. Is that OK?"

Mr. Rosenthal smiles and gives a little nod.

Carlos points to the TV. "May I turn your TV down just a little bit?" he says loudly. The patient nods. "Thank you, Mr. Rosenthal." Carlos gets up slowly and picks out two different shirts from the patient's closet and brings them to the patient. "Would you like to wear your plaid shirt today or your striped shirt?"

Carlos waits as his patient looks back and forth at each shirt; he then looks at Carlos quizzically. "It's your choice, Mr. Rosenthal; do you want to wear your plaid shirt or your striped shirt today?" Carlos knows that he has to get the patient to eat, but he also wants to make sure he is providing person-centered care, keeping Mr. Rosenthal involved in his life. Carlos continues to wait patiently; after a minute, the patient nods and moves his right hand slightly toward the plaid shirt.

Carlos moves the plaid shirt a little closer to the patient. "You want to wear your plaid shirt today?"

Mr. Rosenthal looks at Carlos and nods a bit, saying softly, "Yes."

"Good choice Mr. Rosenthal," Carlos says, "You always get a lot compliments from the ladies when you wear this shirt." Mr. Rosenthal smiles broadly. "You'll be getting calls for dates pretty soon!"

At this, Mr. Rosenthal laughs out loud. Carlos is glad to have connected to his patient. "And how about we put in your hearing aids?" Carlos asks. "You want to be able to hear all those great compliments, right?" The patient gives a small chuckle and nods. Mr. Rosenthal is relaxed and compliant for Carlos to place his hearing aids and get him dressed in time for breakfast.

EATING DISORDERS

Much of our socialization revolves around food ("Let's meet for lunch," "Join us for dinner," or "Come over and we'll call for takeout"). Special food turns an everyday event into a celebration. Food plays a large part in stress management, either by increasing or decreasing intake when we are stressed, and can be an escape from boredom, loneliness, and depression. Children quickly learn to use food in a power play with their parents.

Food, like the substances addressed in the section on use disorders, takes on new meaning when it has a negative impact on our emotions, our health, and our ability to function in areas of our lives. Food is the most commonly used substance to change moods. Eating disorders have nothing to do with the intake of balanced and necessary nutrition and often has little to do with actual flavor and enjoyment of food.

Eating disorders can appear at any time in life, but more frequently manifest in adolescence and young adulthood. They are more prevalent among women than men. Research finds that there is no single cause for eating disorders, but rather there are a combination of behavioral, genetic, social, and psychological factors.

Anorexia Nervosa

The term anorexia means "lack of appetite" and is usually the result of illness. Anorexia nervosa refers to a psychological abnormality in body image perception. Patients with this disorder have such a distorted body image (weight and shape) that they see themselves as obese no matter how thin they are. They have an intense fear of gaining weight or becoming fat and so they restrict food intake. The disorder usually begins in the mid-teens. Women make up the majority of people with this condition. Signs of anorexia nervosa include a weight loss of 25% or more for no apparent reason, with a perceived need to lose even more weight. According to the National Institute of Mental Health, anorexia nervosa has the highest mortality rate of any mental disorder. Although many young women and men with this disorder die from complications associated with starvation, others die of suicide. In women, suicide is much more common in those with anorexia than with most other mental disorders (National Institute of Mental Health, 2016).

Underweight and malnourished patients can present in the health care system with psychological and behavioral features that support a diagnosis of anorexia nervosa. For example, they may have a depressed mood, low libido, irritability, and insomnia. Rather than avoiding the thought of food, this patient can have a food obsession, collecting recipes, watching cooking shows, hoarding food, and cooking for others. They may exhibit a strong need to control their environment, which may add to impaired social function. Some patients with anorexia nervosa are obsessed with physical exercise.

Semistarvation can result in any of several physical affects and symptoms over time, some of which can be life-threatening. Physiologic indicators include vital sign abnormalities, such as low blood pressure, and slowed breathing and pulse. Women may have *amenorrhea*, the cessation of menstruation. Laboratory values may indicate anemia, low white blood cell count, and high cholesterol. The patient may complain of feeling tired and/or cold all the time and may suffer from constipation. Outwardly, emaciation presents with brittle hair and nails and dry and yellowish skin. Deep starvation can cause *lanugo*, the growth of fine hair all over the body to keep warm.

As the body starves, the patient will experience a loss of bone density, damage to the structure and function of the heart, brain damage, and multiorgan failure.

Bulimia Nervosa

A person with bulimia nervosa compulsively eats a large amount of food and then tries to get rid of the food through forced vomiting, fasting, excessive use of diuretics or laxatives, excessive exercise, or any combination of these. This is also known as binge-eating and purging. Patients usually are aware that this is not normal behavior, but are powerless to change it. Patients are typically ashamed of their behavior and keep their eating habit hidden. Bulimics are more frequently are women, adolescents and girls from families that expect a high degree of success. Unlike the patient with anorexia nervosa, those with bulimia nervosa may maintain a normal weight even though they consume large amounts of food; however, they still have an obsession with their body shape and weight. After eating, they usually induce vomiting and/or purge with laxatives.

Physical examination of this patient may reveal foul breath and tooth decay from regurgitated stomach acids. This patient may have swollen salivary glands in the neck and jaw area and a chronically inflamed and sore throat. They may have acid reflux disorder and other gastrointestinal problems, such as intestinal distress and irritation from laxative abuse. Patients who stimulate the gag reflex to vomit may have scarring on the back of their fingers or hands from contact with the teeth.

Severe dehydration from purging of fluids can lead to an electrolyte imbalance (too low or too high levels of sodium, calcium, potassium, and other minerals) that can lead to stroke or heart attack. As with patients with anorexia nervosa, those with bulimia are at a higher risk for suicide.

Treatment

The behaviors related to eating disorders typically are done in secret, thus it is unlikely that patients will volunteer that they are struggling with eating issues. In fact, many patients with an eating disorder will deny that they have a problem and can seem ambivalent about the risks to their health. They can resist treatment and find ways to resist gaining weight.

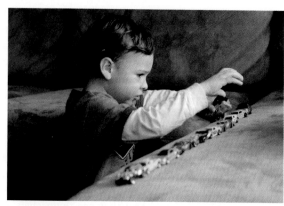

Fig. 6.12 This child with autism spectrum disorder prefers to arrange the cars in a line. (iStock.com/UrsaHoogle.)

Treatment of eating disorders usually involves a team of health care specialists, including a medical doctor, nutritionist, and mental health professional. In extreme cases, hospitalization may be required if the patient's condition cannot be controlled in the outpatient setting. A combination of medications and psychotherapy is common. Gaining control of any of the eating disorders is a life-long struggle, similar to other long-term illness, such as diabetes or heart disease, and all can be handled with proper management and education leading to changes in lifestyle behaviors.

AUTISM SPECTRUM DISORDER

Autism spectrum disorder is a developmental disorder affecting social behavior and communication. Although it can be diagnosed at any age, symptoms usually appear by age 2 years.

According to the diagnostic criteria in the *DSM-5*, a person with ASD has

1. Difficulty communicating and interacting with other people
2. Restricted interests (evidenced, for instance, in an insistence on sameness or routines, fixation on an object) and repetitive behaviors (e.g., repeating patterns of speech, lining up objects [Fig. 6.12])
3. Symptoms that begin at a young age
4. Symptoms that impair the person's ability to function properly in school, work, and other areas of life

Autism is known as a "spectrum" disorder because of the wide range in the type and degree of symptoms people experience, from mild to severe. Although ASD can be a lifelong disorder, treatments and services can improve a person's symptoms and ability to function.

ASD occurs in all ethnic, racial, and socioeconomic groups. Statistics show that in 2014, in 8-year-old children, 1 in every 59 children was identified as having ASD (Table 6.4). Boys were identified as having ASD five times more than were girls. The prevalence of ASD doubled in the 10 years from 2000 to 2010, although sources of data are problematic because of shifting diagnostic criteria over time (Committee to Evaluate the Supplemental Security Income Disability Program for Children with Mental Disorders; Board on the Health of Select Populations; Board on Children, Youth, and Families; Institute of Medicine, 2015). The cause of autism is unknown, although given the range of both symptoms and severity found in individuals, there are probably several factors, both environmental and genetic.

It is important to know some of the typical communication and behaviors persons with ASD may have, as these impact how we can effectively communicate with them. Each person identified as having ASD will present differently. The National Institute of Mental Health (2018) provides the following communication and behavior symptoms.
- Making little or inconsistent eye contact
- Tending not to look at or listen to people
- Rarely sharing enjoyment of objects or activities by pointing or showing things to others
- Failing to, or being slow to, respond to someone calling their name or to other verbal attempts to gain attention

TABLE 6.4   Prevalence of Autism Spectrum Disorder in 8-Year-Olds, 2014

		Prevalence	Percent	About 1 in every "x" children
Overall		16.8 per 1000	1.7%	1 in 59
Sex	Boys	26.6 per 1000	2.7%	1 in 38
	Girls	6.6 per 1000	0.7%	1 in 152
Race/Ethnicity	White	17.2 per 1000	1.7%	1 in 58
	Black	16.0 per 1000	1.6%	1 in 63
	Asian/Pacific Islander	13.5 per 1000	1.4%	1 in 74
	Hispanic*	14.0 per 1000	1.4%	1 in 71

*All other groups are non-Hispanic.
From National Institute of Mental Health. (2018, April). Autism Spectrum Disorder (ASD). Retrieved October 19, 2018, from National Institute of Mental Health Web site: https://www.nimh.nih.gov/health/statistics/autism-spectrum-disorder-asd.shtml. Prevalence data for ASD comes from the CDC's Autism and Developmental Disabilities Monitoring (ADDM) Network.

- Having difficulties with the back and forth of conversation
- Often talking at length about a favorite subject without noticing that others are not interested or without giving others a chance to respond
- Having facial expressions, movements, and gestures that do not match what is being said
- Having an unusual tone of voice that may sound sing-song or flat and robot-like
- Having trouble understanding another person's point of view or being unable to predict or understand other people's actions

People diagnosed with ASD may share some similar symptoms or traits, but each person will be unique in the variance of their social interactions and behaviors. Many of the social communication/behavior interactions, as listed above, make effective communication more challenging because verbal and nonverbal communication may not fit standard associations and verbal verification may not be possible for further clarification. You will need to tailor your communication to each individual, rather than assume the same communication will work with all those identified as having ASD.

COMMUNICATION GUIDELINES

Autism Spectrum Disorder

As stated, the degree of symptoms and level of communication functioning will vary from individual to individual, so you will need to adjust your communication accordingly. The following offer some basic communication guidelines.

- If applicable, speak in advance with the patient's guardian or caregiver to learn how to identify the most effective methods to communicate with this particular patient.
- Arrange to have the patient seen by the same provider and assistants in the same room, to allow for predictable, routine consistency that will alleviate anxiety.
- Have the room be as free from external noises as possible or provide noise cancelling headphones.
- Use indirect lighting when possible, avoiding bright overhead lights.

- Use the patient's name at the beginning of speaking to him so he knows you are talking to him.
- When you talk, place yourself at the person's eye level and in his or her line of vision, but not too close; allow more space between you and the person than usual.
- Use short, concise sentences; say less and say it slowly.
- Use realistic, clear language with no euphemisms.
- Ask as few as possible of the most necessary questions; ask yes/no questions rather than open-ended questions; offer choices.
- Be patient and allow time for the patient to respond.
- Use less mature language with children.
- Do not expect eye contact from the patient.

SOMATIC SYMPTOM DISORDERS AND ASSUMING THE SICK ROLE

At times, with the best of care and the most appropriate medical treatment, certain patients continue to report symptoms similar to other patients who are well on their way to recovery. If tests do not support the patient's complaints, the concern may be either noncompliance or one of several somatic symptoms and related disorders. In somatic symptom disorder, the patient experiences distressing symptoms, most often pain, that causes a disruption in daily life. This individual is preoccupied with his symptoms, spending an inordinate amount of time and energy agonizing over the seriousness of his problem for a long period of time—6 months or longer. Often, the symptoms reported have no physical findings to support the complaint, although the distress is real regardless of medical basis. The term *hypochondriasis* was used for many years to identify those patients who seemed to be consistently "unwell" despite the best medical care. In most instances this is not a conscious choice and patients may not be aware they seem to drift from one vague illness to another with no evidence to support complaints.

The severe anxiety of the patient with somatic symptom disorder dominates that person's life and she will usually dismiss the suggestion that there may be some other source of stress to explain the symptom. These patients access health care with high frequency. They may become very demanding and manipulative and frequently will tell health care workers exactly what they think their symptoms indicate. They can become angry when no diagnostic studies or physical findings agree with their diagnosis. They frequently start and stop treatments as they decide which are the least intrusive, expensive, or likely to make them well. They may complain of excessive side effects to medications that should alleviate their symptoms. When the current provider cannot find a reason for the complaints, these patients frequently "doctor shop" until they find one who will agree to treat them. Patients with somatic symptoms disorder usually dismisses the idea that they should seek treatment for mental health.

Keep in mind that somatic symptom disorder persists for a period of time, usually 6 months or longer. Those who only occasionally escape into the sick role do not consistently demonstrate the deep-seated anxiety seen in patients with true somatic symptom disor-

ders. Much of our behavior is family learned, as is our response to illness and stress. These behaviors may have been formed when a child was able to escape responsibility or gather lots of rewarding attention when he or she was ill. At the least sign of illness some children are put to bed with warm soup, a bed full of toys, and the comfort of a hovering parent. Others are told to take a pill and go on to school. Patients who enjoy the sick role, as opposed to the true somatic symptom disorder patients, usually do well when stress is low. When they are stressed, they truly feel ill, with vague symptoms that on examination have no consistent physical origin. Once the need to escape has passed, these patients playing the sick role usually return to their responsibilities until they are overwhelmed again. If we look and act sick enough, we are excused from taking part in whatever we would rather avoid. Illness can be a very handy escape.

There are almost as many advantages as disadvantages in being just a little bit ill. When we are sick, we may not have to do things we would rather avoid, we may miss work, or not participate in unpleasant social situations, and can let slide unwelcome obligations. However, except for those with somatic symptom disorders, most people eventually move beyond the need to escape into illness; they generally see that they must get better because their friends, families, and those responsible for their care lose patience and begin to reduce the rewards of being sick. The idea of a day or so in bed, being cared for by someone compassionate, may seem a nice rest and relief from responsibilities, but, for most people, the need to be "sick" grows old quickly.

Remember that imagined symptoms (pain, nausea, dizziness) are just as intense and strongly felt as symptoms with a physical origin; we must never treat patients we suspect are playing these roles differently than any other patient. We have a duty to care for patients regardless of the reason for their problems. We must help to determine what these patients need just as we would for any illness with a physical basis. If gently caring for them helps, this may be as therapeutic as any sophisticated medical treatment. Remember also that we are not trained to diagnose illness. This time the patient really may be sick; it is not up to us to decide. Our goal, in these cases, and in all of our interactions, is to assist in finding the reasons for the complaints and to help ensure that each patient achieves and maintains both physical and psychological health.

CHECKING YOUR COMPREHENSION

Write a brief answer for each of the following assignments.

1. What are the unique barriers to communicating with an ill patient?
2. Explain the difference between an advance directive and a POLST form and how they work together.
3. What is the difference between acute and chronic diseases?
4. Explain why communicating with a patient who has cancer is unique to that disease.
5. List the symptoms of depression and things to ask when interviewing a patient you suspect is depressed.
6. How should the health care professional interview a patient suspected of having suicidal ideations?
7. What are the physical manifestations of a patient with anxiety?
8. What clinical markers suggest a patient has a severe substance use disorder?
9. What behaviors would suggest that a patient is looking for drugs from the provider?
10. Contrast the task-centered care model with the person-centered care model.
11. Describe why Alzheimer's disease is a distinctive type of dementia.
12. Explain the difference between the behavior of someone who has bulimia nervosa and someone who has anorexia nervosa.
13. Identify five communication guidelines for working with a person diagnosed with autism spectrum disorder.
14. Explain the difference between someone who "enjoys being the sick person" and someone with somatic symptom disorder.

EXPANDING CRITICAL THINKING

1. Think in terms of quality of life reflected in the following diseases and disorders. In your opinion, list them in order of a negative impact on a person's life. Outline ways the quality of life is diminished. Which do you think would be most difficult to control?
   a. Addiction to controlled substances
   b. Addiction to tobacco
   c. Addiction to alcohol
   d. Obesity
   e. Heart disease
   f. Type 2 or insulin-dependent diabetes mellitus
   g. Hypertension
2. Look again at the problems listed above. Which ones do you think earn the patient more sympathy? Why do you think this is so? Which ones earn the patient more negative reaction? Why?
3. A good friend lost his job several weeks ago, but you know he had been having a difficult time at work for months, feeling unappreciated and often at odds with his manager. Since then he seems increasingly withdrawn. He has canceled several get-togethers and even skipped your tradition of fly-fishing together on opening day. When you call he sounds despondent and seems to be always in bed. You suspect your friend may be depressed and that perhaps this has been going on for a long time, before he even lost his job. How do you help him?
4. Consider any times that you may have felt sad and depressed. What were the circumstances and what was happening in your life at that time? List what they were. Reflect on the various emotions you experienced at that time and write a list. Was there anything that you found helpful to you during that time? A person or persons? Did you seek professional help and did it make a difference? Was there something you read or did or were given by another person? Was it your own belief system? Write these down. How does that experience feel to you now in reflection? Can you use this reflection to help you again if you should feel depressed again? Can you use this reflection to help you empathize with a patient experiencing depression and offer compassionate support?
5. Should a person contemplating suicide be institutionalized or restrained "for his own good"? Explain your answer.
6. Do you think suicide is a crime, a sin, or a personal option? Are there any circumstances conceivable under which suicide is justifiable?
7. Have you ever been tempted to end your life? What were the circumstances? What helped you change your mind?
8. Consider someone you know well whom you think may be an alcoholic, because of how you observe it

affects their work and family life, but they deny that they have a drinking problem. Describe the emotions that come up for you as you consider
a. How they behave socially with you, others, their family
b. How their drinking affects their work
c. How they justifies or makes excuses for their drinking and behavior

9. If drugs were available to improve your quality of life, but would shorten your life by a number of years, how many years would you give up for the following?
a. Physical strength
b. Perfect health
c. Genius intelligence
d. Great popularity
e. Prodigious talent
f. Movie star or model appearance

10. Does it matter to you how much alcohol people drink? How many drinks would it take to make you uncomfortable for the following people?
a. Your pregnant friend
b. Your parents
c. Your date or spouse
d. Your supervisor or employer physician
e. Your pastor or other religious leader
f. Yourself

11. You are reviewing the health history with an 18-year-old female, to see if there are any changes or updates. You notice that she seems very thin, far thinner than the last time she was in for asthma treatment 3 months previously. She is wearing athletic clothes because she came straight from the gym. What behavioral markers could suggest she may have an eating disorder?

12. You are meeting an 84-year-old woman with mid-stage dementia for the first time; she has her adult son with her. Write a scenario for how you establish rapport with the patient and her son.
a. What do you say and to whom?
b. What paralanguage do you intentionally use or avoid?
c. What is your body position and location?

13. You are providing care for a patient with Alzheimer's disease. Describe the specific symptoms and behaviors you would look for to determine if the patient is in the late stage of this disease.

14. At the pediatrician's office, a boy of 11 who has autism spectrum disorder had a difficult time in the waiting room. He covered his ears and howled until his mother asked the receptionist to turn off the television because it was showing a cartoon that bothered him. With no other children in the waiting area, the receptionist obliged. Then the boy gathered all the magazines and opened them to the middle staple, placing one on each empty chair in the room. When the boy and his mother were called back to the exam room, one of the medical billers said to you, "I know it is not his fault, but I wish his mother would discipline him a little better." What do you think? Do you agree or disagree with the receptionist?

Communicating Through the Grief Process

Sharon Campton

CHAPTER OUTLINE

LEARNING OBJECTIVES

On successfully completing this chapter, you will be able to:

1. Define terms related to loss and grief.
2. Discuss the way technologic and medical advances have changed our perspective on death, and the attitudes of health care professionals toward death.
3. Summarize psychological theories about the grieving experience.
4. List specific measures to take when interacting with someone experiencing grief.
5. Describe how spiritual beliefs, cultural perspectives, and age affect the grief experience.
6. Discuss the benefits of support groups and give examples for the grieving patient or caregiver.
7. Describe the function of hospice care and how it differs from other areas of health care.

KEY TERMS

anticipatory grief deep emotions and anxiety felt when an individual becomes aware that a loss will inevitably happen, such as in the case of a patient diagnosed with a terminal illness

attachment theory psychological model stating that the bonds formed by the caregiver–child relationship influences personality development into adulthood, and that grief is felt when a relationship suffers an unwanted separation

bereaved person experiencing grief and mourning

bereavement state of having lost a loved one

complicated grief deep, persistent sadness accompanied by incessant and painful thoughts of the loss that interferes with the ability to function

coping contending with difficulties and overcoming them

dual process model theory of grieving in which the individual at times confronts and at other times avoids the different tasks of grieving

grief normal emotional response to the actual or perceived loss of something valued

grief work in psychology, the notion that individuals feel strong emotions toward a loss and must work through these emotions to reduce their distress

hospice type of care for patients facing the end of life that focuses on pain management and emotional support

mourning outward display of grief

palliative offering comfort, as in pain relief, but not bringing about a cure

respite short interval of rest or relief

? TEST YOUR COMMUNICATION IQ

Before reading this chapter, take this short self-assessment test. Decide which statements are true and which are false.

1. Experiences of loss and grief always follow a specific, sequential progression of stages.
2. It is important to focus your communication more on the patient than on the caregivers' needs.
3. During an illness crisis, a patient's spiritual belief always becomes deeper and more solid.
4. A statement such as "Grandma passed away during her sleep" is comforting and reassuring to a young child.
5. A statement such as "I know how you are feeling right now" is comforting to a patient who has been newly diagnosed with a terminal illness.
6. Patients with terminal illnesses should always be encouraged to attend support groups to discuss their feelings and fears about death.
7. Dr. Elisabeth Kübler-Ross identified the various stages of death or loss and promoted public awareness of this topic.

Results

Statement number 7 is true; all other statements are false. How did you do? Read the chapter to find more information on these topics.

INTRODUCTION

When most of us hear the words "grief" and "loss," the first thought we tend to have is of death, the loss of life. But the experience of loss and grief is much broader than our feelings surrounding death. We experience many kinds of losses throughout our lives, including the loss of life, and we may experience grief for many different kinds of losses. There is *actual loss*, such as the death of a loved one or a pet, the leaving of loved ones or a physical place, loss of a job, loss of relationships, loss of health, loss of ability, loss of memory, loss of home and possessions, and loss of youth. These losses are usually evident to others, in addition to the one experiencing the loss. There is also *perceived loss*, usually apparent only to the one experiencing the loss, such as loss of self-esteem, of identity, of purpose, of belonging or of connection with others, of security or safety, and of opportunities and unrealized dreams. The losses listed above are not comprehensive; you may be able to identify with some of these losses plus additional losses you have experienced.

It is beneficial to all health care professionals to have an understanding about loss and grief. Most of the patients and their families that you will be serving in health care will be dealing with various actual and perceived losses in their lives, especially those losses related to ill health. Some patients and families face death through the diagnosis of a terminal illness, after a short or prolonged illness, or through trauma (e.g., an accident or violent experience). If you will be working in a health care environment where death is part of the care-giving experience, you will receive more specific training for end of life and death; however, all health care workers must have some understanding of what is involved with loss and grief. This chapter introduces the grieving experience, and outlines the strategies for therapeutic communication with patients who are facing loss in its many forms.

Terminology

Terms used to describe the process of dealing with loss vary through the health care community. We are using the definitions discussed overleaf for the commonly used terms related to loss.

Grief and Coping

Grief is the normal emotional response to an actual or perceived loss of something we value or of any kind of change. The degree to which we feel grief is often related to the degree of value we placed on what was lost. When we experience loss, we may or may not recognize that what we are feeling is grief; our response to certain losses may be expressed more readily as anger, sadness, disappointment, guilt, regret, depression, and/or a philosophic approach to just accept it and move on with our lives. But the deeper, underlying emotion is grief, whether recognized as such or not.

Feelings of loss are not limited only to the moment of the loss; these feelings can also be experienced in anticipation of loss, such as when patients or family members learn of the terminal or life-changing nature of an illness in which they may have years, months, days, or hours to live before the event of the loss. If there is time to prepare for the loss and the grieving process can begin early, this is called anticipatory grief – the deep emotions and anxiety felt when an individual becomes aware that a loss will happen, such as in the case of diagnosis with a terminal illness (Fig. 7.1). Anticipatory grief, whether by the sick or dying or by those who care for them, may have an impact on emotional connections as each person prepares differently for the loss or the change. Family dynamics play a large role in this as well. During this time communication with family members and between family members can be particularly challenging.

If grief begins with the loss of a loved one through death with no warning, as in sudden or accidental death, or the sudden loss of a body part or personal health, there is no time emotionally to prepare and we cannot protect ourselves from emotional overload. Grief is just as heartfelt and real no matter the circumstances, but it may be easier to process when spread over time.

Complicated grief is a persistent, intense grief that is much stronger than normal; it is characterized by chronic sadness and constant thoughts of the person who has died. An individual with complicated grief suffers increased pain and delayed healing, with a preoccupation on the loss so great that it interferes with normal function (Shear, 2012).

As discussed in Chapter 5, stress is a physiologic burden on the body. The deep emotions and anxieties of grief can be a major source of stress. Physical responses to grief may include increased blood pressure, exhaustion, insomnia or sleep disruptions, altered eating patterns, as well as other symptoms. Physiologic and emotional manifestations, such as depression, significantly lower resistance to opportunistic diseases, which in turn may lead to physical illness in addition to emotional stress. Because everyone experiences grief at some time, our minds have adapted by developing a means of adjusting to loss. Coping refers to the actions we take to overcome difficulties caused by stressors and it is essential to maintaining the health of the body. From infancy through young adulthood, we develop strategies to reduce distress, learning by watching those around us as well as by trying various coping mechanisms to see what works (Skinner & Zimmer-Gembeck, 2010).

Mourning and Bereavement

Mourning, the outward, external expression of grief, is also very personal. Our individual and shared social responses, behaviors, and rituals are usually influenced by our spiritual and cultural beliefs, as addressed later in this chapter. Often mourning involves action, symbolism, ceremony, and/or ritual, such as visitations, wakes, funerals, memorials, and celebrations of life.

Bereavement is particularly related to loss of life. It usually refers to the state occurring after having lost a love one—a period of both grief and mourning. The person experiencing grief and mourning may be referred to as the bereaved.

SHIFTING PERSPECTIVES ON DEATH

As we have discussed, people experience grief for many different kinds of losses, not just death; however, it is

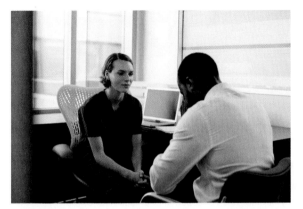

Fig. 7.1 This doctor had just delivered bad news about the patient's health. Anticipatory grief is felt when we know that a loss is impending. (iStock.com/Monkeybusinessimages.)

helpful to understand how our relationship with death has evolved. At the beginning of the 20th century, approximately 1 in 5 children in the United States died before age 5. A person who lived until his or her fifth birthday could expect to live until about age 55 (Human Mortality Database). Most people died at home with very little medical intervention and no technologic life support. Death was usually the result of accidents or acute contagious or infectious diseases; there was little that medicine could do to keep people alive for very long. Families kept their dead at home until burial, which was usually in a private family graveyard or the local church cemetery. Burying the dead nearby kept them as close as possible to their family and allowed the family to visit and continue the relationship after death. The rituals and public displays of mourning and the support of close communities comforted survivors. Most families consisted of several generations – aunts, uncles, and cousins living nearby or with each other, so that everyone experienced the death of family members as a natural part of life.

When physicians had few remedies and resources to save patients from disease or death, doctors, patients, and families seemed more willing to accept that death or disability was inevitable. As medical technology advanced and antibiotics cured many of the infectious illnesses that killed our ancestors, the median age for death in the developed world extended to the late 70s and is still rising (Fig. 7.2). With the science of medicine extending life by decades, death and disability were no longer seen as acceptable options. The dominant attitude among clinicians and patients shifted to provide interventions as long as the technology allowed (Fuchs, 1974). For many health care professionals, to acknowledge death, or even loss of an acceptable health status, was to admit defeat. Many physicians felt it was a personal failure on their part if a patient died—a failure of both medical technology and the doctor's proficiency—and were reluctant to discuss end-of-life care options (Price, 2016). This may be difficult to understand because we currently encourage open communication and patient empowerment.

Modern society has put distance between everyday life and the experience of death.

Care of the dying is now primarily the responsibility of institutions, not families. Many Americans have never lived with a person who is terminally ill. Mortuaries handle our dead and bury them away from us in generic public

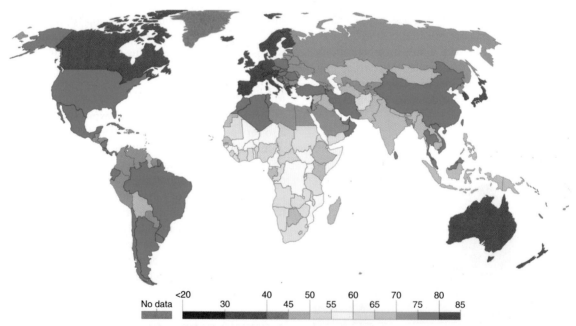

Fig. 7.2 Life expectancy, 2015. Shown is period life expectancy at birth. This corresponds to an estimate of the average number of years a newborn infant would live if prevailing patterns of mortality at the time of its birth were to stay the same throughout its life. (From Roser M. Life expectancy; 2019. Published online at OurWorldInData. org. Retrieved from https://ourworldindata.org/life-expectancy [Online Resource]. Accessed June 17, 2019.)

cemeteries. Many people no longer see death as part of life but as something to be avoided at all costs, even if those costs are quantity of days versus quality of life. The definition of death has changed from simply "an absence of life" and is measured by complex technologic means such as cerebral and brainstem function. Hearts are restarted, pulmonary function is maintained, and organs are transplanted.

In the past a patient with cancer usually did not die from the cancer, but from a more immediate infection to which the patient succumbed in his/her weakened state. Today we can treat many of the opportunistic infections common to various types of cancer, but this may result in prolonged suffering before death from the disease itself. Some health care professionals, caregivers, families, and patients feel that we are delaying dying, rather than prolonging life. This has led to professional and ethical dilemmas surrounding the degree to which we should intervene with life support at the end of a patient's life or to allow patients to determine when they die through physician-assisted death in states where this is legal. Many families and medical practitioners are thinking harder about whether to allow the terminally ill to die without intervention or decide to remove all life support, such as ventilators to help the patient breathe (Fig. 7.3), medications to help the heart work, and food and water through feeding tubes or intravenously. The question of how to define the end of life is not simply a medical determination; it is strongly impacted by cultural, political, and spiritual beliefs and practices.

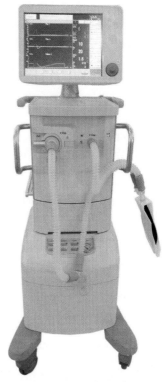

Fig. 7.3 A ventilator provides life support that enables a patient to breathe. Ventilation and other measures sustain the patient until the body is ready to resume functioning, but when the patient is unconscious and there is no chance for recovery, physicians and families must decide whether to continue this intervention. (iStock.com/tigristiara.)

⊹ LEGAL EAGLE

Advance directives, POLST forms, and related health care documents are addressed in Chapter 6. As a health care professional, you are legally obligated to follow the patient's directive. You may not agree with the patient's decisions or wishes, but failure to follow the directives can result in fines and legal action against you and the health care setting. You must stay abreast of new laws pertaining to completing and documenting advance directive forms both at the national level and in your state.

A significant contributor to the current active discussion of the role of medicine and the quality of life is Dr. Atul Gawande's *Being Mortal: Illness, Medicine and What Matters in the End (2014)*. He addresses the impact of medicine on life and death, which was prompted by his experience with his dying father. Dr. Gawande posits that our current, common medical approach to end of life does not consider a person's quality of life. As with a growing number of health care professionals, Gawande advocates a palliative care model, one that attempts to comfort and relieve pain rather than try to cure, to improve quality of life for the time a person has left.

The public is beginning to see that while saving lives is a noble purpose, prolonging life without quality is a questionable achievement that may need to be considered on a case-by-case basis. This text will not attempt to address ethical, legal, and spiritual issues, but it will concentrate on understanding and communicating with those experiencing losses and those responsible for their care. Remember that in the medical setting, great loss may involve degrees of illness and may not necessarily mean that death is imminent. Your more direct involvement in dying and death will depend on your specialty and your career choice, but dealing with the loss of health is common to almost all areas of medicine. The mechanics of death as it pertains to your specialty will be covered in other areas of your training.

THEORIES DEALING WITH LOSS AND GRIEF

The study of dying and death is as old as the practice of medicine, but its credibility as a separate topic is fairly recent. In 1917, Sigmund Freud (1856–1939), the Austrian neurologist and founder of psychoanalysis, wrote about the subject in his essay "Mourning and Melancholia." Freud cautioned that grief and loss should be faced head on to avoid long-term depression. Freud called this grief work, the notion that individuals feel strong emotions toward a loss and must work through these emotions to reduce their distress.

Dr. Elisabeth Kübler-Ross (1926–2004), a Swiss-born American psychiatrist, is credited as being the pioneer who brought the discussion of dying and death into popular culture. Dr. Kübler-Ross wrote extensively on end-of-life issues in the 1970s and 1980s on a level that the public could understand. Her most popular contribution is her identification of five stages of grief that a dying person experiences in reaction to receiving news that he/she has a terminal illness: denial, anger, bargaining, depression, and acceptance (Kübler-Ross, 1969). She wrote that a person needs to pass through these stages to process grief. Like Freud, Kübler-Ross' theory is grounded in grief work, positing that the bereaved must address his emotions in order to reduce distress. Her work found a wide audience among both health care professionals and laypeople, and her grief theory became the traditional model for many decades. Although Dr. Kübler-Ross' stages as written applied to the experiences of terminally ill patients, these stages have since been adopted by others to address loss and grief that people experience *after* a death occurs, and then again to grief owing to losses *other* than death.

Dr. Kübler-Ross's writing gave rise to misconceptions, however, namely that a grieving person must pass through these stages in a certain order or that a person must experience all five stages. Later in her career she was careful to note that the stages she named were not intended to fall in a sequential pattern. In fact, during her own end of life, Dr. Kübler-Ross personally experienced grief to be fluid, not the linear stages she had written about. Her stages remain very popular in our culture, even though her scholarship has since been dismissed by professionals owing to a lack of empirical evidence and research.

More recent research and writing attempt to address the complex and fluid nature of loss and grief. In 1991 J. William Worden described the process of grief as a task model based on developmental psychology in his book, *Grief Counseling and Grief Therapy*. Worden conceptualizes four tasks for the grieving person to complete the mourning process and reestablish emotional equilibrium. His four tasks take one from grief through mourning, the inward to the outward expressions of loss, emphasizing that these tasks are fluid, not sequential stages.

Task 1: To accept the reality of the loss

Task 2: To work through the pain of grief

Task 3: To adjust to an environment in which the deceased is missing

Task 4: To find an enduring connection with the deceased while embarking on a new life (Worden, 1991)

Another stage-oriented approach is the work of John Bowlby and his collaborators, whose study of infants and children led to a theory of attachment (Bowlby, 1960). Attachment theory describes the bond-building that takes place between an infant and its caregiver or caregivers from an evolutionary standpoint and also describes grief as the feelings experienced when that bond or attachment is involuntarily severed. Later theorists expanded the scope of attachment formation into adult relationships, both familial and romantic. Psychiatrist Colin Parkes built on Bowlby's attachment theory to identify four overlapping phases of adult grief.

- **Numbness**, which may last hours or days
- **Pining**, a deep searching coupled with intense anxiety for what was lost
- **Disorganization and despair**, characterized by poor concentration, loss of appetite, and a fixation on the deceased
- **Reorganization**, the return of appetite, sociality, and normal living

Importantly, these phases are understood to be nonlinear; they are fluid, merging, and replacing one another as the individual processes the loss. Phases can sometimes return again and again when a person is reminded of the loss, such as when visiting an old neighborhood, or on certain dates, such as birthdays and anniversaries. As wth other grief work theories, working through these phases allows the grieving individual to adapt to the loss; however, Parkes also acknowledges the role of avoiding the loss and suppressing grief in the healing process.

Much empirical evidence supports the claims of the psychoanalytic school that excessive repression of grief is harmful and can give rise to delayed and distorted grief—but there is also evidence that obsessive grieving, to the exclusion of all else, can lead to chronic grief and depression. The ideal is to achieve a balance between avoidance and confrontation which enables the person gradually to come to terms with the loss (Parkes CM, 1996).

In 1999 Margaret Stroebe and Henk Schut also recognized some core problems of the grief work models, arguing that they do not specifically identify the stressors faced by the bereaved (Stroebe and Schut, 1999). In addition, grief work models fail to account for the complexity of grieving and underestimate the importance of avoiding the loss. Their dual process model posits that a grieving person must cope with the loss on one hand, adjust to lifestyle changes on the other, and rest from both of these types of stressors at times (Fig. 7.4). For Stroebe and Schut the grieving individual does not always confront the stressors' loss directly, but rather oscillates between processing the loss and avoiding the loss in an attempt to adapt. The class of loss-oriented stressors in the dual process model draws on traditional grief work theories, whereas restoration-oriented stressors include the new things the bereaved must do in the wake of the loss. For example, a spouse must not only process the loss of his or her loved one, but also handle the stressors of the new living situation. A man whose wife had always paid the bills must now take on responsibility of paying bills, filing taxes, and managing finances following her death. He will also face many other stressors related to living without his wife, such as reframed relationships with friends, neighbors, and family, going out to dinner or to movies alone or with others, and so on. For Stroebe and Schut, the grieving individual handles both types of stressors in doses, taking a break from the loss on occasion. In this way, the dual process model attempts to provide a more comprehensive view of grief.

No consensus exists among grief counseling professionals as to any definitive grief process and mental health professionals employ a wide variety of theories to conceptualize their patients' grief. As you can see, many theories expand on each other and overlap. If there is a prevailing view among professionals in the field, it is that grief is so individualized no one can pigeon-hole people in how they grieve. No specific road map exists for grief; each person grieves differently depending on many factors in her life at any given time. What now is understood is that each person experiences grief over varying lengths of time, which may include some or all of the phases or "tasks" stated in the various grief theories. Just as Dr. Kübler-Ross came to understand in her own personal experience, we know grief to be more fluid, moving around and sometimes returning to different phases or tasks. The grief experience is intensely personal and inconsistent, and cannot be hurried.

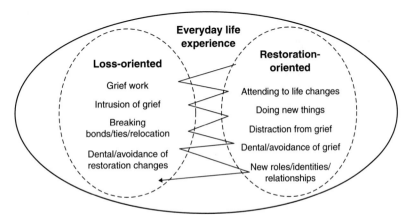

Fig. 7.4 In the dual process model, the grieving individual must cope with loss-oriented stressors and restoration-oriented stressors. (From Stroebe M, Schut H. The dual process model of coping with bereavement: rationale and description. *Death Studies.* 1999;23(3):197–224.)

🗨 COMMUNICATION GUIDELINES

Theories of Loss and Grief

Loss, grief, and mourning should not be placed into any specific or generic formula; it is not your place to psychoanalyze the patient's or family's responses. Be compassionate and present, and refer patients or caregivers to professionals and/or resources for them to get more specific support, as addressed later in this chapter.

COPING WITH LOSS AND GRIEF

How we cope with stress throughout life can have an impact on how we cope with grief. As we discussed in Chapter 5, "Communicating Through Barriers," when a person finds a coping mechanism that works, he or she tends to return to it again and again. Someone who has coped through denial all of his or her life may now spend more of the grieving time in denial. The person who reacts with anger to any frustration will become enraged at this thing so beyond personal control. Likewise, someone who is easily depressed may remain in the depression phase without journeying beyond that phase or task. In terms of the dual process theory much depends also on how many restoration-oriented stressors are being juggled at the same time. For example, will the cost of treatment or care-giving be a major problem or will the needs of the survivors be covered? Will a parent be left with young children to rear alone (Fig. 7.5)? Will physical modifications be necessary in the home or will the patient need to be moved to a facility to receive the level of care necessary? Is an adult child left with a complicated estate and many debts? If loose ends are tied up and realistic plans have been made, grief usually progresses more smoothly.

For many of us, moving forward in our grief depends on how we attribute meaning.

It is natural for us to desire or to feel the need to know the meaning, purpose, or reason for our loss. This is particularly true when loss occurs suddenly, perhaps violently, and appears to be "senseless." Sometimes there is a clear cause and effect reason for loss; sometimes we derive meaning for our loss after the fact, on reflection; sometimes we must come to accept that there may be no reason and choose to live with the lack of resolution. Our life experiences, culture, and spiritual beliefs can significantly influence how we derive meaning of our losses, as discussed later in this chapter. Psychiatrist Colin Parkes identified risk factors that can lead to complicated grief, such as when the loss occurs to someone especially vulnerable or under traumatic circumstances (Box 7.1).

BOX 7.1 FACTORS INCREASING RISK AFTER BEREAVEMENT

Traumatic Circumstances
- Death of a spouse or child
- Death of a parent (particularly in early childhood or adolescence)
- Sudden, unexpected, and untimely deaths (particularly if associated with horrific circumstances)
- Multiple deaths (particularly disasters)
- Deaths by suicide
- Deaths by murder or manslaughter

Vulnerable People
General
- Low self-esteem
- Low trust in others
- Previous psychiatric disorder
- Previous suicidal threats or attempts
- Absent or unhelpful family

Specific
- Ambivalent attachment to a deceased person
- Dependent or interdependent attachment to a deceased person
- Insecure attachment to parents in childhood (particularly learned fear and learned helplessness)

From Parkes CM. Coping with loss: bereavement in adult life. *British Medical Journal.* 1998;316(7134):856–859. Retrieved October 8, 2018, from https://www.ncbi.nlm.nih.gov/pmc/articles/PMC1112778/.

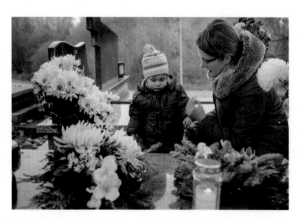

Fig. 7.5 Coping is more difficult when there are more restoration-oriented stressors, such as becoming a single parent when one spouse dies. (iStock.com/Pawel Czaja.)

When the pain of loss is accepted, healing begins. If the loss is not death but is health and mobility, new skills must be learned, new roles assumed, and new life directions determined by the patient, family, and caregiver. If the loss is death, these adjustments are to be experienced by the living. Although waves of grief return at times and, for some people, grief never fully goes away, the bereaved eventually begin to feel hope and joy again without the same intense feelings of loss and emptiness.

Earlier in this chapter, we discussed the physiologic changes that accompany stress, such as increased blood pressure, exhaustion, sleep disorders, and altered eating patterns. These may be the types of symptoms patients and family members bring to health care workers when they become overwhelmed and may be signs that coping mechanisms may not be working. Our responsibility as health care workers involves offering compassion to patients and caregivers as they learn to cope with grief.

COMMUNICATION GUIDELINES

Coping With Loss and Grief

As we have discussed, grief is a highly individualized process felt and expressed differently by each one of us. Many of us are attracted to helping professions because of our desire to help others in need. Although interventions can be therapeutic in much of our work as health care professionals, the appropriate response is to listen and support, rather than try to "cure" the bereaved.

- *Never presume to educate or provide care to patients or family beyond the scope of your practice.* Make your health care team aware of your observations if a patient is struggling with grief so they can refer patients to the appropriate specialists.
- Establish trust and a good rapport early, so that patients and family feel comfortable talking with you.
- Listen actively. Look for nonverbal cues that may provide further meaning to what the other is feeling, especially how those cues may inform you as to what is not being said.
- Withhold judgment through your own verbal and nonverbal communication. All patients must be treated with compassion and respect. The reason for the patient's loss of health is not your concern. If the person's loss of health is caused by poor personal choices, your own personal convictions are not to be displayed in any way.
- Take note of any urge you have to "fix" a patient's or caregiver's situation; if you have this urge, pause, slow down, and do not attempt to "fix." Instead, acknowledge what the individual is feeling. A person will feel heard and validated by a statement such as, "I hear that you're having a hard time."
- You do not always have to do or say something to be helpful. *Simply sitting in silence and just being present can be very comforting.* If welcomed and permitted, a gentle touch on the person's hand or shoulder may convey compassion. Be present for them, or allow them as much privacy as they need. Be alert for cues for either need.
- Seek clarification if you are unsure of what the person wants. "Is it your desire to just have me listen or do you want help with solutions?"
- Simply say, "I am so sorry for your loss." Do not try to be profound or philosophical. Statements such as, "He would not want you to grieve." "She is in a better place." or "You'll eventually get past this." are not helpful and may even be hurtful.
- Seek out practical ways to help in addition to medical measures. In an inpatient situation, help patients and families gather laundry, tend gift flowers, and plan for home care; in an outpatient situation, you may help arrange transportation or make care simpler for home treatment.
- Help the family and patient gather resources for all available support, such as medical social workers, support groups, spiritual care, hospice, and grief counselors.
- Encourage **respite**, a short interval of rest or relief, without guilt. Caregivers need time to themselves and patients may also need time without hovering caregivers. A break from closeness helps caregivers avoid burnout and reduces anger and depression.
- Talk with the provider if the patient or caregiver feels that needs are not being met, such as pain relief or anticipatory education. Take advantage of every resource available to you and to patients for assistance.

WORDS AT WORK

In this example, the health care professional seeks clarification to determine if the patient merely wants to share or is asking for solutions.

Patient: I'm having a rotten day.

Medical assistant: I'm sorry to hear that. Do you want to tell me about it?

Patient: I feel awful. I need you to help me get out of this funk.

Medical assistant: What I hear you say is that you want me to fix your problem or lead you out of your funk. Is that right?

Caregivers

When the patient experiences a loss of health or is dying, the family and survivors are experiencing many of the same phases of grief or tasks of mourning. Remember the caregivers as you tend to the patients. There may be a loss of security, great financial and physical demands, added responsibility, and major life changes to accommodate the patient's care, particularly if the situation involves a long, debilitating illness. Although some patients and families fight death to the last breath, in other cases, death may be a release and a relief for patients and caregivers.

Show you care by mentioning the deceased and remembering good things. You may say, "Mr. Jones, I am so sorry about Mrs. Jones. We always enjoyed visiting with her. It appears that you miss her terribly." This will not renew Mr. Jones's grief—it never went away—but will reaffirm that other people miss Mrs. Jones also. Never say, "I know just how you feel," because you do not, even if you have experienced a similar loss; each grief is intensely personal. And even though it may be so, never tell the survivor, "It was for the best." He may come to realize this, but it is not your place to point it out.

Compassion Fatigue

At times, the unrelenting pain of certain patients is overwhelming. This can be either the patient's emotional pain or physical pain that does not seem to respond to anything we, or other health care providers, do to help. For some people, grief, in particular, is so devastating that the process is intensified beyond our ability to offer comfort directly or by providing resources; some physical pain is so unbearable that our strongest medications are ineffective. We may

dread contact with the grieving or suffering patient or family because we believe there is nothing substantial we can do to help. In these instances, when our professionalism and all we have to offer is not enough, we may doubt ourselves and pull away from the sufferer. We look for reassurance in other situations that make us more comfortable; we turn to other patients who we know we can help. In these instances, you should step back emotionally, take a deep breath, and be present for whatever compassion you can offer. Under no circumstances should you abandon a patient or caregiver who seems beyond your ability to help, no matter how slight that aid may be.

It is possible to experience "compassion fatigue" when we are off-balance with the care we provide to others and the care we provide to ourselves. This can have both physical and emotional consequences, affecting our physical and mental health. The nature of our work can also lead to "burnout," a term that implies that your fire to help has gone out. This loss of enthusiasm for your profession is a high price to pay for caring. What can you do to provide self-care and make it easier to go back every day and practice your passion?

- Develop outside interests that direct your mind away from health care.
- Make time for yourself. Do things you enjoy away from the professional setting and do not feel guilty about it.
- Take care of yourself: relax, exercise, eat right, and hydrate with water.
- Work some form of self-care into your daily life inside and outside of work, such as take a minute or two to breathe deeply; take a ten-minute walk or listen to a favorite piece of music; read something that brings you enjoyment; journal; spend time with family and friends.
- Explore spiritual practices that may help you maintain balance, perspective, and clarity of purpose, such as prayer, meditation, studies.
- Read available literature and visit websites dealing with compassion fatigue and grief and "letting go." You will find helpful suggestions for yourself and your patients.
- Ensure that you have your own support system of family, friends, and interest groups.

As we do everything in our power to help our patients, we must remember to care for ourselves. There may be a realistic time to leave our profession and move on to something different, but we want to do that for the right reasons. If we leave the profession because we can no longer give what it requires, not only do we lose, so do our patients.

GRIEF AND DIVERSITY

Although our responses to loss are personal, contemporary thinking on grief holds that each person's way of grieving is informed by his or her own experiences and culture. What we think about loss, dying, and death, and how we behave in response to loss, is shaped by elements of our culture, including our spiritual belief systems and cultural perspectives.

Spirituality

During and after a great loss, many patients and caregivers may need spiritual assistance as much as they need medical attention. To communicate effectively, you must respect a wide variety of spiritual needs. Rather than defining and outlining each religion's focus on death, we suggest that you familiarize yourself with the predominant beliefs in your area that differ from your own, and then expand your research to include other spiritual practices not represented locally. Knowing about other religious beliefs should not threaten your own beliefs; rather, it should broaden your acceptance of different cultures, which is vital to understanding and effective communication.

The importance of respecting patients' spiritual beliefs is addressed in Chapter 4. Remember that spiritual beliefs can be independent of established religions and, although people may use similar vocabulary in different beliefs, it is important never to assume you know what the person means. Asking, "Can you please tell me what [term] means to you?" is a good way to allow the other person to clarify what he or she may believe. Many Americans now define themselves as *spiritual but not religious*, in that they believe in something or someone beyond themselves but do not adhere to a particular religion.

Most spiritual beliefs and religions reflect and focus on the purpose of being and the meaning of life. Our spiritual beliefs may help us determine how we cope with dying, death, and nonbeing, because all religions address end-of-life issues and immortality. Those who accept death as the end of existence or the beginning of a continuing form of life may find that comforting as they experience grief. On the other hand, spiritual beliefs that include judgment and the possibility of a torturous afterlife for some may add significant stress and distress to the personal grief process.

Spiritual beliefs take on new and stronger meanings when our concepts of "being" are challenged. The crisis of illness may either shake or deepen faith as it brings about great change. Some people may believe that if their faith is strong enough, there will be no suffering or death, that there may or will be physical healing; when suffering continues or death occurs, it can test even a strong faith. Health care professionals know that unexplainable cures can and do happen in medicine, but they are infrequent and not expected. Be prepared for even deeper grief reactions if faith is shaken or lost in the midst of the grief process.

From a practical standpoint, spiritual beliefs frequently affect medical practice. Patients and families come to us with strong beliefs about the right to life versus the right to die. Patients may refuse blood transfusions even if death is probable without replacing blood loss; they may demand or reject surgery; they may refuse to be organ donors or receive organ transplants; and they may refuse an autopsy for a deceased member. All of these issues may become magnified if some family members believe one way and others believe differently.

As health care professionals, we do not make choices for our patients or families but we do have to respect and abide by the decisions made by others that may differ from or even be contrary to our own spiritual beliefs. How you may feel about suffering and loss, dying and death, and however much you may want to guide the bereaved to your spiritual view, *you must never impose your beliefs on patients or family members*. Introducing conflicting beliefs is never appropriate. Watch for cues during this difficult and fragile time; it may not be appropriate for you to offer spiritual comfort and may increase stress rather than relieve the situation.

Most hospitals and long-term care settings have a chaplain, recommended by Joint Commission standards, who is specially trained to provide emotional support and spiritual care to patients from a variety of faiths (Fig. 7.6). Chaplains listen to patient concerns, support faith exploration, and help provide peace through illness and hospitalization. The chaplain has specialized training to help patients who are in despair, who have experienced

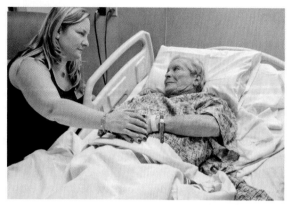

Fig. 7.6 A chaplain provides spiritual care to a patient according to her wishes. (iStock.com/JodiJacobson.)

trauma, who are struggling with meaning, and those who are dying. Many facilities provide interfaith spiritual support, enabling them to address the spectrum of spiritual practices and needs. Chaplains can also refer patients to clergy within the area or contact the patient's or family's spiritual advisor. With the patients' or families' permission, having a trained professional offer spiritual comfort frees us to attend to physical and medical needs.

COMMUNICATION GUIDELINES

Spirituality
What may we do to ensure that spiritual needs are met during the grief process?

- Approach people's beliefs with humility and respect. Avoid any sense of judgment.
- Be open to learn about a variety of faiths and spiritual practices, directly from the other and/or from your own explorations.
- Ask clarifying questions if you are uncertain what the person means by using certain terminology. Also, if they use terminology that is familiar to you, do not assume you know what they mean; ask, "What does prayer mean to you?" to allow them to explain in their own terms.
- Allow for the patient's or family's time alone with the spiritual leader and work around those who are grieving without intruding. Remain available to tend to physical needs as necessary.
- Never, by any communication cues, verbal or nonverbal, imply that you question someone else's spiritual beliefs. Respecting everyone's freedom to believe what he or she chooses is one of our most basic rights and is never more important than during the crisis of bereavement.

TAKING THE CHAPTER TO WORK

Engaging a Chaplain
Carlos is a personal care aide with a home health agency that helps people who need assistance with daily living activities, often older adults. He has been a caregiver for Mrs. Sweeny for three years, and her health is beginning to decline. Mrs. Sweeny has come to trust and care deeply for Carlos because of his gentle, friendly manner and genuine care for her. She has trusted sharing many things about her life with Carlos, including more recently her readiness for death. She states that she's lived a long, full life and doesn't desire to linger in a weakened state. Mrs. Sweeny has shared with Carlos previously that she does not believe in God or any higher power. "When I die, that's it," Carlos remembers her saying, "We only get one chance, the end of this life is the end, and the afterlife is just a fairytale." She seemed quite accepting and matter of fact about it.

Carlos has, however, noticed some new things during Mrs. Sweeny's more recent conversations as she talks about her readiness for death. She tends to fidget with her blanket, she doesn't maintain eye contact as readily, and she states emphatically with a monotone voice about being okay with the complete end of life. Carlos suspects that Mrs. Sweeny may be experiencing a spiritual struggle. His particular Christian faith believes in an afterlife, which gives him great comfort, and he believes that Mrs. Sweeny would find comfort in that as well; however, he knows he cannot impose his beliefs on Mrs. Sweeny, nor is he trained to address a spiritual need, so Carlos asks his patient if she would be open to a visit with the agency's interfaith chaplain. He explains that the chaplain has no spiritual agenda; she is available to support the patient in what Mrs. Sweeny determines she needs. Carlos knows that the chaplain will not persuade the patient to any particular belief, including his own, which he'd prefer for the patient but he respects the patient and the chaplain and their independent beliefs and approaches to life and death. Mrs. Sweeny agrees, and Carlos puts in a request for the chaplain. Carlos continues to provide gentle, friendly, skillful care to Mrs. Sweeny, wanting what is best for her, not what he thinks may be best for her.

Cultural Perspectives

As we noted in Chapter 4, learning as much as you can about other cultures will help you communicate more effectively in every area of medicine, including loss, grief, dying, and death.

Culture is a significant factor in the way people address loss, but that does not mean individuals within the same culture behave the same way when grieving. As noted earlier, culture informs our value systems and provides us with guidelines for acceptable and/or expected behavior, but the countless variations across and within cultures leave us largely unable to categorize how people of different cultures deal with dying, death, and grief.

Thinking back to the terminology at the beginning of this chapter, recall that grief is personal, but mourning is the external expression of grief. Mourning rituals help the living pay tribute to the dead. They are influenced by our social customs and/or spiritual beliefs and help in the healthy processing of grieving. Some cultures expect very vocal and demonstrative mourning. Some require large gatherings of family. Some place emphasis on displaying the deceased and others prefer to remember their loved one in health. Some mourn silently; still others may celebrate death with joyful singing and dancing. Those who weep loudly do not necessarily feel grief any more deeply than those who were taught to display only discreet emotion. As with all care interactions with our patients, health care professionals should aim to identify cultural differences and become informed about the values of those we treat, working within their value systems to provide culturally competent care.

Grief and Loss Across the Lifespan

How we experience loss and grief changes from childhood through adulthood. As with different cultures and religions, individuals within each age group have many different coping skills, making it difficult to predict with certainty how any age will respond to grief and loss. The stages of development are addressed in Chapter 4 and they have an impact on how perceptions of loss, death, and grief change as we grow and mature. There is a difference between cognitive developmental understanding and an individual's actual experience of loss, death, and grief at any age and throughout a lifetime.

Children

In the recent past, children lived with extended families of many generations and were aware of the death of family members at an early age. Many lived on farms and witnessed the deaths of livestock as a part of life. Today, death is often initially "experienced" by children as part of an animated movie or video game. Thinking they are protecting their children from grief, some well-meaning parents hide the death of a well-loved pet or quickly provide a replacement before the child has a chance to actively grieve for the one that died. They may tell children that Grandmother is "sleeping" or "passed away," when the idea of passing away means nothing to the child, and the child may become anxious about sleeping and not waking up. Trying to protect children from the reality of loss may prevent them from developing effective coping skills to withstand the intensity of loss when it inevitably occurs.

With limited or unrealistic comprehension of the finality of death, young children may have more difficulty working through the task of grieving. As with adults, how well children cope with grief depends on many factors including their developmental age, how much support they receive from caregivers and other resources, the child's life experiences with other forms of losses, and how many other stressors they may have at this time.

The recognition of death and the grieving process must be reexamined with each new level of development, maturity, and understanding. Preteen children may continue to wonder about death, with questions such as, "Does it hurt?" or "Are animals there?" Some children and young people may think death is a reversible process. At each new stage of development and awareness, children need to reconsider loss until they have matured through the process to acceptance.

Helping children cope with the loss of someone or something significant in their life, even a loved pet, is challenging no matter what the child's age. *Always check with the parent or legal guardian and take your lead from them because you can support and perhaps supplement what they choose to present to the child.* You are not likely to provide direct care related to loss, grief, and death for children without special training. Specially trained professional health care workers, such as child life specialists and medical social workers, in hospitals and other health care settings can support children by using terminology that is developmentally appropriate (Box 7.2). Health care professionals may refer professional psychological help.

COMMUNICATION GUIDELINES

The Child in Grief

You are not likely to communicate grief support for children without specific training, especially when death is involved; again, stay within your scope of practice. However, you may provide care to children experiencing other types of loss and grief.

- **All** communication related to death must be addressed with the parents or legal guardians before addressing this topic with the child. Their views and beliefs must be known and supported.
- Be cautious of using euphemisms; they can be very confusing.
- Encourage questions, but do not press; simply be available when the child feels the need to talk.
- Explain that it is normal to feel sad, lonely, or angry with loss.
- Help parents/guardians to understand that regression to more dependent stages is not uncommon, such as bedwetting or fear of being alone.
- Grieving may manifest in headaches, nightmares, phantom illnesses, decreased school performance, and social challenges.

BOX 7.2 HEALTH CARE SPECIALISTS FOR HELPING CHILDREN DEAL WITH LOSS

Medical social workers assess patient and family emotional, physical, and psychological needs to recover from and/or adapt to illness. This may involve coordinating equipment, transportation, counseling, referrals, support groups, and much more, depending on need. Medical social workers are employed by hospitals; residential treatment centers; skilled nursing, assisted living and memory care facilities; retirement communities; hospice; and veteran treatment centers, among others. They require either a Master of Social Worker (MSW) or Licensed Clinical Social Worker (LCSW) degree.

Child life specialists are pediatric health care professionals who provide age-appropriate preparation for children and families facing illness, recovery, and disability in hospital settings. They tend to the psychosocial needs of children, allowing the medical professionals to tend to the medical needs. They require being a Certified Child Life Specialist (CCLS).

Adolescents

Developmentally adolescents are better able to conceptualize death than younger individuals. Loss and grief are more common in teen literature and movies about adolescents. Some adolescents directly experience or are indirectly influenced by violence and death in their communities, perhaps also in their schools. Deaths in this age group tend to be more unexpected, sudden, and traumatic. Almost half of the deaths among those aged 12 to 19 years are caused by accidents, with one-third of all teenage deaths owing to motor vehicle accidents (Fig. 7.7) (Miniño, 2010). This age group is more likely to experience the loss of a classmate than of a family member, other than a grandparent. Because so many adolescents utilize the internet and social media in their daily lives, they also are inclined to use these sources for support when grieving; depending on the health level of their coping skills, they may access healthy online resources or unhealthy online resources. Referrals and supportive resources for this age may be fewer than those targeted to younger children and adults. Teens may be more withdrawn or private in their grief, not sure how to identify or separate the grief from the many other normal developmental changes they simultaneously are experiencing in their lives. Communicate patience, presence, genuine care, seeking clarification and referrals for additional support.

The Dying Child/Adolescent. Coping with anticipated and actual loss and grief of a dying child is especially challenging and health care professionals who work in pediatrics will have specific related training. Referrals to health care professionals, such as child life specialists, medical social workers, chaplains, or other trained professionals or support groups, can be sources of comfort and support for the child and family. Families cope better when they know what to expect, such as how much pain the child will experience, whether pain can be managed and how it will be managed, how debilitating it will be, and how long it may last. The child also needs age-appropriate explanations.

Your most effective and therapeutic measure is to support and comfort parents to cope with the situation as calmly and with as much preparation as possible, within your scope of practice. Calm acceptance also helps soothe the child, who may pick up on his parents' anxiety or sadness.

Remember the siblings and families of a dying child. Other children in the family may resent the time and attention denied them and feel guilty about these perfectly natural

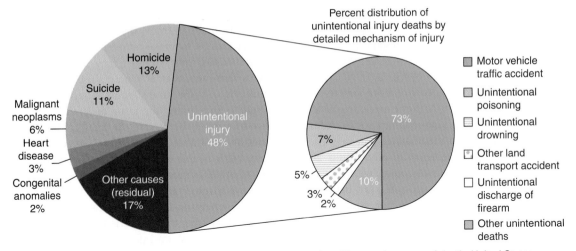

Fig. 7.7 Percent distribution of all deaths to teenagers age 12 to 19 years, by cause of death: United States, 1999–2006. (From Miniño AM. *Mortality among teenagers aged 12–19 years: United States, 1999–2006.* Hyattsville, MD: National Center for Health Statistics; 2010. Retrieved October 9, 2018, from https://www.cdc.gov/nchs/data/databriefs/db37.pdf.)

▶▶ TAKING THE CHAPTER TO WORK

Concern for a Family Member

Let's meet Hyun, a certified nursing assistant (CNA) at a children's hospital on the oncology floor. She is assigned to care for 10-year old Toby, who is dying of leukemia. Toby's parents are very attentive and one or the other parent is with Toby at all times. When both parents visit together, they bring Toby's siblings, who are 6-year old Anna and 13-year old Troy. The floor has a separate room for patient siblings that includes a variety of toys, puzzles, books, art materials, and video screens. When the entire family arrives, Hyun notices that after kissing Toby, Anna immediately runs to the sibling room and begins to draw pictures and play with some of the toys and occasionally another child. Hyun notices that Troy greets Toby with high energy, a smile and fist bump, talks animatedly with Toby for a bit and teases him, then when he leaves Toby's room, Troy slowly slumps down the hallway with low energy and no discernable expression on his face. Troy often walks past the sibling room to another sitting area, not designated for children, and becomes absorbed in his smartphone, often wearing earpieces.

The hospital encourages the CNAs to engage with patient families as part of their overall care. Hyun frequently observes CNAs sitting with Anna, who readily laughs and chats with them as she draws or plays; Anna rarely seems to be alone. Hyun has not observed CNAs engaging with Troy, so she decides to do so and stands near the adolescent, who eventually looks up at her without any expression.

"Hi. I'm Hyun, and I help care for your brother. You're Troy, right?"

"Yeah."

"I like your phone case. I have the same one in red."

"The red one is cool."

"Do you mind if I sit down, Troy?"

Troy shrugs his shoulders and returns to his phone screen. "I don't want to interrupt you if you're listening to something."

"Nah, it's okay," and Troy removes one earpiece, leaving the other in, but still keeps his focus on his phone screen.

Hyun is careful to keep the conversation focused on Troy and not Toby or Anna. "Do you live nearby?"

"No, about an hour away."

"Wow, that's far. Is it hard for you to make that long trip?"

"I miss hanging out with my friends."

"I can imagine that would be hard."

"Yeah."

Troy continues to look at his screen and Hyun sits in silence. She is pleased to have established some contact with Troy, but senses this encounter isn't going to go any further. She thanks Troy for chatting with her and says that she'll see him another time. Troy nods silently and reinserts his other earpiece. Hyun is concerned that Troy's needs during this challenging time in his family are not being addressed. She decides to inform the hospital's child life specialist about her encounter with Troy and to ask him to meet Troy during the family's next visit.

feelings. Every family member, no matter how strong he or she appears to be, needs comfort. Again, child life specialists and medical social workers are an invaluable resource.

Adults

Compared with children, adults have more time to plan and anticipate their mortality as they experience the loss of health or death among their contemporaries. Adults have typically experienced many losses and may have worked on coping with them realistically. Adults also may choose unhealthy means of coping with loss and grief, such as substance abuse (addressed in Chapter 6), risky behavior, and poor choices. Where adults are in their life span has an impact on how they process loss and grief and their readiness to accept mortality.

Younger adults often think they are "immortal" and have often had fewer direct experiences of significant grief. Young adults are more likely to die of accidents or acute diseases with little or no time to plan. They may leave young children and complicated family affairs, which magnifies the grief response and makes survivor grief more intense. Family and caregivers may feel that their loved one's life was cut short.

Middle-aged adults may have accomplished many of their life plans and have a more realistic view of life and loss, and often of death. Many middle-aged adults are sandwiched between caring directly or indirectly for ill and/or aging parents while still providing care to their own children; they may be experiencing anticipated grief at the loss through death of a parent as well as the loss of their children leaving home. These adults have more direct experiences of loss and grief and in establishing a means of coping with and mourning their losses.

Most older adults have fewer pressing obligations, such as young children or career objectives. However, they experience an acceleration of loss and grief in their lives, such as loss of friends, health, ability, meaning and purpose, autonomy, independence, mobility, and physical living space. They may have fewer available support resources, finances, friends, and available family members. Many may also have less fear of death and some may even welcome death if they feel they have lived a full life or desire to avoid any more illness, pain, or suffering.

SUPPORT RESOURCES

Most communities have valuable active groups to support patients and families who are experiencing loss

and grief. If the loss involves health, but the patient is not terminally ill, most diseases and disorders have support groups to make adjustment to the condition less traumatic. Such support may be in the form of groups that meet regularly on a drop-in or registered status (Fig. 7.8). Because support groups are composed of people undergoing the same or similar losses, they serve to remind the grieving individual that he or she is not alone. Rather than feeling isolated, the support group helps people identify similar experiences in the lives of others. Often the support group has members who have adapted to their new circumstances following loss, which helps instill hope in newer group members. Besides discussing their experiences emotionally, support groups also share information, coping strategies, and resources that help the healing process; some even engage in outside activities to promote social growth.

Identify the various grief support groups in your area to recommend to patients, families, and caregivers. Community-based agencies and some health care facilities may offer free or low-fee grief support and individual grief support sessions. Some people will prefer to process their grief one-on-one; others will choose to process their grief in the company of others. Grief support groups may include those addressing the loss of a parent, a child, a sibling, a spouse/partner, or a pet; age-related groups for children, adolescents, adults, and seniors; groups for different gender identification; and groups for death by homicide, suicide, and specific types of illnesses/diseases. Grief support workshops may include art therapy with certified art therapists, play acting, surviving the holidays and/or significant anniversaries, and many more.

The internet also provides many options to find information and support, especially for unique and rare illnesses and losses. Before you divulge personal medical information and experiences use discretion and take time to research websites and support groups carefully, getting referrals when possible, to make sure that the sites are legitimate. So many official-looking scamming and phishing sites will misuse your information. Types and levels of support groups are covered more fully in Chapter 3, "Educating Patients."

Support does not necessarily need to be an organized group; as noted in Chapter 3, a strong group of close friends can be just as effective. This is seen in groups of widows or widowers who meet and share grief and joy in their mutual circumstances. Many times these groups are more supportive than formal groups of strangers,

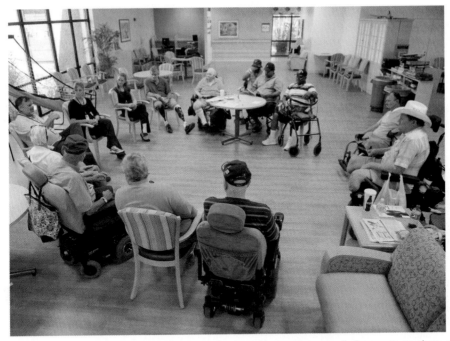

Fig. 7.8 An amputee support group for Veterans who have lost one or more limbs meets to share experiences. The group also participates in recovery-based recreational activities, such as fishing and sports. (Photo by Jason W. Dangel/U.S. Dept. of Veteran Affairs.)

even with the common interest of illness. The familiarity of shared history with friends is very comforting.

As with all other coping measures, patients must make decisions that bring them comfort. Trying to promote what we think is best for patients will only increase stress. Also, as previously mentioned, referrals to trained health care professionals within many health care systems include child life specialists, medical social workers, as well as chaplains and possible grief support counselors.

HOSPICE

Hospice is a specific type of care for patients facing the end of life that focuses on pain management and emotional support. This care provides palliative comfort measures, not curative treatment. Medicare, which covers most hospice costs, pays for this type of care when the patient has a prognosis of 6 or fewer months. Hospice provides holistic care, respecting patient's choices for medical, emotional, social, and spiritual needs and support. Comfort and compassion are provided with no medical measures against the patient's wishes and within the guidelines of Medicare. Hospice patients

may reside in skilled nursing facilities, memory care facilities, independent living facilities, assisted living settings, and licensed residential board and care facilities, as well as at home.

Hospice interdisciplinary teams consist of providers, nurses, medical social workers, home health aides, nutritionists, pharmacists, grief counselors, and volunteers, as well as others. They provide medical, psychosocial, and spiritual care to patients, family members, and caregivers (who may be hired personal caregivers or those employed by facilities) to support their adjustment to the approaching loss. They address what to expect in the death process, funeral arrangements, financial concerns, and grief. Many hospice organizations train volunteers to provide respite care, allowing for temporary time off/away for the caregiver. If the dying patient is at home, a hospice provider may arrange inpatient respite care where the patient stays at a hospital or other facility for up to 5 days to give the caregiver time to rest. Some volunteers provide music and pet therapy (Fig. 7.9) (see Spotlight on Success box).

After a death, at a time when many friends of the family have said their goodbyes and returned to their normal life, hospice provides grief support services

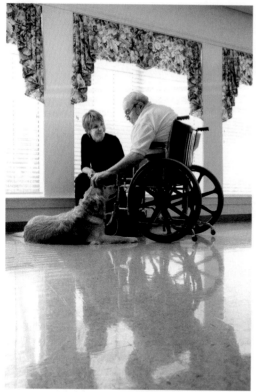

Fig. 7.9 A therapy dog and his volunteer visit a patient in hospice care. (iStock.com/iophoto.)

that may include individual and group counseling, art therapy, and many other support services mentioned above to assist with grieving and mourning. Many not-for-profit community-based hospices provide grief support services education programs for the community that are not limited to only hospice patients and their families.

CHECKING YOUR COMPREHENSION

Write a brief answer for each of the following assignments.

1. Explain the difference between an actual and a perceived loss. Give an example of each.
2. Define grieving, mourning, and bereavement and explain how they differ.
3. In the dominant U.S. culture, how have perspectives on death changed from 1900 to today? How would physicians from 1900, 1965, and today differ in their discussion of death with patients?
4. What do all the theories of loss and grieving discussed in this chapter have in common? How does the dual process theory differ from other conceptualizations?
5. List things you should *not* do when caring for a grieving patient, family member, or caregiver.
6. Describe how a 5-year-old's understanding of death differs from that of an adolescent.
7. Describe how a young adult's understanding of death differs from that of an older adult.
8. List two health care specialists who can be particularly beneficial in helping patients/families/caregivers address matters of loss and grief.
9. Explain the function of hospice care and how it differs from other areas of health care.
10. List six members of the hospice interdisciplinary team.

EXPANDING CRITICAL THINKING

1. If you found studying this chapter difficult or unsettling, describe your feelings as you worked through the subject.
2. In 50 words or fewer, explain how you feel about death. Consider death for yourself or for those close to you. Do you see death as a natural part of life or do you avoid considering the prospect?
3. Do you fear the unknown or do you have faith that only good will come to you after death?
4. If you knew the day of your death, would you live differently? If so, what would you do?
5. What do you want to accomplish before you die?
6. How would you say "goodbye" to those you love?
7. How would you want those you love to say "goodbye" to you?
8. What technologic measures would you refuse at the end (i.e., endotracheal tube, IVs, automated external defibrillator [AED] chemotherapy), or would you request that every measure be used to keep you alive? Would you make the same choices for those you love?
9. How do you think your view of death differs from your parents, grandparents, or younger siblings?
10. Write your own obituary and epitaph.
11. How does your family grieve? How does this differ from your friends or classmates?

Communicating in the Workplace

Linda Boyd

CHAPTER OUTLINE

LEARNING OBJECTIVES

On successfully completing this chapter, you will be able to:
1. Explain the characteristics of professionalism.
2. Explain the provisions of HIPAA regarding patient privacy.
3. Explain the purpose of a case conference.
4. Describe the format of a meeting.
5. Describe common communication challenges and the strategies to overcome them when communicating with coworkers, physicians, managers, and regulatory agency personnel.
6. Discuss the best practices for communicating as a manager.
7. Demonstrate professionalism when communicating over the telephone.
8. Demonstrate professionalism when communicating over email.
9. Demonstrate professionalism when writing business letters.

KEY TERMS

agenda in meeting, a list of what will be discussed and in what order

blind carbon copy (bcc) a sending option used in email when the sender wants to include someone on the email for information only, but the individual's identity is not shared with other recipients

business associate Classification under HIPAA for a contracted vendor who uses protected health information to perform a service on behalf of a covered entity.

covered entity Classification under HIPAA for an organization that collects and manages health information, such as a provider.

carbon copy (cc) sending option in emails when the sender wants to include someone on the email for information only and are not expecting that individual to respond

case conference cohesive group of interdisciplinary professionals coming together to coordinate patient treatment

consultation to obtain advice or another opinion from a specialist regarding any aspect of patient care

emergent condition or situation that needs immediate attention

Health Insurance Portability and Accountability Act (HIPAA) passed into law in 1996 by Congress and enforced in full in 2003 to ensure equal access to certain health and human services and protects the privacy and security of health information

interdisciplinary combination of two or more specialties working together to meet a specific goal

minutes summary record of what took place at a meeting

protected health information (PHI) under the law, any health information, such as medical history or current status, that can be linked to an individual

professionalism skills, judgments, and behaviors that are expected in the workplace

referral formal contract between two or more health care team members to provide services to a patient

STAT requiring an immediate response

Triage a process of determining the degree of sickness and placing the patient into an appropriate level of care

💡 TEST YOUR COMMUNICATION IQ

Before reading this chapter, complete this short self-assessment test. Decide which statements are true and which are false.

1. It is permissible to call a physician "Doc"; this is friendlier.
2. You should never communicate with a regulatory agency investigator without the permission of your supervisor.
3. When discussing problems with coworkers, it is important to tell them how their behavior makes you feel and how it affects your ability to work.
4. Any sudden deterioration in a patient's condition is an example of an urgent situation to communicate to a physician.
5. As a manager, you should communicate sympathy and, not empathy, to your staff.
6. Phrases such as "that won't work" should be avoided when speaking to your manager.

Results

Statements 3 and 6 are true; all the other statements are false. How did you do? Read the chapter to find more information on these topics.

INTRODUCTION

The previous chapters have focused on communicating with patients. However, you will also be communicating with coworkers and other members of the health care team. Workplace communication must be professional and courteous and should be based on ethical and legal integrity. In this chapter we discuss behaviors and skills of successful health care professionals, specifically the importance of professionalism, team collaboration, and respecting patient privacy when discussing their care with others. We discuss the display of professionalism through effective communication. Not only are professionalism and good communication important to learn now, they are attributes and skills that can continually improve throughout one's career.

Being able to communicate effectively with other health care professionals is critical because poor and ineffective communication can harm patients' lives. Better communication in patient care leads to better health outcomes and improved overall quality of care for patients, as well as increased patient satisfaction, greater patient safety, and fewer medical errors and malpractice lawsuits. Effective communication skills can be learned and continuously improved through professional commitment and practice. Working environments where colleagues effectively communicate see better relationships and less staff turnover. Furthermore, there is a direct relationship between job satisfaction for health care professionals and their ability to show compassion and warmth to patients. Health care professionals are more satisfied in work environments where they feel supported, respected, and valued, where they have clearly defined job roles and experience work equity and fair compensation. By extension, those health care professionals who have effective communication skills are more likely to have successful careers.

PROFESSIONALISM

Professionalism is defined as the skills, judgments, and behaviors that are expected in the workplace. Health care professionals must be honest and show integrity in the work that they do. Each health care professional must be responsible for his or her own behavior and work products or outcomes. In a health care setting, professionalism may include, but is not limited to the following.

- Showing respect for the humanity of others
- Being polite and dependable
- Safeguarding patient privacy
- Following ethical guidelines
- Maintaining accurate and timely health records

A hallmark of professionalism is the characteristic of being respectful to others, no matter who they are or why they are in the workplace. From patients and their families, to support services personnel of all types, peers, providers, and facility administrators, everyone must be treated with dignity and respect. Accept each person's contribution to the health care team. No one person or position is more important than another. This means listening to others and valuing their concerns and ideas. It also means being honest with others in the workplace about where things stand; your coworkers will decide their actions based on the information you provide them; therefore, dishonesty can be disrespectful to their efforts at work. Honesty also directly influences your reliability as a person. The importance of dependability is the fostering of trust, which is at the center of all types of relationships. When people follow through on promises and commitments, they become more trustworthy. Dependability at work affects behaviors, both large and small. Simply returning a phone call when promised or completing tasks in a timely manner promotes trust in work relationships. Showing up late makes you an unreliable individual and is disrespectful to others expecting you to be in a certain place at a certain time. In the bigger picture, your dependability reflects how you carry yourself at work. Are you pleasant and positive, even when the job gets trying and difficult? A person who becomes irritable, pessimistic, or scattered when stressful situations arise does not display dependability.

Another characteristic of a professional is being helpful to others. When you notice a coworker struggling with too many tasks, offer to pitch in. Share your experience and understanding of the best ways to get things done. Support new team members by slowing down and showing them what to do.

Professionalism also means staying work-focused and, in health care, this means staying patient-focused. You can show respect by responding to the patient as a person using the guidelines presented throughout this text. In their actions, health care professionals must put the patients' needs and safety above all other priorities. This means that responsiveness to patient needs supersedes not only self-interest, but also the operations of the health care setting. There are times when putting the patient first is not the easiest option. For example, consider a difficult patient with whom the nurse has developed a good rapport. Right before her lunch break, the nurse discovers he has soiled himself and will need a sponge bath and new dressings. The nurse knows this care will go most smoothly if she is present, so she takes the extra time to introduce the nurse on the next shift and assure the patient he is in good hands. When health care professionals consistently behave in a way that puts the patient's needs first, they display a work-focus that will in turn earn them the respect of their coworkers.

COMMUNICATION GUIDELINES

Professionalism
Listed below are guidelines to remember for communicating professionally in the workplace.
- Be pleasant, polite, and optimistic. Greet others, be energetic, and smile. Patients, especially, should never see anything but your best self.
- Mind your use of words and phrases. Do not swear or cuss, do not talk about inappropriate topics, and do not make vulgar jokes. Avoid any type of communication that may alienate or offend a coworker or patient.
- Do not gossip with other team members or patients. For example, it is unprofessional to say, "Did you hear that Dr. Raymond is getting a divorce?" or "I heard that he is involved in a big malpractice case."
- Never criticize or question a peer's performance or professionalism in front of other colleagues or patients. Instead say, "Before we leave today, I would like to talk with you about something. Can we meet in the lounge at 3 pm?" and bring the discussion into a private area.
- Do not let your private life detract from your performance at work. Confiding in a coworker is common and acceptable, but do not let your personal problems dominate the workplace.
- Accept everyone. Value individual skills and strengths and accept weaknesses and, in turn, others will accept your strengths and weaknesses.
- Stay within your boundaries. It is not your job to discipline or reprimand another employee. The supervisor must handle these tasks.

WORDS AT WORK

The following phrases promote communication and dialogue. Do use these phrases.
"Let's talk about it."
"You did a great job with …."
"Let's try it this way."
"I need some advice."
"How would you handle this problem?"
"How can I help you?"
"I'll be free in 5 minutes to help you."
    The following phrases hinder communication and halt dialogue. Do not use these phrases.
"Are you out of your mind?"
"You're lazy."
"You're crazy."
"You don't know what you are talking about."
"I can't help you."

THE HEALTH INFORMATION PORTABILITY AND ACCOUNTABILITY ACT

Health care professionals are legally bound to be confidential and not share information, discuss, or disclose patient information with anyone, including family, friends, or another health care professional, without the consent of the patient. Although parts of the law are aimed at other facets of health care, the Health Insurance Portability and Accountability Act (HIPAA) of 1996 is the primary legislation protecting individuals' private information. HIPAA limits the communication of all protected health information (PHI), defined as health data that can be identified with an individual. This means that any information concerning the patient's health status connected to the patient's name, address, telephone number, date of birth, or other identification must be kept strictly confidential. The identifying information must be associated with the health information, such as on a laboratory report or hospital bill. These documents would contain a patient's name and/or other identifying information associated with the health data. It is important to note that identifying information alone would not be designated as PHI. Violations of HIPAA, even accidental, can result in termination of employment and large fines.

Under Title II of HIPAA, the Privacy Rule provides protection for the privacy of health information, but does not interfere with patients' access to health care or the quality of health care delivery. It governs the use of patient personal information by covered entities—any organizations that obtain and manage health information—in the way health information is held, stored, or transmitted. Covered entities include health care providers, health plans (insurers), and health care clearinghouses (Table 8.1). It also affects business associates—vendors who contract with covered entities and use health information in the course of providing a service. Some examples of business associates might be a transcription or translation service, accrediting agency, or software vendor. It stipulates who may access the information and under what conditions access is given. The Privacy Rule encompasses all modes of communication, including electronic data, paper documents, and oral communication.

When disclosing or using PHI, health care professionals must only use or disclose the minimum amount of PHI necessary to meet the request or the intended purpose. Further, they should have limited access to only the PHI they need to fulfill their task or duties. For example, imagine a medical assistant sees a friend in the waiting room one afternoon, but is not involved in her friend's care. The medical assistant is not permitted to seek out any information about his health status or treatment. She cannot look at her friend's health record to see why they were in the office today and she cannot ask her coworkers for any information about her friend unless

TABLE 8.1	**Covered Entities**
Type	**Examples**
Health plan	• Dental insurance provider • Vision insurance provider • Health insurance provider • Employer group plan • Medicaid • Medicare • Military or veterans group plans
Clearinghouse	• Billing entity • Repricing company • Any business that facilitates or processes protected health information (PHI)
Provider	• Doctor • Dentist • Psychiatrist • Psychologist • Chiropractor • Pharmacy • Nursing home • Clinic

From Elsevier. *Introduction to Health Services Administration.* St. Louis: Elsevier; 2018.

the medical assistant needs this information to provide patient care. Discussing the patient's complaint or condition is a violation of patient privacy and an improper disclosure of health information because the patient did not authorize the disclosure and the medical assistant did not need the information to care for the patient. A physician caring for a patient, on the other hand, can and must see a patient's entire medical record to perform his or her job.

The law protects health information even between spouses and close family relations. A husband may not know about his wife's health condition unless his spouse lists him as an authorized person. If a patient's father is a doctor within the health system, the doctor may not view his child's health record without his child's consent.

Remember that not all communication about a patient's health is PHI, however. In many cases, a patient is not identified by name; conversely, a patient may be identified, but nothing about his or her health is discussed. For instance, patients in a waiting room are commonly called by their first name and, in hospitals, patient names are sometimes placed on charts outside hospital rooms.

To protect patient privacy every effort should be made for health care professionals to speak with patients in a private space and to avoid discussions with colleagues in public areas, such as hallways, elevators, parking lots, and the waiting room.

Of course, there are many occasions when health information can or must be shared. Patients are routinely referred to other doctors, they may get transferred to a different facility, or they may want a second opinion. In these cases the patient will authorize the release of information (ROI), discussed in greater detail in Chapter 9.

INTERDISCIPLINARY COMMUNICATION

Communicating with various health care workers is termed *interdisciplinary communication.* Interdisciplinary is the combination of two or more specialties working together to meet a specific goal. The main goal of interdisciplinary communication is to promote optimal patient care. Table 8.2 lists medical specialties; Table 8.3 lists licensed health care professions; and Table 8.4 lists the various allied professions recognized by the American Medical Association. Each specialty provides a unique viewpoint and treatment plan for the patient and family. Interdisciplinary communication also

- Promotes teamwork, therefore improving staff productivity and efficiency
- Improves the patient care environment
- Meets the requirements of various regulatory agencies
- Helps to create or revise policies and procedures that affect more than one department

Referrals

Patients are often referred to specialists for specific health care issues. A referral is a formal contract between two or more health care team members to provide services to a patient. Patients can be referred to specialties, such as those listed in Table 8. Other common referrals include home care agencies, social services, and various financial support

TABLE 8.2 Common Medical Specialties and Subspecialties	
Physician Specialty	**Description**
Allergist	Diagnoses and treats patients who have strong reactions to pollen, insect bites, food, medication, and other irritants
Anesthesiologist	Administers substances that cause loss of sensation, particularly during surgery
Cardiologist	Diagnoses and treats patients with diseases of the heart and blood vessels
Dermatologist	Diagnoses and treats patients with diseases of the skin
Family practitioner	Delivers primary health care for patients of all ages
Gastroenterologist	Diagnoses and treats patients with diseases of the digestive system
Gynecologist	Diagnoses, treats, and provides care to women with disorders of their reproductive system
Hospitalist	Employed by a hospital; medical practice focuses on patient care situations specific to acute care settings
Neonatologist	Diagnoses and treats diseases and abnormal conditions of newborns
Obstetrician	Cares for women before, during, and after delivery
Oncologist	Diagnoses and treats patients with cancer
Ophthalmologist	Diagnoses and treats patients with diseases of the eye
Orthopedist	Diagnoses and treats patients with diseases of the muscles and bones
Pathologist	Studies changes in cells, tissue, and organs to diagnose diseases and/or to determine possible treatments
Pediatrician	Delivers health care to children
Psychiatrist	Diagnoses and treats patients with disorders of the mind
Radiologist	Uses radiography and other tools to diagnose and treat a variety of diseases

From Davis NA. *Foundations of Health Information Management*, ed 4. St. Louis: Elsevier; 2017.

TABLE 8.3 Licensed Health Care Professions

Title	Credential	Job Description
Certified nurse midwife	CNM	RN with additional training and certification; performs physical examinations; prescribes medications, including contraceptive methods; orders laboratory tests as needed; provides prenatal care, gynecologic care, labor and birth care; and health education and counseling to women of all ages
Diagnostic cardiac sonographer or vascular technologist	DCS or DVT	Assists in the diagnosis and treatment of cardiac and vascular diseases and disorders; performs noninvasive tests, including echocardiographs and electrocardiographs
Emergency medical technician	EMT	Progresses through several levels of training, each providing more advanced skills. EMT's medical education encompasses managing respiratory, cardiac, and trauma cases and often emergency childbirth. Some states also recognize specialties in the EMT field, such as EMT-Cardiac, which includes training in cardiac arrhythmias, and EMT-Shock Trauma, which includes starting intravenous fluids and administering specific medications
Licensed practical or vocational nurse	LPN or LVN	Provides bedside care, assisting with the day-to-day personal care of inpatients; assesses patients, documents their progress, and administers medications and intravenous fluids when allowed by law; often works in hospitals or skilled nursing facilities and in physicians' offices.
Medical technologist	MT	Performs diagnostic testing on blood, body fluids, and other types of specimens to assist the provider in arriving at a diagnosis.
Nurse anesthetist	NA	Registered Nurse (RN) who administers anesthetics to patients during care provided by surgeons, physicians, dentists, or other qualified health professionals.
Nurse practitioner	NP	Provides basic patient care services, including diagnosing and prescribing medications for common illnesses; must have advanced academic training, beyond the RN degree, and must also have extensive clinical experience.
Occupational therapist	OT	Assists in helping patients compensate for loss of function.
Paramedic	Paramedic	Specially trained in advanced emergency skills to aid patients in life-threatening situations.
Physical therapist	PT	Assists patients in regaining their mobility and improving their strength and range of motion. They devise treatment plans in conjunction with the patient's physician.
Physician assistant	PA	Provides direct patient care services under the supervision of a licensed physician; trained to diagnose and treat patients as directed by the physician and, in most states, are allowed to write prescriptions; take patient histories, order and interpret tests, perform physical examinations, and make diagnostic decisions.

TABLE 8.3 Licensed Health Care Professions—cont'd

Title	Credential	Job Description
Radiology technician	RT	Uses various machines to help the provider diagnose and treat certain diseases; machines may include x-ray equipment, ultrasonographic machines, and magnetic resonance imaging (MRI) scanners.
Registered dietitian	RD	Thoroughly trained in nutrition and the different types of diets patients require to improve or maintain their condition. They design healthy diets for patients during hospital stays and can help plan menus for home use. They also teach patients about their recommended diet.
Registered nurse	RN	Provides direct patient care, assesses patients, and determines care plans; they have many career options.
Respiratory therapist	RT	Commonly uses oxygen therapy to assist with breathing; also performs diagnostic tests that measure lung capacity. Most RTs work in hospitals. All types of patients receive respiratory care, including newborns and geriatric patients.

From Proctor D, Niedzwiecki B, Pepper J, Bhattacharya Madero P. *Kinn's the Administrative Medical Assistant*, ed 13. St. Louis: Elsevier; 2017.

TABLE 8.4 Allied Health Occupations Recognized by the American Medical Association

Title	Credential	Job Description
Anesthesiology assistant	AA	Functions as a specialty physician assistant under the direction of a licensed and qualified anesthesiologist; assists in developing and implementing the anesthesia care plan.
Art therapist	ATR	Uses drawings and other art and media forms to assess, treat, and rehabilitate patients with mental, emotional, physical, and/or developmental disorders.
Athletic trainer	ATC	Provides a variety of services, including injury prevention, assessment, immediate care, treatment, and rehabilitation after physical injury or trauma.
Audiologist	CCC-A	Identifies individuals with symptoms of hearing loss and other auditory, balance, and related neural problems; assesses the nature of those problems and helps individuals manage them.
Blood bank technology specialist	SBB	Performs routine and specialized tests in blood center and transfusion services, using methods that conform to the accepted standards in the blood bank industry.
Diagnostic cardiovascular sonographer/technologist	RDCS, RVT	Using invasive or noninvasive techniques (or both), performs diagnostic examinations and therapeutic interventions for the heart and blood vessels at the request of a physician.
Clinical laboratory science/ medical technologist	MT, MLT	In conjunction with pathologists, performs tests to diagnose the causes and nature of disease; also develops data on blood, tissues, and fluids of the human body using a variety of methodologies.

(Continued)

TABLE 8.4 Allied Health Occupations Recognized by the American Medical Association—cont'd

Title	Credential	Job Description
Counseling-related professional	LPC, LMHC	Deals with human development through support, therapeutic approaches, consultation, evaluation, teaching, and research; practices the art of helping people to grow.
Cytotechnologist	CT	Works with pathologists to evaluate cellular material from all body sites, primarily through use of the microscope; examines specimens for normal and abnormal cytologic changes, including malignancies.
Dance therapist	DTR, ADTR	Uses the psychotherapeutic properties of movement as a process that furthers the emotional, cognitive, social, and physical integration of the patient as a tool for healing.
Dental assistant, dental hygienist, dental laboratory technician	CDA, RDH, CDT	Performs a wide range of tasks, from assisting the dentist to teaching patients how to prevent oral disease and maintain oral health.
Diagnostic medical sonographer	RDMS	Uses medical ultrasound to gather sonographic data, which can aid in the diagnosis of a variety of conditions and diseases; also monitors fetal development.
Dietitian, dietetic technician	DTR	Integrates and applies the principles of food science, nutrition, biochemistry, physiology, food management, and behavior to achieve and maintain good health.
Electroneurodiagnostic technologist	REEG-T	Records and studies the electrical activity of the brain and nervous system; obtains interpretable recordings of patients' nervous system function.
Genetics counselor	IGC	Provides genetic services to individuals and families seeking information about the occurrence or risk of a genetic condition or birth defect.
Health information management professional	RHIA, RHIT	Provides expert assistance in the systems and processes for health information management, including planning, engineering, administration, application, and policy making.
Kinesiotherapist	RKT	Provides rehabilitation exercise and education designed to reverse or minimize debilitation and enhance the functional capacity of medically stable patients.
Massage therapist	MT	Applies manual techniques, and may apply adjunctive techniques, with the intention of positively affecting the health and well-being of a patient or client.
Medical assistant	CMA, RMA, CCMA, CMAA	Functions as a member of the health care delivery team and performs both administrative and clinical procedures and duties; a multiskilled health professional.
Medical illustrator	MI	Specializes in the visual display and communication of scientific information; creates visuals and designs communication tools for teaching both medical professionals and the public.
Music therapist	MT-BC	Uses music in a therapeutic relationship to address the physical, emotional, cognitive, and social needs of individuals of all ages; assesses the strengths and needs of clients and patients.

TABLE 8.4 Allied Health Occupations Recognized by the American Medical Association—cont'd

Title	Credential	Job Description
Nuclear medicine technologist	RT	Uses the nuclear properties of radioactive and stable nuclides to make diagnostic evaluations of anatomic or physiologic conditions of the body; also provides therapy with unsealed radioactive sources.
Ophthalmic laboratory technician, medical technician/technologist	COT, COMT	Collects data and performs clinical evaluations; performs tests and protocols required by ophthalmologists; assists in the treatment of patients.
Orthoptist	CO	Performs a series of diagnostic tests and measurements on patients with visual disorders; helps design a treatment plan to correct disorders of vision, eye movements, and alignment.
Orthotist/prosthetist	RTO, RTP, RTPO	Designs and fits devices (orthoses) to patients who have disabling conditions of the limbs and spine and/or partial or total absence of a limb.
Perfusionist	CCP	Operates extracorporeal circulation and autotransfusion equipment during any medical situation in which the patient's respiratory or circulatory function must be supported or temporarily replaced.
Pharmacy technician	CPhT	Assists pharmacists with duties that do not require the expertise or judgment of a licensed pharmacist.
Radiation therapist, radiographer	RRTD	Delivers prescribed dosages of radiation to patients for therapeutic purposes; provides appropriate patient care and maintains accurate records of the treatment provided.
Rehabilitation counselor	CRC	Determines and coordinates services to assist people with disabilities in moving from psychological and economic dependence to independence.
Respiratory therapist, respiratory therapy technician	RRT, CRT, RPFT, CPFT	Evaluates, treats, and manages patients of all ages with respiratory illnesses and other cardiopulmonary disorders. Advanced respiratory therapists exercise considerable independent judgment.
Surgical assistant	CSA	Assists in exposure, hemostasis, closure, and other intraoperative technical functions that help surgeons carry out a safe operation with optimal results for the patient.
Surgical technologist	ST, CST	Helps prepare patients for surgery and maintain the sterile field in the surgical suite, making sure all members of the surgical team follow sterile technique.
Therapeutic recreation specialist	CTRS	Uses treatment, education, and recreation services to help people with illnesses, disabilities, and other conditions develop and use their leisure in ways that enhance their health.

From Proctor D, Niedzwiecki B, Pepper J, Bhattacharya Madero P. *Kinn's the Administrative Medical Assistant*, ed 13. St. Louis: Elsevier; 2017.

services. Physicians often speak to other physicians about specific care issues. For example, an internist may refer a patient to a cardiologist for evaluation and management of the patient's cardiac pathologies. The cardiologist will then treat the patient for his heart problems and the internist will continue to treat the patient's other conditions.

A consultation is different. In a consultation the patient goes to a specialist for an evaluation. Then, the consultant recommends a treatment plan to the primary care doctor. The patient's primary doctor will then treat the condition.

Referrals and consultations are made after discussing the problem with the patient. The patient has the right to accept or refuse another's professional services. For example, the physician may choose to refer the patient to a home care agency for home health aide services, but the patient can refuse the service. However, there are exceptions to this rule. If the physician or other health care provider feels the patient or family member needs the services from a protective service agency, the patient or caregiver cannot refuse these services without a court order.

Guidelines for Referrals

You will be involved with assisting the provider in making referrals. Referrals begin with a physician's order. In the order the physician will communicate to you the following information.
- Type of services needed
- Date services should begin
- Duration of service or goals of the service
- Specific instructions. For example, the physician may refer a patient to a physical therapist for crutch-walking education, but may specify the patient is to be "non–weight-bearing for 3 weeks, then begin progressive weight-bearing as tolerated."

Depending on the health care facility where you work, there may be "standing orders" allowing you to make certain referrals. For example, a standing order may state, "Refer new patient with type 2 diabetes to a diabetes educator for glucose monitoring instruction." In this case, the order is already written and you may begin the referral process without consulting the physician.

Follow all HIPAA regulations and make sure the patient has signed an ROI form. The ROI should include the patient's name, date, signatures, and any specific guidelines regarding who can and cannot be given patient information (see Chapter 9).

After the order is written and the ROI is completed the referral request can be made. Either an oral or a written report should then be sent to the appropriate agency. If a report has been written use the appropriate agency form. Watch your spelling. Attach any documents, as necessary. Written referrals are generally faxed to the agency. It is important to follow up on written referrals to be sure they were obtained and to determine the progress of the referral.

COMMUNICATION GUIDELINES

Referrals

You can use the acronym **CONSULT** to remember practical tips when referring a patient.

Clarify: Clarify terms that you do not understand before making the call. For example, if the physician wrote, "PT to help with gait training," you should know that PT refers to a physical therapist and understand the basics of the term "gait training." Clarify to which agency the referral is to be made. And finally, clarify that the referral agency can assist you with this case before you start to give a lengthy report only to find that the agency does not offer those services or they cannot meet your time constraints. For example, you may say, "Hello, This is Dr. Robert's office calling with a referral for a patient who needs a physical therapist for gait training in her home. Is this a case that you could help us with?"

Objective data: Give the agency the appropriate demographic data such as the patient's name, age, sex, address, and phone number and then the objective data stating the reason for the referral. For example, "Mrs. Santelgo, an 87-year-old woman, had a fractured ankle 2 weeks ago and needs a home physical therapist to help her."

Necessary past history: Give the agency the patient's pertinent past medical or surgical history. For example, "She has insulin-dependent diabetes and has a short leg cast on her left leg." It is not necessary to list past surgeries or medical conditions unless they affect the plan of care. Additional information regarding past surgeries or medical conditions (e.g., appendectomy, 1974) can be sent on the referral form.

Symptoms/signs: Provide the agency with a list of the specific symptoms or signs the patient is experiencing in relation to the referral need. For example "Her toes on the left foot are ecchymotic, but they are warm and have good capillary refill. She becomes short of breath with minimal exertion."

Unusual circumstances: You should alert the agency to any situations or circumstances that would or could hinder its ability to care for this patient. For example, "She has three big dogs and eight cats." This information is relevant for a home care agency to know so they can select an appropriate physical therapist who is not afraid of dogs or allergic to cats. However, this information would not be necessary to communicate if you were calling an outpatient physical therapy department and the patient was going to be seen inside their facility for gait training.

Looking: Explain in detail what services the patient is looking to obtain. Include any information about time constraints. For example, "She needs to have the physical therapist come in the afternoon. She goes to the outpatient clinic in the mornings for her chemotherapy. She is home by 1 p.m."

Time: Explain to the referring agency when you want or need the services to start. For example, "The doctor would like the services to start this week. Is this possible?" If the agency personnel cannot reasonably guarantee the services, you need to communicate that to the physician so other arrangements can be made.

Stick to the facts. Provide only the facts in a professional, nonjudgmental manner. Do not hide or conceal issues regarding the patient. Do not exaggerate the patient's conditions. Never gossip.

Case Conferences

When communication is based on meeting the needs of a particular patient, it is termed a *case conference*. A case conference is a cohesive group of interdisciplinary professionals coming together to coordinate patient treatment. Case conferences start with each health care worker giving a summary of his or her clinical findings to the rest of the group. Discussion follows. The team works together to prioritize the patient's needs and to create a plan of care.

A case conference can be formally organized or can be an impromptu meeting between professionals from different specialties. Formal case conferences are often planned and organized by the designated team leader. Generally the team leader is the physician, case manager, or social worker. The team leader invites appropriate members of the health care team. Depending on the situation a clergy representative, administrative staff, or regulatory personnel may be invited. In most cases the patient or family is not present. However, depending on the case and the issues, the patient and/or family may be asked to attend a later portion of the conference.

Case conferences can occur anywhere in the health care environment. They occur within hospital settings as well as in ambulatory care settings. The hospital's ethics committee may hold a case conference to discuss the removal of life support devices. In these situations, nonbiased, objective persons are designated to represent and speak on the patient's behalf. Legal council may also be invited to these conferences.

There are certain situations in which a case conference must be held. For example, in a long-term care facility, the Centers for Medicare and Medicaid Services (CMS) require an interdisciplinary case conference to be held periodically for any patient who is receiving Medicare benefits. There are specific guidelines for when and how often these conferences need to be held and who must attend. Medicare requires that a family member or significant other be invited to the meeting. Family members may decline to attend the meeting. Failure to hold these conferences and to document them properly can result in fines and potential loss of the right to bill for certain services.

During any case conference, communicate your clinical findings in an objective manner. It is never appropriate to gossip about the patient or family members or to let your own personal feelings or biases affect your clinical judgment. Any communication or discussion occurring in the meeting must stay in the room. It is not appropriate to discuss the meeting with anyone not associated with the case.

> ## ▶▶ TAKING THE CHAPTER TO WORK
>
> ### A Productive Case Conference
>
> Sue is working in a pediatrician's office. She has been asked to come to a case conference regarding the Flash family. The Flash family consists of a single mother with four children. The father of two of the children is in jail and the paternity of the other children is unclear. The pediatrician begins the case conference by

asking Sue to report on the number of appointments Ms. Flash has cancelled. Sue communicates the information and mentions that Ms. Flash has told her "she does not have a car and transportation is a problem." A social worker mentions that the Flash family is eligible for free bus passes to doctor's appointments. The members discuss the bus pass policy and agree that this is a good solution. The pediatrician directs the social worker to get the passes and have them mailed to Ms. Flash. Then, the pediatrician asks Sue to communicate the bus pass information to Ms. Flash. Sue's ability to communicate the facts in an organized manner allows the team to identify and correct a problem. This improves patient care.

Meetings

One of the most important opportunities for communication is during meetings. Meetings are successful if they are well-organized, well-led by a chairperson, and serve a necessary and focused purpose. Attendees need to be considerate of others and make sure everyone is heard. It is highly recommended that all businesses establish a policy for the use of cell phones during meetings. Cell phones often provide distraction from the meeting and what is being discussed and should always be on silent during a meeting. All attendees should agree not to send or read text messages during the meeting because it is disrespectful to others who may be speaking. If a call needs to be taken, it should always be taken outside the meeting room. Table 8.5 list several common terms used in formal meetings.

Agenda

Every meeting should have an agenda. An **agenda** lists what will take place and be discussed during the meeting. Ideally, the agenda should be sent with the meeting invitation. Agendas promote meeting efficiency because participants can prepare ahead of time for the topics to be discussed. Productive meetings are those that are focused on what needs to be achieved and an agenda can help do this. Figure 8.1 provides an example of an agenda.

Agendas generally include the following items.
- Date and time of the meeting
- Location of the meeting
- List of meeting invitees and any materials they should bring

TABLE 8.5   Terms Used in Meetings

Term	Meaning
Ad hoc	Arranged for a single purpose or work product
Adjournment	Closing or ending of a meeting
Amendment	A proposal to make a change
Quorum	The minimum number of attendees needed to proceed forward with the meeting
Subcommittee	Small subgroup of meeting attendees to deal with a specific project appointed by a larger committee
Unanimous	When all meeting attendees (or members) vote in favor of something

From Elsevier. *Introduction to Health Services Administration.* St. Louis: Elsevier; 2018.

- Topics to be discussed. Topics that were previously discussed should be referred to as "old business"; topics that need to be discussed at the meeting should be referred to as "new business."
- List of any guest speakers
- Attachments may also be added if there are background materials that participants should read ahead of time. If attachments are used, it is helpful to identify on the agenda which attachment goes with which topic to be discussed.

Minutes

During a business meeting, a staff member should be assigned to "take minutes." Meeting **minutes** are a summary record of what took place and what was discussed at a meeting (Fig. 8.2). Meeting minutes typically show
- Who attended and participated in the meeting, as well as those who were absent
- Date and time the meeting was called to order
- Documentation that minutes from the previous meeting were approved and accepted, identifying any amendments made to those minutes
- A summary record of issues that were discussed
- A description of announcements and decisions that were made
- Time the meeting adjourned

AGENDA
Internal Medicine Specialists
Thursday, January 5th, 2020 at 8:00 AM
Conference Room A

CALL TO ORDER

I. Opening Remarks—Dr. Smith

II. Approval of December 21, 2019 minutes—Judy Milton

III. Further discussion of draft inventory survey—Louise Parker

IV. Presentation of most recent Administrative Report—Louise Parker

V. Presentation of most recent Budget Report—Tim Wilton

VI. Announcements—Dr. Smith

VI. Discussion of next steps and confirmation of next meeting date/time
—Dr. Smith

VII. Other Business

ADJOURN

Fig. 8.1 Agenda. (From Elsevier. *Introduction to Health Services Administration.* St. Louis: Elsevier; 2018.)

Meeting minutes serve multiple purposes, including the following.

- Creating documentation for any potential auditing, accrediting, or regulatory purposes with a signature of the person who created the minutes
- Allowing those invitees who missed the meeting to see what happened
- Providing a resource for the next meeting's agenda, including the date, time, and location of the next meeting, if a follow-up meeting is needed. Specifically, the minutes will highlight any outstanding action items to be covered at the next meeting.

The staff member who takes the minutes may be asked to perform duties, such as

- Arrange the meeting date, time, and place
- Send the invitation to potential attendees
- Draft the agenda
- Circulate the agenda to attendees (ideally with the meeting appointment)
- Take notes at the meeting
- Draft, proofread, and get approval of the minutes
- Circulate minutes to all invitees (including those who did not attend the meeting)

Physicians/Providers

All types of health care workers must communicate effectively and professionally with physicians and other patient care providers. Other providers include nurse practitioners, nurse anesthetists, and physician assistants. These professionals are ultimately responsible for patient care. As a newcomer to the medical field you may feel intimidated speaking with a provider. This is understandable and very common among new graduates. These feelings will subside as your experience level increases, your comfort level grows, and you become more acquainted with the physicians and providers in your workplace. Each physician is an individual with a unique personality. Some physicians are very outgoing and happy to answer your questions, whereas other physicians may appear to be short-tempered. Do not allow personality

January 2020 Staff Meeting Minutes
Internal Medicine Specialists

CALL TO ORDER
An Internal Medicine Specialists' staff meeting was held in Conference Room A on Thursday, January 5, 2020. The meeting was called to order by Dr. James Smith at 8:05 a.m.

ATTENDANCE
Dr. James Smith, Dr. Anna Cambell, Dr. Madison Anders, Louise Parker, Tim Wilton, Judy Milton, Pamela Sota, and Mike Layton were in attendance. Dr. Anthony Kasik and Amber Ryder were absent.

I. Opening Remarks - Dr. Smith thanked all staff members for their assistance in transitioning the last portion of patient records into the new database.

II. Approval of December 21, 2019 minutes - The minutes from the month of December were read by Judy Milton and approved.

 III. Further discussion of draft inventory survey - Louise Parker presented the latest changes made to the draft inventory survey. Tim Wilton suggested that the cost of inventory items be totaled and reported at each staff meeting in the future. It was agreed that this information will be added to inventory reports for staff meetings beginning in February 2020.

IV. Presentation of most recent Administrative Report - Louise Parker presented the Administrative Report for December 2019. The only notable item in the report was longer call hold times. Louise recommended that the staff consider why the call hold times were longer for this month and come back to the next staff meeting with ideas for improvement.

V. Presentation of most recent Budget Report - Tim Wilton presented the Budget Report for December 2019. During the presentation, Tim reminded all staff that budget requests for 2017 are due to him no later than January 6, 2020.

VI. Announcements - Louise Parker announced that Amber Ryder will continue to be out on medical leave until January 12, 2020.

VI. Discussion of next steps and confirmation of next meeting date/time - Dr. Smith stated that the next meeting will be held on Thursday, February 2, 2020.

VII. Other Business - Louise Parker reminded staff members that the office will be closed on January 16, 2020 in observance of Martin Luther King Day and on February 20 in observance of Presidents Day.

ADJOURN
Dr. Smith convened the meeting at 8:49 a.m.

Fig. 8.2 Meeting minutes. (From Elsevier. *Introduction to Health Services Administration.* St. Louis: Elsevier; 2018.)

issues and reputation to interfere with the need to contact a physician. If you find yourself avoiding a physician, speak to your manager and create a resolution plan. You must work to overcome any communication obstacle.

Treat the provider with respect. Respect is a two-way process. If you respect the provider for his or her knowledge and skills, the provider in turn will respect you and your skills. Respect is a trait that grows with time.

When deciding to contact the provider about a patient concern, prioritize the nature of the problem. Triage is a process of determining the degree of sickness and placing the patient into an appropriate level of care. In certain situations, you should contact the provider *STAT*, whereas in other cases you may be able to leave a message. STAT is a situation that requires immediate attention. The nature and type of emergencies that you will experience depend on your job title, place of employment, job setting, and specialty. It is important for you to be able to determine the emergent situations in your particular job and the appropriate method of communication. Your clinical supervisor or preceptor will teach you specifics as related to your duties. However, there are some general guidelines that affect every health care worker.

Contact the provider STAT for situations such as the following.
- Life-threatening change in a patient's condition
- Sudden deterioration in a patient's condition
- Laboratory or radiology results that require immediate interventions
- Patient care concerns that require emergent care

Contact the provider (non-STAT) for situations such as the following.
- Clarification or changes to medications that are not life-threatening. For example, a patient may call the physician's office and tell you that his morning blood sugar was 210. The patient wants to know if he should increase his evening insulin dosage. This situation is not an emergency, but it must be handled in a timely fashion. If the patient had called the office reporting a very high or low blood sugar or was experiencing symptoms, then the physician would need to be contacted STAT.
- Some patient care concerns do require urgent care. For example, a nurse from a skilled nursing facility has called a physician's office and told you that a patient has developed a new skin ulcer. This patient deterioration does not warrant an emergent page, but needs to be handled in a timely manner (Box 8.1).

BOX 8.1   TRIAGE LEVELS

Emergent: A condition or situation that needs immediate attention. The failure to act quickly will probably result in a serious or untoward event.

Urgent: A condition or situation that needs quick and prompt attention. The failure to act within a reasonable timeframe could result in the patient's condition deteriorating.

Nonurgent: A condition or situation that needs to be addressed, but it is not time-dependent. The outcome will not be worse if the condition is not resolved promptly.

Leave a message (email, voice mail, or answering service) in situations such as the following.
- Normal laboratory or radiology results
- Positive patient care updates
- Patient or family/caregiver requests to speak with the physician about a nonurgent matter

---

COMMUNICATION GUIDELINES

Physicians and Providers

Before the provider can make changes to the patient's medical regimen, he or she needs a thorough understanding of what is happening to the patient, when the change occurred, and what treatments have worked or not worked. When communicating with a provider, use the acronym **DOCTOR**.

Describe (describe the problem): Use terms that you are comfortable using. For example, "Mrs. Brown came into the office for her weekly blood pressure check. She was complaining of feeling very weak."

Observation (explain what/when you observed this problem): "She arrived at 10 a.m. and was very unsteady on her feet."

Clinical signs/symptoms (explain the clinical signs that you are seeing): "Also, I noticed that she was slightly confused and very diaphoretic. She was pale. Her pulse was 84 and blood pressure was 100/60."

Treatment (explain any treatments you have started or performed): "Because she is diabetic, I checked her blood sugar and found that it was 40. I gave her a glass of orange juice."

Observations (describe any changes since the treatments): "She is more alert now and her blood sugar is now 80."

Request (ask the provider for treatments or changes to the plan of care): "Her daughter drove her to the office. Do you want her to stay until you come back into the office or can she leave with her daughter?"

It is very poor and unprofessional communication to say to the physician, "Mrs. Brown does not look good. Something is wrong." Physicians who feel they must draw each piece of information from you will become irritated and frustrated. Frustration is a barrier to positive communication.

By following this acronym, you will provide the necessary information to the provider in an organized and professional manner. On hearing this information, the provider can then decide to order tests, change medications, or initiate other treatment options.

▶ TAKING THE CHAPTER TO WORK

An Emergent Event

Ramona is working at Mayhew's obstetric and gynecology office. The receptionist calls her and states that a young woman has just arrived and is bleeding. Ramona talks to the woman and determines that she is 28 weeks' pregnant and started vaginally bleeding about 20 minutes ago. Ramona recognizes this is an emergent situation and contacts the physician STAT. The physician returns the call and Ramona communicates the patient information in a calm, concise manner. The physician tells Ramona that she is in the office elevator and will be there in a moment. Ramona tells the patient that the doctor is coming and offers her reassurance. The physician examines the patient and decides to have her transported to the hospital via an ambulance. Ramona calls for the ambulance and communicates with the dispatcher. Then Ramona tells the receptionist to direct the ambulance personnel into the appropriate examination room. Ramona and the physician communicate the patient information to the emergency medical technicians. Lastly Ramona calls the patient's spouse and alerts him to the situation. She communicates with the spouse in a calm manner and offers reassurance.

This emergent event was handled smoothly because Ramona communicated with the receptionist, physician, patient, ambulance dispatcher, and technicians. She also took the time to talk with the patient's spouse. Ramona's communication skills improved patient care.

Managers/Supervisors

You must be able to communicate openly and freely with your manager or supervisor. You should feel comfortable speaking about many different topics, such as policy and procedural issues, staffing problems, or workplace environment concerns.

Although some medical settings have established business hours, with employees and employers on site at the same time, many medical facilities operate 24 hours a day, 7 days a week. You may work nights, or just weekends, and have very limited access to your supervisor. Some supervisors are responsible for various site locations and you may work at a satellite office and rarely see him or her. It is difficult to develop a communication rapport with someone when time and access are limited. Failure to overcome this barrier affects your ability to communicate successfully with your supervisor.

At times, you will need to discuss personal information with your supervisor. Personal issues that may affect your ability to work at your best level should be discussed with your supervisor before your work is affected. Discuss scheduling changes as soon as possible.

Before entering the manager's office, knock on the door and ask permission to enter. Be aware of your kinesics and nonverbal cues. When you speak to your manager, have a list of key points that you wish to discuss. Start the conversation by saying, "I would like to talk about three things. They are …" and then begin with the main issue. Do not sound vague or unclear; for example, do not say, "I think there is a problem with this schedule." If you think you need more than 15 minutes to discuss your concerns, schedule an appointment with your manager. Scheduling an appointment demonstrates courtesy and allows for the manager to give you his or her full attention.

👤 COMMUNICATION GUIDELINES

Managers/Supervisors

Sometimes you will need to discuss a problem at work with a supervisor. You can use the following guidelines to discuss an issue with your manager in a professional manner. Keep in mind that you should not try to explain someone else's problem.

- Present your problem. For instance, say "I noticed I am scheduled to work the evening shift 5 days next month and it is always on a Friday." Avoid stating the problem in an accusatory manner, such as asking, "Why does no one else have to work Friday evenings?" Keep the conversation focused on your needs.

- Communicate the effects of the problem. Say, "I understand that afternoons need to be covered, but it is hard for me to work late on Fridays because I can never find a babysitter on a Friday night." Do not use words or phrases such as "This is not fair."
- Offer a solution that will meet everyone's needs. "My daycare is open late on Mondays, so I would like to offer to switch my Friday for someone's Monday. Can I post a note on the bulletin board to switch a few shifts this month?" Do not demand that the problem be resolved or make a statement such as, "You need to fix this problem or else!"
- Never blame particular individuals for problems. State the facts. For example, "The last 3 days I worked, I did all the inventory sheets. It makes me feel frustrated." Avoid accusing anyone, such as "Michele has not done the inventory sheets in over a week."
- Trust your manager to understand and take action.

⚡ WORDS AT WORK

The following phrases promote communication and dialogue. Do use these phrases.
"You can count on me."
"You have a good point."
"Thank you for this opportunity."
"I have given some thought to our problem and this may work…"
"I have an idea on how we can better use our resources."
The following phrases hinder communication and halt dialogue. Do not use these phrases. "It's not my job."
"It's not my fault."
"I've had it."
"This is a waste of time."
"I'm only human."
"I know who did that."
"It won't work that way."

Regulatory and Accreditation Agencies

To ensure consistent, quality patient care the health professionals and their institutions (clinics, offices, hospitals) are among the most highly regulated agencies. Standards of operating can come from government entities or accreditation agencies. See Table 8.6 for a list of common regulatory agencies.

These agencies make site visits to monitor compliance with regulations and standards. Certain agencies send investigators on a regular basis (annually, semiannually), whereas others send an investigator only after a complaint has been filed. Some agencies visit without prior notice and others send documentation stating the date and time of the visit. Failure to prove compliance during a visit (unannounced or planned) can have serious repercussions for the health care setting. Fines can be assigned and facilities can lose their licensing or accreditation. It is your job to communicate to the investigator that your health care setting is in compliance.

Guidelines for Contacting Regulatory Agencies

After you are hired take the initiative to learn what regulatory agencies affect you and your position. Ask your manager questions such as, "What agency or agencies supply us with a license to operate?" "What is our accreditation agency?" "When can we expect to be inspected?" "What regulations/laws should I be familiar with?" A policy and procedure manual will answer most of those questions. If you are hired into a hospital setting you will be required to attend a hospital-wide orientation process where most of this information will be explained in detail.

Most agencies have a list of "reportable incidents" and the timeframes for making reports. For example, the Centers for Disease Control and Prevention (CDC) has a specific list of communicable diseases that must be reported. Your local health department also has a list of communicable diseases that need to be reported and their timeframes.

Each state has a division responsible for receiving and investigating suspected and confirmed cases of child or elder abuse or neglect. There are time constraints on these reports as well. Generally an oral report is required within 24 or 48 hours, followed by a written report within 5 to 7 days. Failure to report and fill out these forms within the specified time can result in fines to the health care agency and to you personally and, in certain cases, even a reprimand on your professional license.

Each agency has its own forms that need to be completed and has instructions on how to make a report. Most agencies have a 24-hour number available for questions. All agencies have contact information on their internet site. Remember, it is your job to know the regulations that affect you and your position and it is your responsibility to remain current on any changes.

TABLE 8.6 Types of Regulatory Agencies

Centers for Disease Control and Prevention (CDC)	Federal (Atlanta, GA) www.cdc.gov	Responsible for tracking all types of diseases and illnesses. Also promotes education programs and preventing diseases. Good resource for vaccine-related information.
Centers for Medicare and Medicaid Services (CMS)	Federal with state offices www.cms.hhs.gov	Regulates Medicare and Medicaid funding programs. It also monitors and controls HIPAA and CLIA regulations.
Department of Public Health (DPH)	State, local: To find your state's Department of Health, go to a search engine and type the name of your state and then "health department"	Responsible for tracking various diseases in the state, promoting and ensuring safety of health care institutions within the state, regulating licenses of health care providers.
U.S. Food and Drug Administration (FDA)	Federal (Rockville, MD) with regional office www.fda.gov	Responsible for drug manufacturing, prescription control; regulates medical devices.
The Joint Commission (TJC)	Private (Oakbrook, IL)	Sets and enforces standards for health care institutions. Issues accreditations to health care institutions
Occupational Safety Health Administration (OSHA)	Federal: With state offices. Federal office located in Washington, DC. www.osha.gov	Responsible for ensuring workplace safety for employees.

SPOTLIGHT ON SUCCESS

Networking

Creating a good working relationship with various referral agencies can be advantageous to your career and your advancement. Many health job opportunities are never advertised. They are spread through networking. Networking grows by communicating with your colleagues inside your office and outside your setting. Every time that you speak with a referral agency, think of it as a networking opportunity. You never know when an exciting job will arise. Being in the right place, at the right time, and having the right friends can make it happen.

Communication Challenges

You will face many challenges when communicating with a regulatory agency investigator or representative. The first challenge is understanding the standard and the language within the standard. A standard is a specific regulation or statement that is written by an agency and it depicts the minimum level of expected care. Standards are sequentially written and organized by a series of numbers and letters. For example, the investigator may say to you, "I need to see your action plan for compliance with standard 256B, subsection 67.39, Part III, version B." Unless you are very proficient with the standards, you may feel overwhelmed. Ask for clarification if necessary.

Most investigators are very serious about their responsibilities. They often have years of experience that can cause you to feel anxious when communicating with them. This is understandable. If you are well prepared and aware of the facilities' compliance sources, you will feel less intimidated. Fear is a barrier to communication. Fear may be based on potential fines, loss of licensure, or repercussions from your manager. However, if your health care setting is up to date and follows all regulations, fear should not be a factor.

There may be times or situations during your career that make you feel the need to report an incident without your manager's approval. For example, you may feel the health care setting is overbilling for claims, conducting Medicare fraud, or writing illegal prescriptions. No matter what the situation, follow your own ethical standards and always work within the law.

COMMUNICATION GUIDELINES

Regulatory and Accreditation Agencies

All of these challenges can be difficult to overcome. However, you will be able to overcome them using these tips. Use the acronym AGENCY.

Answer: Answer the investigator's questions in a professional, nonhostile manner. For example, do not make a comment such as, "Of course we follow all your rules"; instead, calmly and politely say, "We follow all of the regulations within your guidelines."

Give only the appropriate data or information. Give investigators the information they need, but do not offer additional information or data that are not requested. Let investigators lead the investigation.

Encourage open dialogue. Offer your assistance and show your enthusiasm for helping. For example, you may say, "If you have any questions, please let me know. I will be in the next room." This statement shows your cooperative spirit and opens the communication line.

Never hide or conceal any information. Hiding or concealing information can be perceived as a criminal act and you can be held responsible for your actions. If the investigator is looking for certain information and you know that it's being concealed, do not participate in concealing its existence.

Confidentiality: Know what information must be released and to whom. For example, a patient diagnosed with tuberculosis must be reported to your state's public health department, even if the patient does not want it reported. Before you give investigators patient information, you need to know what agency they represent and to what parts of the chart they are allowed access. For example, an investigator may have access to the chest x-ray report, but not to the patient's HIV status. Give only the necessary information. Also remember to follow the HIPAA regulations.

Your attention: It is important that you communicate to investigators that they have your full attention and participation. For example, comments such as, "Yeah, I'll get that for you in a minute," does not communicate professionalism or respect.

- Know the regulations and stay abreast of them. It is easier to stay current than it is to play catch-up. Ask the investigator "What changes can we expect to see in the next few years?"
- Never offer an investigator a bribe.
- Federal and state agency investigators will always have an official identification badge. Ask to see the badge. Ask for credentials before releasing any information. Some health care settings issue temporary badges for investigators to wear during their visit. If you are assigned to wear a badge, make sure you have it on and it is visible. Badges communicate professionalism and credibility.

WORDS AT WORK

The following phrases promote communication and dialogue. Do use these phrases.
"Can I answer any questions for you?"
"If you need me I'll be in my office."
"I think you can find everything you need in here."
"That's a good idea. We will try that here."
"Thank you for your suggestions."

The following phrases hinder communication and halt dialogue. Do not use these phrases.
"That's a dumb rule."
"So, what are you looking for?"
"Hurry up."
"There is nothing wrong here"
"We do it our own way."

COMMUNICATING AS A MANAGER OF PEOPLE

Numerous challenges exist in being in charge. You are no longer "one of the gang." Usually your first management position will be in a middle management or supervisory role. This means that you will have a title such as "assistant office manager" or "assistant clinical coordinator" and will be given some administrative duties but will have limited power to change or revamp existing rules.

Peer competition may also exist. A newly hired manager often receives this promotion after a selection process from which other coworkers who had applied were excluded. You may feel challenged by those who also wanted the position. To receive their respect you need to communicate that you respect your former colleagues and welcome their support.

One of the most important rules in communicating from a position of authority is to know your department, recognize the problem areas, and understand why they exist. Get to know your coworkers. It is very difficult to communicate effectively when you lack background information.

COMMUNICATION GUIDELINES

Staff and Employees

- Always communicate positive and encouraging news and information. Celebrate the victories. For example, "Last week we reached 100% compliance. Great job everyone." Praise coworkers as often as possible. This increases self-esteem and has been proven to increase work output.
- Actively listen to what your coworkers tell you; think before you speak.
- Avoid phrases such as "calm down." Instead you may say, "I see you are upset, let's talk about what is going on." Let the other person talk while you actively listen. Listen between the lines. Allow periods of silence. Recap conversations, such as, "If I understand correctly, this is the problem." Then, rephrase the problem. Ask for resolution ideas. This helps your team feel part of the solution rather than part of the problem.

When there is a problem, you can communicate it to the staff remembering the acronym **BOSS**.

Behavior: Explain the behavior that you have noticed. Do not accuse or place blame. For example, state " I have noticed that the quality controls are not being done on a regular basis."

Objective: Provide the staff with objective findings, not subjective comments. For example, "According to this sheet, we are only 75% compliant." Use the word "we" to show that this is a team problem, not an individual's problem.

Spreads: Explain how this spreads and affects other people, patients, or staff. For example, "It is important that we are compliant with these checks for the safety of our patients, and it is a regulatory requirement."

Suggest/search: Provide some suggestions for resolving the problem or ask your staff for ideas. For example, " I have two ideas on how we can improve this. We could rotate the responsibility to different times or I could assign a person to do it. Does anyone have any other suggestions?" Another possible sentence would be "We haven't had this issue before; what has changed to cause it?" By searching for the root of the problem you will be able to resolve the problem more quickly and easily.

Support and Compassion

When you are in charge you will be confronted with staff's personal problems. Examples of personal problems are death of family members, financial problems, or divorces. It is easy to become absorbed in such problems, but you need to keep everything in perspective. When you are in

charge you need to communicate empathy and not sympathy. Chapter 1 discusses these terms with a patient focus. Below you will find some additional information about applying these skills when you are in charge.

Sympathy is understanding and caring about another person's problem. It requires that you suspend judgment or avoid jumping to conclusions. With empathy you must try to walk in another person's shoes for the moment. It does not mean that you need to agree, but that you emotionally understand their feelings. Once you understand the situation, then you can give support and encouragement. Here are some phrases that promote empathy: "Let's talk about what is happening," "Tell me about your situation." Use the power of silence to let the other person tell you what is happening. Give the conversation your full attention and work toward a thorough understanding.

Empathy means that you feel the same emotions the other person feels. If someone is sad, you feel sad; if someone feels anxious, you feel anxious. If you empathize with every staff member's problems, you will be unable to work as a manager effectively. You need to be able to understand the problem but also consider how it will impact the team.

Consider the following situation.

Manager #1: "I understand that you are going through a divorce; let's talk about how we can meet your needs and the needs of the department."

Manager #2: "I am sorry that you are going through a divorce. You must be very upset. Let me know what I can do to help."

Which statement makes a bigger impact?

Manager #1 communicates sympathy. She demonstrates that she understands the problem and is working to resolve it as it pertains to the workplace. Manager #2 communicates sympathy, but sounds insincere and does not work toward a solution.

Conflict Management[*]

Conflict is an unavoidable part of almost any job or workplace. Conflicts in a health care setting can range from everyday disagreements to major controversies that can lead to litigation or, in rare cases, even violence in the workplace. They can arise between physicians, between physicians and staff, and between the staff and the patient or

---

[*] The editors are grateful to the Carol Colvin, whose work in *Introduction to Health Services Administration*, St. Louis, 2018, Elsevier, forms the basis of this section of the chapter.

patient's family. Whatever the nature of the conflicts, they almost invariably have an adverse effect on productivity, efficiency, and patient care, and can lead to miscommunication, poor morale, and a high rate of staff turnover.

Conflict is between opposing sides created by incompatible needs, drives, or interests. It is often the result of differences from varying perspectives. For example, a health care professional reacts to a situation or conflict based on his or her training and life experience. He or she may also manage daily situations from the standpoint of office policy or precedents set by previous situations. When employees face the same problems in different ways, conflict often results.

In health care, as in any other industry, conflict can be valuable when managed properly. Despite being viewed as negative and something to be avoided at all costs, conflict can produce multiple positive outcomes in the workplace. Diverse attitudes and backgrounds can produce creative approaches to solve problems and reach goals in an organization. Additionally conflict can often trigger critical thinking as a team effort to seek resolution. An effective health services administrator should be able to manage conflict in a way that produces positive outcomes and steers the team toward the goals that support the mission of the business.

Conflict that is well managed can improve team effectiveness and cohesiveness. Meaningful conflict can also produce the following results.

- **Employee engagement:** Employees who feel free to disagree or offer different viewpoints are more likely to engage in workplace problem-solving and discussions.
- **Increased understanding:** When a team learns to resolve conflict, it often helps them better understand their goals, both individually and as a team.
- **Team focus:** Conflict focuses team members on the task at hand and allows them to stay zoned in and moving toward the goal.
- **Team cohesiveness:** Stronger relationships between employees can develop when honesty is promoted and divergent perspectives are respected.
- **Employee morale:** When employees feel free to speak freely in a professional manner, without fear of repercussions or retaliation, they are more likely to feel like a respected and valued part of a team.

Effectively managing conflict allows a team to identify problems and seek solutions. A team that learns to embrace conflict by respecting the ideas of others can increase efficiency, effectiveness, and employee satisfaction.

Conflict management in the health care industry is commonly associated with the management of information, both before and after patient care takes place. Communication is vital in providing effective services to patients in an efficient and effective manner. When unresolved conflict exists in a health care setting communication becomes the unfortunate victim, which has a direct effect on patient care, employee satisfaction, and customer loyalty.

When it comes to conflict, communication is both the cause and the resolution. Therefore, a manager should take steps to address conflict and improve communication. For example, a common method is establishing a professional code of conduct that includes all health care providers and staff. Clearly written established rules make it easier for all employees to follow rules and guidelines while taking personality out of the equation, which is often at the root of conflicts.

With communication at the center of both conflict and conflict resolution, it is important to develop a business culture conducive to teamwork and collaboration. Being able to reduce the frequency and intensity of workplace conflicts and empower employees with skills to address conflict has multiple benefits to the health care organization, including

- Employees who understand how to communicate internally are more likely to communicate effectively externally, leading to fewer complaints.
- Decreased employee turnover, which leads to decreased training costs. Additionally, long-term employees tend to produce more work in shorter timeframes with fewer errors compared with new employees.
- Increased patient loyalty, fewer medical errors, fewer costs in follow-up treatments, lower costs of compensation to patients in cases where there are losses caused by medical errors, and lower administrative costs owing to legal fees.
- Creating breakthrough ideas. Allowing team members to work through conflict in a professional, respectful manner can lead to breakthrough ideas as everyone works toward a common goal through honest feedback without fear of negative repercussion. Conflict often produces ingenuity.

Notice that throughout this communication the speaker emphasized "I." Starting a conversation by saying "You are loud," immediately sets the person referred to as "you" on the defensive. Focus on how it makes you feel and how you perceive the problem.

COMMUNICATION GUIDELINES

Conflict Management

You can use the acronym **PEER** to work through conflicts with staff, colleagues, and others.

Present the problem (explain the problem as you see it): "Today I was trying to teach a patient how to use a home glucometer. We could hear your laughter in the hall."

Explain (explain how the problem makes you feel): "I felt really embarrassed when I was talking to the patient."

Effect (explain the effect the problem has on your ability to do your work): "It bothers me because I have to repeat my message and I feel that I have to apologize for the loud noise."

Resolve (explain that you want to resolve this problem so that you can work together better): "I really enjoy working with you and I want us to be able to work as a team, so I would like to resolve this problem. Can you try to lower your voice when sitting at the desk?"

TELEPHONE COMMUNICATION*

One of the most frequently used forms of verbal communication in health care is used over the phone. Often, communication by phone provides the patient the first impression of a health care organization; it all begins with how the phone is answered. Whether the phone call is to schedule an appointment, refill a prescription, or provide critical health information regarding treatment, the phone call can have a positive or negative impact on the organization. Put yourself in the patient's shoes and consider what happens when the phone rings and rings. One begins to question whether the medical office will ever answer the call, whether the practice is understaffed, and what the quality of patient care and attention provided will be. If patients have to leave a message, it will be their expectation that their message will be returned.

Answering the Call

A good rule of thumb is that all phone calls should be answered by the third ring. All employees in the health care organization should work toward this

goal, not just the front desk receptionist. Otherwise, if the call is not answered, the patient may hang up and call again, which just creates another call for you to handle later. Once you answer and have to put the caller on hold, always ask first and wait for a response before doing so. Just pausing that extra moment indicates that you care about the caller and his or her time.

The telephone greeting should be friendly and professional. It helps to smile when answering calls as this improves the likelihood that your voice conveys the same friendliness and energy. It has been shown that people can sense whether a speaker is smiling or frowning. Make sure to speak clearly using a moderate volume and speed. Although people like to hear the sound of their own name, health care professionals need to exercise discretion when mentioning the name of the caller and/or patient to protect confidentiality. At a minimum, avoid using both the patient's first and last name over the phone in case your conversation is overheard.

Offer to take a message if you cannot handle the call immediately. For example, if you are going to need to have another staff member answer the patient's questions, take a message. Otherwise the caller may be placed on hold and waiting for a long period of time. This may create extreme frustration for the patient. This also helps health care providers work more efficiently because calls can be addressed in batches, therefore avoiding interrupting work flow, which can often be a cause of medical errors. If you have taken a message, ensure that the call has been returned. Remember the importance of following through on promises and the role of dependability in building patient trust. The worst situation is not returning calls, which suggests the business does not care about its patients, thus leading again to patient attrition. Therefore, the more efficient the work process is, the more quickly you can help patients get the care they need.

Confirming Appointments

Using reminder calls or emails can reduce the number of no-shows and cancellations. However, do not include too much information in these communications. For example, if you must leave a voicemail message, keep it brief and succinct. If the message is too long, key pieces of important information may be lost or perhaps not even heard.

---

* The editors are grateful to the Meredith Robertson, whose work in *Introduction to Health Services Administration*, St. Louis, 2018, Elsevier, forms the basis of this section of the chapter.

Test Results

Often patients will call the medical office for their test results. Make sure that the health care provider has seen the test results first and given permission to share them with the patient. Office policies should indicate which health care personnel can deliver test results and other medical information to patients. If the test results are unfavorable the health care provider should share the results directly with the patient and give further instructions to the medical staff. Any questions regarding test results should be addressed by the health care provider and the staff should show caution on not crossing the line of practicing medicine without a license. As a general rule of thumb the best approach for handling positive or abnormal test results is to schedule an appointment for the patient with the health care provider; serious news is best delivered in person rather than over the phone. Sensitivity and tactfulness must be used in answering and managing these types of calls.

Health care professionals should also be careful that they properly identify patients before giving out any test results over the phone. All health care personnel need to be aware of federal and state laws and regulations regarding the release of any medical information to someone other than the patient, including patients who are minors. Sharing information with individuals other than the patient may be considered a breach of confidentiality and violate the privacy rules of HIPAA.

Some health care organizations may use the patient's date of birth or other types of personal information known only to the patient to be used as a form of identification. Other organizations may even use a special password or code that patients must provide before confidential information is released. It is recommended that health care professionals obtain at least two methods of identification before sharing confidential medical information.

Billing

Patients may be calling to discuss their billing concerns. If billing matters are handled by another staff member or external company, tell the patient that the call will be transferred. (Some facilities use external agencies; in which case, you may need to provide the caller with that entity's phone number.) If your organization is responsible for billing, politely ask patients to hold while you obtain their billing record. Once you have their information in front of you, thank them for waiting and tell them that you can answer their question(s) now. If there was an error, apologize and let them know that a corrected statement will be sent in the mail as soon as possible.

Ideally, patients should be given information on charges and fees prior to or when services are rendered. This practice will reduce the number of billing calls. However, fees vary widely among different facilities and it is often impossible to quote an exact fee before services are incurred. So, in these situations, patients should be given a good estimate of what they may expect to pay overall at the time of the initial visit. After giving patients an estimate remind them that the rate may vary based on any tests ordered and their results and the diagnosis made by the health care provider. If the facility requires the copayment to be paid at the first visit, make sure this is communicated to the patient. If it is office policy to regularly discuss fees over the phone, it is best practice to create a script that staff members can use when needed.

Closing the Call

When closing the call, use the same friendly tone you used to begin the phone conversation. Ensure that any instructions or medical information has been understood by the patient. Remember to avoid using any medical terms or abbreviations that the patient may not understand. Repeat key pieces of material discussed during the call to confirm the caller has understood the information. Make sure to ask if the patient has any other questions and thank the caller for the phone call before saying goodbye.

Triage

Health care professionals who work in outpatient centers or physician offices are often involved in telephone triage. Telephone triage is very tricky because the health care professional must rely only on the information that the caller is giving. After determining the nature of the problem, you often need to give advice on handling the problem. In other courses, you will learn specific skills for triaging and giving advice, but be aware that this practice is highly risky and must be carefully documented. Document the following information.

- Date and time of the call
- Name of the caller

- Name and age of the patient (if different than the caller)
- Nature of the problem
- Severity of the problem
- Length of time the problem has been ongoing
- Any interventions that the caller has tried and the results of those interventions
- Any instructions that you gave to the caller
- Follow-up plan for the problem along with the timeframe: for example: "If the vomiting does not stop within 24 hours, call the office for an appointment".

This information is charted in the patient's medical record. If you are working at a clinic and the caller is not a patient, follow your office's policy. Some policies state that you cannot triage or give advice to nonpatients, but other facilities allow you to do so. If the clinic allows nonpatients to call, there should be a telephone triage log that documents the calls.

EMAIL

As with other business settings, the health care industry continues to transform and move toward more advanced technology. One of the more significant examples of this is the way health care professionals interact with patients by email and online. Email is universally used for both professional and personal reasons to communicate and exchange information quickly and effectively. Therefore, poor email etiquette has the potential to sabotage both your personal and your professional reputation. If you are a new employee, it is always beneficial to talk with your supervisor about any specific email etiquette used by your health care organization. Just as any other forms of communication, emails are a reflection of you and your employer.

This section will further discuss common mistakes that are made in email communication and ways to avoid damaging your business' reputation when you are using it.

Email or Phone Call

The first consideration when writing an email is to decide whether email is the best method of communication for the information you are sharing. When a message has multiple pieces of information that require explanation or negotiation, you should pick up the telephone instead. Otherwise, an email may generate several "back and forth" emails and create added confusion and wasted time. If timing of communication is critical, such as last-minute cancellations of meetings or appointments, a phone call may be warranted to ensure a timely delivery. Additionally, other instances when an email may be inappropriate is when bad news needs to be communicated.

Replying to Incoming Email

In general, you should reply to any incoming email. Even if you do not know how to respond to the email immediately, it is better to send a note to the sender that the email has been received than to send no response at all. Without a reply or an email-received receipt, the sender is left wondering whether you received it, whether you have forgotten it or ignored it, or why a response is taking so long. If more time is required to answer the sender's email, the best approach is to respond with an estimated timeline as to when you expect to reply, such as: "I should have an answer for you by early next week." Response times will vary based on the content of the incoming email, but often email responses should be sent within 24 to 48 hours.

If an incoming email triggers an emotional response from you, such as anger, it is recommended that you do not respond immediately. If time permits, "sleep on it" and wait until the next day to respond; at a minimum, take a moment to catch a breath to prevent an emotional or inappropriate response. Remember emails last forever. When responding, make sure to address all issues from the incoming email and answer all questions.

Before hitting "send," consider whether the information being conveyed is related to the business or is it personal. Emails coming from the health care staff should always be business-related. You should ask yourself whether you would be comfortable putting the message on company letterhead or whether the information should be shared outside of the office.

Subject Line

When sending an outgoing email, it is a good practice to ensure your subject line conveys a summary of the email message. The subject line should be descriptive, but short and concise. If the email contains a date or deadline, include this in the subject line. Make sure to proofread your subject line as closely as the contents of your overall email. Table 8.7 shows examples of poor and effective email subject lines.

TABLE 8.7 Examples of Email Subject Lines	
Poor Email Subject Lines	**Effective Email Subject Lines**
Greenville Healthcare Conference	Invitation: Greenville Healthcare Conference: Aug. 12–14
Monthly Report Due	Monthly Budget Report: Due to John Smith Jan. 2
Interesting Article	FYI: Article with Tips on Healthcare Communication with Elders
Action Needed!	Action: Decision on Billing Vendor Needed by Oct. 1

From Elsevier. *Introduction to Health Services Administration.* St. Louis: Elsevier; 2018.

Message Content

The goal of your email is to convey accurate and timely information to the reader. When creating your email, the communication should be clear, with the most important points at the top of the message. The reader should not have to dig through the full email or, even worse, have to reread the email to get the main information. The purpose of the email should be stated in the first or second sentence of the email. Later in the email, you can provide more detailed information or additional context. You may even indicate that "the background of the issue is described below." When creating the email content, here are a few additional tips.

- Indicate at the beginning of the email whether or not the recipient needs to take some action.
- Avoid responding with "OK." For example, if your supervisor emails you about an office issue and you respond with "OK," you may come across as flippant or curt. If you are trying to respond quickly from your phone, it may be better to wait until you are at a computer before responding so you can provide a more thorough response.
- Avoid jargon, medical terminology, and abbreviations in emails to readers who may not be as familiar with the health care industry as you are. Be aware of your audience and write out abbreviations.
- Avoid emoticons, emojis, text abbreviations (i.e., LOL, OMG), and using multiple exclamation points.

Using these will make the sender and the employer appear unprofessional.

Most readers appreciate the use of bullet points for more detailed information and easier reading. This allows readers to do a quick skim of the email and to get its main points if they are short on time. It is also easier to read if the writer includes space between main points of information. A good rule of thumb is to limit paragraphs to no more than five sentences.

One of the most common pitfalls to emailing is interpreting a writer's tone of voice in an email. So, be cautious when using sarcasm and/or humor in emails. If you have any question about how something might be received, it is better to leave it out or choose different words. Always go out of your way to ensure an email is polite, professional, and courteous with the use of "please" and "thank you." Also, avoid using all caps or lower case letters; all caps may be interpreted as the sender yelling and the use of all lowercase may imply a lack of urgency or laziness of the sender.

Health care professionals must be aware that much of the information they are communicating is confidential in nature. Therefore, you should always check with your supervisor regarding your organization's policy for emails to ensure compliance with the HIPAA guidelines. Some health care facilities may have standard privacy language included in all email correspondence that provides contact information in the event that the email is sent to the wrong address.

Closing and Signature

Professional emails should always include a closing signature that provides your full name, title, company, and other contact information, such as a phone number. A more formal business closing may use "Sincerely" or "Best regards" before your signature. Alternatively, "Thanks" is often an acceptable way to close a business email.

Proofreading

Before sending the email, best practice is always proofread it. A well-written email is one that has been proofread and uses appropriate capitalization, punctuation, grammar, and spelling. One tip is to read your email out loud before sending it. Health care personnel should also double-check the spelling of names and addresses to ensure accuracy and to avoid sending the email to either the wrong person or having it "bounce" back or be returned.

Carbon Copy and Blind Carbon Copy

Professionals will often use carbon copy (cc) when they want to include someone on the email for information only and are not expecting the cc'd recipient to respond. Similarly, blind carbon copy (bcc) may be used to include someone for informational purposes, but his or her identity is not shared with the other recipients. Oftentimes, "bcc" is used to send an email to the entire list of recipients, but keeps the identity and email addresses of those recipients hidden.

Reply to All

The "reply all" should only be used when, in fact, everyone on the email truly needs the information in the response. It may be appropriate to reply only to the sender and then manually add the addresses of only some of the other recipients. Also, never "reply all: on an email where you were blind copied (bcc'd). The original sender used bcc: to keep your identity confidential. If you reply all, then you reveal your identity. The bottom line is it is important to take the extra time to be cautious about sending your emails to the right people.

Forwarding Emails

When forwarding an email, your message, with your signature, should be above the forwarded email. Do not mix your text with the forward message, which can be confusing. Avoid making any changes to the forwarded email, unless you want to reduce the length of the text in which case you can use "..." to let the reader know you have removed a portion of the text. It is also important to "clean up" the forwarded email by removing any unnecessary carets, such as ">," or poorly formatted line breaks. Also, consider removing any email addresses from the forwarded email to protect the initial sender's privacy.

Attachments

When it comes to adding attachments to an email, such as a document or a photo, consider the size of the attachment. It may be appropriate to provide a warning if you are sharing a significantly large file (e.g., something over 10 MB). You may want to ask the recipient if it is okay to send a file that large or whether there is a better time of day when there is less email traffic. It can also be helpful to use email tools that ensure your emails always include subject lines and attachments if you include the text "attachment enclosed."

PROFESSIONAL AND FORMAL BUSINESS LETTERS

Health care professionals frequently use **business letters** as a form of written communication with patients, colleagues, and other professionals. It is important that these letters are courteous, written clearly, and articulate the main points of the communication at the beginning of the letter. In the workplace, you should be prepared to draft the following types of business letters.

- Appointment reminder letters
- Patient billing letters
- Referral letters (referring patients to another provider)
- Excused absence letters (for students or employees to document the reason for absence from school or work)
- Office announcement letters (e.g., changes in staff, insurance, hours, or other office protocols)

All formal business letters should be written on letterhead stationery and typically have one-inch margins on each side. Spacing throughout the letter should be consistent, either using single-space or double-space. To ensure readability, the letter should use a simple font, such as Times New Roman or Arial. Avoid overusing bold and italics for emphasis. Each letter should include seven key pieces, in order from top to bottom, as listed below.

- Business's address
- Current date
- Recipient's address
- Greeting
- Main body
- Closing
- Signature

Figure 8.3 shows an example business letter.

Business Address

It is common practice for businesses to have their address on the letterhead. However, if this is not the case, the letter should include the sender's address at the left margin, one inch from the top of the letter. Use single spacing and include the clinic or business's name, street or P.O. box address, city, state, and zip code. It is not necessary to include the individual health care provider or employee's name because the author will be signing the letter at the end.

Sender's Address in the header of the document	**WALDEN-MARTIN** **FAMILY MEDICAL CLINIC** **1234 ANYSTREET I ANYTOWN, ANYSTATE 12345** **PHONE 123-123-1234 I FAX 123-123-5678** (1 blank line)
Date	March 23, 20XX
	(1 to 9 blank lines so body of letter is centered vertical on the page)
Inside Address	Ms. Celia Tapia 12 Highland CT Anytown AL 12345-1234 (1 blank line)
Salutation	Dear Ms. Tapia: (1 blank line)
Body of the Letter	You were seen on March 20, 20XX for a sore throat. As you know, the rapid strep culture came back negative. We did a 24-hour culture and that test result was also negative. (1 blank line) If you continue to feel ill and are not improving, please do not hesitate to call our office at (123) 123-1234 for an appointment. (1 blank line)
Closing	Sincerely, (4 blank line)
Signature Block	James A. Martin, M.D. (1 blank line)
Reference notation Copy notation	JAM/bn c. Joan Smith, M.D.

Fig. 8.3 Example business letter. (From Proctor D Niedzwiecki B, Pepper J, Bhattacharya Madero P. *Kinn's the Administrative Medical Assistant,* ed 13. St. Louis: Elsevier; 2017.)

Date of Letter

The date of a letter should reflect the date the letter was written and it should be spelled out, such as December 15, 2020. If using letterhead, it should be inserted on the second line following the letterhead. Or if not using letterhead, it should be on the second line below the business address.

Recipient Address

The address of the recipient should be left justified. Allow for one blank line between the date line and the recipient address. This address should include the recipient's name and title on one line and then, on separate lines, the department or agency where they work, then the street address, city, state, and zip code. Two-letter state abbreviations should be used. Always include the recipient's name or the guardian's name in the case the letter is going to the household of a minor.

Greeting

The greeting is also left justified and placed on the second line below the recipient's address. The greeting should always be formal in business letters beginning with "Dear" and followed by the person's title (i.e., Mr., Ms., Dr.), his or her name, and a colon. When addressing letters to women, try to use the recipient's preferred title. If you do not know her preference, use "Ms." For example, "Dear Dr. Jones:" may be the greeting. If the gender is unknown, you may use the first and last name without a title or use the generic phrase "To Whom It May Concern."

Main Body

Two lines below the greeting is where the main body of the letter begins. In general, business letters tend to be short. The first part of the letter is a gracious opening clearly defining the purpose of the letter. Any remaining paragraphs should support the main point of the letter, with any action to be taken described at the end of the letter.

Closing

The closing of the letter should be left justified and formal. It should be two lines below the body of the letter. Generally, letters close with "Sincerely." The closing should always be capitalized and followed by a comma. If the closing has multiple words, only capitalize the first word, such as "Best regards."

Signature

Formatting should include four line spaces where the sender will sign. Under the signature should be the typed name, title, and credentials of the sender. The title should be capitalized and placed directly below the name.

Form Letters

In this digital age, health care offices may use form letters to save time. Form letters created by different word processing software can be personalized with patients' names and addresses and even personal case notes. However, if you are using a form letter, it should be personally signed if possible.

CHECKING YOUR COMPREHENSION

1. Define the term professionalism. Give three examples professional behaviors.
2. According to privacy laws, with which persons in the health care setting can you share patient information?
3. List three benefits of interdisciplinary communication.
4. Define the terms emergent, urgent, and nonurgent. How does provider notification vary for each setting?
5. What are the benefits of a meeting agenda?
6. How do regulatory agencies monitor health care organizations?
7. What acronym can help you resolve conflict in the workplace? Explain each letter.
8. Why are telephone skills an important part of communication?
9. When using email, what are the considerations for patient privacy and HIPAA regulations?
10. What occasions require a written business letter? Name three.

■ EXPANDING CRITICAL THINKING

1. You suspect that the physician for whom you are working is overbilling Medicare for procedures that were not done. How would you discuss this issue? With whom would you discuss it? What are the legal implications of not reporting Medicare fraud?

2. During your job orientation, you notice that your new employer is using an outdated blood pathogen standard. How would you go about discussing this with her?

3. Think about your best friend. Could you work effectively with her or him? Why or why not? Assume that you have developed a conflict working together. How would you feel about communicating this problem? What steps can you take to increase your comfort level?

4. How do you feel about communicating with physicians? Do you feel intimidated? What steps can you take to improve your comfort level?

9

Documenting Patient Care

Linda Boyd

CHAPTER OUTLINE

The editors are grateful to the Betsy Shiland, whose work in *Introduction to Health Services Administration*, St. Louis, 2018, Elsevier, forms the basis of this chapter.

LEARNING OBJECTIVES

After completing this chapter, the student will be able to do the following.

1. List the information found in the record.
2. List the uses of the information in the health record.
3. Discuss ownership of the health record and the release of information.
4. Explain the features and benefits of EHR technology.
5. List best practices for documenting patient care.
6. Explain the purpose of medical coding and list the transaction code sets required by law.

KEY TERMS

advance directive legal document that provides guidance about the patient's desired treatments to sustain life when he or she becomes incapacitated

algorithm step-by-step procedure for solving a problem using logical progression

audit trail feature of the electronic health record that tracks users who accessed a patient record and when they did so

authentication assumption of responsibility for the data collected

clinical decision support (CDS) function of the electronic health record that recommends approaches for diagnoses of specific diseases, guides selection of the correct diagnostic tests, and assists in the treatment and monitoring of patients

coding representation of diagnoses and health care services using alphanumeric characters

computer-assisted physician order entry (CPOE) software featuring decision support through which a provider selects medications and sends orders electronically

continuity of care provision of care for a patient over a period of time

contraindication reason not to pursue a treatment

countersignature evidence of the supervision of a subordinate's documentation

discharge summary documentation of a visit given to the patient at check out

durable power of attorney (DPOA) type of advance directive that allows the patient to name another individual who legally makes health care decisions on the patient's behalf

electronic health record (EHR) system that maintains patient demographic and clinical information digitally and offers computerized physician order entry, e-prescribing, and decision support

health record report of the care a patient received and the relevant facts, findings, and observations about the patient's health

informed consent patient's authorization to receive treatment following the provider's discussion of various treatment options and risks

interoperability capacity for different computer systems to communicate, exchange data, and use the information that has been exchanged

notice of privacy practices (NPP) plain-language document given to patients by the provider that details how a patient's information will be used and disclosed, the organization's duties to safeguard patient information, and a patient's rights concerning privacy

patient portal website on which patients can interact and communicate with their provider, view laboratory results, and track, monitor, and send information regarding their personal health data

protected health information (PHI) under the law, any health information, such as medical history or current status, that can be linked to an individual

protocol guideline for the treatment of a disease or disorder

release of information (ROI) authorization by the patient to disclose his or her protected health information to another person or entity

❓ TEST YOUR COMMUNICATION IQ

Before reading this chapter, complete this short self-assessment test. Decide which statements are true and which are false.

1. Documenting in the health record is optional.
2. Patient education is documented in the health record.
3. The health record is used for billing purposes.
4. The health record can be used as evidence in a court of law.
5. Electronic health records are always available to any provider in the country.
6. Computers will soon make medical coding obsolete.

Results

Statements 2, 3, and 4 are true; all others are false. How did you do? Read the chapter to find more information on these topics.

INTRODUCTION

Documentation is central to the health care industry and it is the primary means by which health care professionals communicate their care of the patient to one another. Physicians and providers must record and communicate the care plan to nursing staff; nursing staff must monitor progress and report their interventions to the provider; medical billers must communicate to insurers and other payers what services were provided to the patient and why; and government overseers and accreditation agencies must ensure the facility and its staff adhere to laws and guidelines. All this communication and much more relies on the careful documentation of patient care. This chapter explores the means and methods of health care documentation, including digital advances that allow us to locate, store, send, and receive information, as well as the uses for that information in the delivery of patient care.

THE HEALTH RECORD

All the information we gather from the patient interview—all the findings, orders, and actions of the provider, and all the instruction we dispense to patients over the course of their care—is recorded to communicate what has been done and should be done for the patient. Along with the patient's name, contact information, age, ethnicity, marital status, financial data, and other information, the details of each encounter are documented in the patient health record, sometimes referred to as a *medical record* or *patient chart*. A health record is a report of the care a patient received and the relevant facts, findings, and observations about the patient's health. It is a chronologic assemblage of all the data about an individual patient, recorded so that medical and legal professionals can refer to the information later, if needed. Regulatory and accrediting agencies review documentation because health records are the central means of communication in health care. Failure to document in the heath record properly can result in fines and loss of licensure.

Health records include demographic information (the patient's name, address, social security number, etc.), legal consent forms, financial information, and clinical data, such as the chief complaint, history and physical examination, imaging and laboratory results, provider orders for treatments and medications, nursing progress notes, and any referrals.

Medical information was traditionally kept in paper files and charts (Fig. 9.1). Today, however, the electronic health record (EHR) is far more common. An EHR stores medical information digitally, and, as we will discuss later in this chapter, has many more features besides simple storage.

Clinical Content

One method of documentation in the health record is the "SOAP" method, which stands for subjective, objective, assessment, and plan. As discussed in Chapter 2, the *subjective* section includes the symptoms that the patient is experiencing—such as nausea, pain, confusion—that

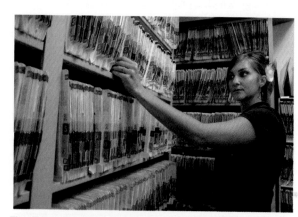

Fig. 9.1 Paper files have been used for decades to store patient information, and it is still the common practice in many facilities. (iStock.com/DenGuy.)

cannot be objectively measured. *Objective* signs are the other pieces of the complaint—those that can be measured or observed, such as fever, weight gain, or a rash. The *assessment* piece is the provider's compilation of signs and symptoms and evaluation to determine a diagnosis. The *plan* is the provider's action plan or treatment regimen for the given diagnosis. As part of the treatment, any medications prescribed will be documented in the health record, along with the prescribing order to the pharmacy, and any consultations or referrals.

Signatures

Specific sections must be *authenticated* by the provider or clinical staff when documenting in the patient's medical record. The term authentication means that the provider's name and title are present and legible for each entry or notation in the patient's health record, signifying responsibility. A countersignature is an additional signature on a document that may be required in some states, such as for physician assistants and nurse practitioners who practice under a physician.

Imaging and Laboratory Documentation

As part of the diagnostic process, the physician may write an order for additional testing that includes imaging or laboratory work. The results of these tests must be entered into the medical record because they are integral to the substantiation of the diagnosis and patient's treatment plan. Laboratory results, whether they are completed on- or off-site, are directly entered into the patient's medical record and should include the normal ranges for each laboratory test. Imaging studies, such as x-rays, CT scans, and MRIs, are incorporated in the record using a software application, such as a *picture archiving and communication system*, that digitizes images and allows for their electronic storage and transmission (Fig. 9.2). Because of this technology, images can be taken in one facility and sent and interpreted by physicians hundreds (and sometimes thousands) of miles away.

Operative Reports

If the health care organization offers ambulatory surgeries, a report will be generated that includes the preoperative assessment and postoperative management or instructions. Any findings during the surgical procedure, such as images from a colonoscopy or biopsy results, will be included and the entire report will be

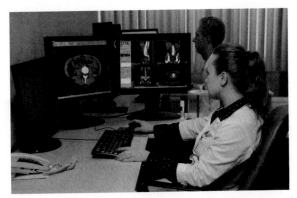

Fig. 9.2 A radiologist, who specializes in the interpretation of diagnostic images, studies an MRI using the picture archiving and communication system (PACS). (iStock.com/Medvedkov.)

reviewed and signed by the physician responsible for the procedure. Anesthesia reports may be documented separately and are often found in hospital medical records.

Patient Education

Depending on your job and title, the amount of patient education that you will be involved with will vary. Chapter 3, "Educating Patients," discusses patient education in detail. Although most patient education sessions are informal, it is important to document patient education in the health record. The following points should be communicated.

- Who was present (e.g., patient and caregiver and the relationship of the caregiver to the patient)
- What was taught (e.g., medications, diet, exercise, self-care)
- How it was taught (e.g., demonstration, return demonstration, video, handouts)
- Length of teaching (e.g., 10 minutes, 30 minutes)
- Level of understanding (e.g., "Patient verbalized or demonstrated understanding")
- Plans for additional teaching/support groups (e.g., "Patient referred to diabetes support group." "Handout with additional information given to patient.")
- If an interpreter was present, his/her name and the language translated

Discharge Summary

The discharge summary, also called a discharge report, is provided to the patient when he or she is discharged or checks out after a medical visit. The discharge summary includes the patient's diagnoses; any procedures that were performed; the patient's diagnostic studies, including laboratory and imaging; progress notes; physician's orders; consultation reports; and any discharge instructions.

SPOTLIGHT ON SUCCESS

If the patient is being discharged from an inpatient care unit Against Medical Advice (AMA), follow your medical center's policy manual. Most settings have a form the patient needs to sign that advises him or her of the risks of leaving AMA. Physicians must be notified of the patient's decision. Document all communication that took place between you, the physician, and the patient regarding this decision. Patients who are discharged AMA still must be offered education and resources for follow-up care. All attempts to offer these services must be documented, even if the patient refuses the services. The physician may opt to send a patient–physician relationship termination letter.

Legal Forms

Several pieces of documentation are collected to legally protect the patient, the provider, and the health care organization. These include the patient's consent to receive treatment, consent to send health information to the patient's insurer or other payer, and any advance directives.

Informed Consent

First, to receive treatment, a patient must consent or agree to be treated by the providers at the health care organization. Introduced in Chapter 6, a current informed consent form must be signed by the patient and appear in his or her health record before any services can be provided. Informed consent involves a full explanation of the plan for treatment; the potential for complications, risks, and side effects; a discussion of alternate treatments, if any; and the consequences of not performing the treatment at all. The provider—and no other member of the health care team—must make sure the patient understands the treatment or procedure and answers all questions before the patient signs a consent form. Once the patient has enough information to decide to undergo the treatment, she can sign the form, which is maintained in her health record.

✳ LEGAL EAGLE

Without consent to treat the patient, the provider could be charged with the crime of *battery*. Battery can mean the patient was physically harmed or injured, developed an illness because of the provider's intervention, or even felt violated because of not consenting to the provider's touch. If the patient refuses to consent to treatment—and the treatment is performed anyway—the patient can then sue for battery.

Notice of Privacy Practices (NPP)

The **notice of privacy practices (NPP)** details how a health care organization may disclose or use a patient's protected health information (PHI) both with and without her authorization, the patient's rights concerning her privacy, and the organization's responsibility to safeguard her information. The NPP is required to be presented to the patient in clear, easy-to-understand language. It is usually given to new patients at their first appointment. The patient signs a form indicating that she has received the NPP, which is placed in her health record.

Because payment for the patient's treatment is often contingent on third-party payers, such as a health insurance company, the information regarding the specifics of the diagnoses and treatments must be sent to these payers. In other words, the patient must authorize the health care organization to share his or her health record with the payer so that the payer can compensate the provider for any services. The NPP makes the patient aware that it will share information regarding the patient's diagnosis and treatment with his or her third-party payer.

Advance Directives

As discussed in Chapter 6, the **advance directive** details the types and limits of care if a patient is unable to communicate his or her wishes. For example, using an advance directive, patients may elect, in advance, to forego feeding or breathing tubes when, for example, they are in an irreversible coma or a condition that requires life support. Another legal document that may need patient authorization is a *do not resuscitate (DNR)* order. A DNR order is a document signed by the patient specifying that, if the patient has no heartbeat or is not breathing, no life-saving measures should be performed, such as cardiopulmonary resuscitation (CPR). A **durable power of attorney (DPOA)** specifies who will make medical decisions for the patient and under what type of circumstances. Each of these legal documents is maintained in the health record. These may be subject to state law and you should be familiar with the state laws that apply.

Uses

Health record documentation helps physicians and other health care providers monitor the patient's health, plan the patient's treatment, and evaluate the patient's health. This communication is crucial to providing quality care in both the short and longer term. It also has important uses in billing, research, legal matters, quality improvement, and facility administration.

Patient Care

One of the most important reasons for documentation is to facilitate the patient's continuity of care, or the providing of the individual's health care over time. Being able to access the reasons for the patient's previous medical visits, his medical history, laboratory and imaging results, past and current medications, and treatment plan is critical in maintaining and continuing the patient's care. The health record is the means by which this information is communicated.

For example, a patient goes to sees his primary care provider (PCP) because of symptoms of a severe cold. The medical assistant measures the patient's height, weight, and vital signs. The PCP examines the patient, diagnoses a sinus infection, and prescribes an antibiotic. All this information is recorded in the patient's health record. Several weeks later the patient finishes his prescribed course of antibiotics but is still feeling ill. He returns to the medical office where his vital signs are taken again. The PCP reviews the patient's health record, including the information from his last visit (Fig. 9.3). Because the details of the patient's previous visit were carefully documented, the PCP can see the previous diagnosis and the specific antibiotic prescribed. The PCP can also see that the patient's body temperature was normal 2 weeks ago, but is now measured at 103.1°F! Based on this patient history, the PCP can confirm that the patient has not been improving, and may provide a different antibiotic or pursue a different diagnosis and treatment plan.

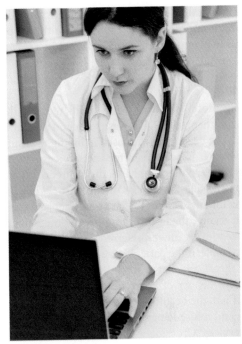

Fig. 9.3 A physician reviews the patient's medical record before the visit to see the prior diagnosis and treatments for this patient. (iStock.com/Rich Legg.)

As you can imagine, this communication becomes even more important should the patient see a different provider over the course of his care. Different health care professionals can examine the patient's health record to learn about the patient's condition over time. They use this information to help the patient. Continuing the example above: For instance, the physician orders laboratory testing—a complete blood count (CBC)—to get more information about why the patient is still ill after the antibiotic treatment. The results from the laboratory are entered into the patient's health record. They show that his white blood cell count is below the normal range, which is unusual for a patient fighting an infection. The PCP decides to refer the patient to a hematologist, a specialist who has more training and experience diagnosing and treating disorders of the blood. The hematologist refers to the patient's health record to see all his symptoms as well as all diagnostics test and treatments that have been done for the patient so far. Because of having all this information, the hematologist knows, for example, that there is no need to order the same testing and that prescribing the same antibiotic would not be therapeutic. In this way, the health record serves as a tool for health care professionals to communicate about a patient in a way that is accurate and comprehensive.

Billing

Among those who work with health records, there is a maxim that states, "If it wasn't documented, it wasn't done." The health record is used in billing to ensure that the provider is being paid for the services rendered to the patient. On the other hand, the insurer or other party paying the bill uses the record to ensure they are not paying for any services that are not necessary. Using the health record, the health care provider must document the need for treatment, referred to as *medical necessity*. For example, if the patient is treated with antibiotics for strep throat, the diagnostic justification should include a patient history of a sore throat and a positive strep test. If not, the health insurance company may deny the claim and refuse to pay the health care organization for the services. Ordering a chest x-ray for a patient who presents with a sore throat would not be justified unless other signs or symptoms warrant the procedure, such as accompanying abnormal lung sounds, pain in the chest, or difficulty breathing. Without proper documentation, no care is considered to have been performed and, therefore, is not paid.

In the hospital setting, *peer review organizations* (PROs) will examine records to determine whether the patient's length of stay was appropriate. Unless documentation supports the hospital stay, the institution or setting will not be compensated. Medicare and other insurers base the amount they will pay hospitals on *prospective payment*, a system in which hospitals are paid for services based on a precalculated structure. Under this system hospitals are paid a set fee for treating a patient regardless of the actual cost. The fees are determined by the patient's diagnosis, age, gender, and the presence of complications. Each diagnosis is assigned a "standard" length of hospital stay and a "standard" dollar amount. If the hospital spends more money than the "standard," the hospital loses that difference. Unless the documentation supports the need for the hospital stay, these payers will not compensate the hospital. Health care professionals must document everything in the patient's health record, including any change in the patient's condition that would warrant a change in the plan of care.

> ## ▶ TAKING THE CHAPTER TO WORK
>
> **Prospective Payment**
> Paula Morello is an 82-year-old woman on Medicare who was admitted to the hospital for pneumonia. After 2 nights in the hospital, her attending physician intended to discharge her on the third day. On the morning that Paula was to be discharged, the certified nursing assistant (CNA) noticed a severe rash had begun to spread on Paula's side and back. The physician decided it would be best to keep Mrs. Morello in the hospital for another night. According to Medicare, patients with pneumonia should be discharged in 3 days. Medicare will not cover the extra day in the hospital for an allergic rash, the treatment of which could have been managed at home. The hospital will not be paid for their care of Mrs. Morello on her fourth day.

Legal Matters

There may be occasions when the patient's medical care can become a legal matter. Patients who feel a provider's actions adversely affected their health may seek damages in a court of law. A patient's health record is considered a legal document and may be used as evidence in court either to support the patient's case against the provider or to help defend the provider's actions. Thus, every clinical staff member is trained to document patient information in health records completely, accurately, consistently, and in a timely manner.

Risk Management

The health record documents patient-related events that occur within the health care facility, but only the facts of an incident as they are related to the care of the patient. For example, if the patient is given the wrong medication, the documentation in the health record includes the date and time of the occurrence. It would also communicate the medication and dosage given and any actions taken to remedy the situation. Note that the health record does not contain the incident report.

Management/Administration

Health services managers and administrators evaluate documentation to make business decisions. By looking at patient records, administrators can monitor compliance with regulations and laws, staffing levels, patient care, and the use of equipment and technology. Information from facility documentation is used to monitor how well the facility is functioning and to make decisions regarding services. For example, the health services administrator may look at records to identify the sources of revenue for the clinic. The health services administrator may also use the data in medical records to track the number and types of patients seen in the clinic to help negotiate contracts with insurance companies and monitor the number of referrals to determine whether an in-house service is cost-effective or not.

Staffing and budgetary needs can also be evaluated based on documentation. For example, assume that you are working in an outpatient mental health clinic that has two shifts (days and evenings). By comparing the number of patient visits and procedures done on various shifts, the supervisor can request more staffing during peak hours.

Quality Improvement

Health care professionals look at health record documentation for quality improvement purposes. Quality improvement is the process of identifying a problem, educating staff about the problem, and then reevaluating to see if the problem has been improved or resolved. Quality improvement programs are required by many regulatory agencies.

▶▶ TAKING THE CHAPTER TO WORK

Performance Improvement

Alyssa, a supervisor at an urgent care clinic, is always looking for ways to improve quality. Alyssa has reviewed patient records and identified that whether the patient is taking vitamin supplements is not being documented. She decides to create a quality improvement program to fix this problem. She starts by communicating this problem to the medical assistants and explains why recording this information is important. After a period of 2 weeks, Alyssa reviews new health records to see if the staff are recording whether the patient takes supplements and what kinds. She decides to do additional staff education for the medical assistants whose record-keeping is still lacking before imposing disciplinary action.

Research and Public Policy

Documentation is also important for research purposes, such as for monitoring diseases and deaths and taking policy action to reduce them. Once a patient's diagnosis is documented in the medical record, this information will be translated into ICD-10-CM codes, discussed

later in this chapter. These codes are used to communicate health data and are indicators of the overall health of a general population. Specifically, this coded information can be used in research to study disease patterns, manage health care, monitor outcomes, and allocate resources. For example, if data from the ICD codes show an increase in the new cases of a sexually transmitted infection, such as syphilis, the state or county health department may increase funding to the health departments to hire more staff and provide free testing services to the community.

Ownership

Ownership of the medical record is an interesting topic and the cause of some confusion among patients and even those within the health care industry. There is no consensus on who owns health records; both federal and state laws are unclear or inconsistent. However, the common thinking is that the patient owns the *information* in the record, but not the *medium* on which the information is kept. For example, in the case of paper records, the physical paper belongs to the health care organization, whereas the information belongs to the patient. This means that the patient may request certain changes be made to the information in the medical record, such as change of address and name, and how this information is used and shared outside of the health care organization; however, the organization owns the medium that the patient's information is on. Further, the health care organization is responsible for maintaining those medical records and protecting them against data breaches. The data in the health record are owned by the patient; however, the storage and maintenance of this data are the responsibility of the health care organization that collected the data.

Release of Information

A patient's health record must be protected from unauthorized disclosures. This means that no individual or entity may have access to the patient's protected health information (PHI) unless the patient allows it, with some exceptions for matters of law enforcement or emergency situations. It is the responsibility of the health care organization to keep this information safe and secure. Releasing or sharing such information without the patient's consent is a breach of confidentiality and a Health Insurance Portability and Accountability Act of 1996 (HIPAA) violation.

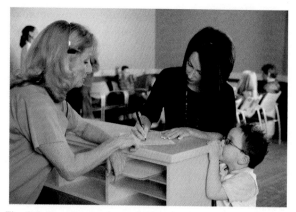

Fig. 9.4 A mother at the pediatrician's office signs a release of information form to obtain a copy of her son's health record. (iStock.com/Vitali Mitchkou.)

At times a patient may wish to have his records sent elsewhere. For example, the patient may switch providers, see a specialist, or want to have another medical professional review their problem. In all these cases, the patient must sign a **release of information (ROI)** form authorizing the provider who is maintaining the record to disclose the heath record (Fig. 9.4). A patient will also be asked to sign an ROI if they are being transferred to another facility so that the new provider can see their history and plan of care. If a patient is hospitalized, they may be asked to sign an ROI on their discharge to have the records from their hospital stay sent to their primary care provider. Even if the patient wishes to view their own records, they must sign an ROI form. Usually, the record is sent by secure fax, although sometimes the patient may pick up paper copies to deliver them to another provider by hand. All signed ROI forms are kept in the patient's health record.

The use of the patient's PHI for the purposes of billing the health insurance company for the cost of the care is listed in the NPP and patients state in writing that they received this notice. A separate ROI form is not required for this disclosure.

Electronic Health Records (EHRs)

Because health care is an industry that relies on multiple parties having the most current information delivered quickly, it should be no surprise that communication technologies have become central to the work of health care professionals. For most of modern medicine, however, medical offices and health care facilities have maintained medical information in paper files and charts, and many providers still do. As computers and technology became more advanced and affordable, the health care industry recognized the benefits of being able to record, store, and retrieve patient information electronically. As a result, more and more health care facilities are moving away from paper-based records to a digital or electronic format. This trend toward adopting EHRs has been heavily boosted by incentives from federal and state governments.

An EHR is a digital version of the patient's paper chart that records and maintains demographic and clinical information about the patient that can be quickly retrieved and shared with multiple providers and staff. Often, the terms EHRs and electronic medical records (EMRs) may be used interchangeably, although a distinction should be made. Like the EHR, the EMR contains the standard demographic and clinical data, but the information is gathered in one provider's office or during a specific encounter.

EHR technology is capable of much more than simply storing medical data. Current EHR systems are highly sophisticated and, for example, can send prescriptions directly to pharmacies, alert providers to potential drug allergies, order tests, and suggest treatment plans to providers. Box 9.1 lists the features of a fully functional EHR system.

Benefits of EHR Technology

There are multiple benefits and advantages to the EHR system for patients, the provider, and the health care facility. The first benefit is timely access to the health record from many different places. When patient data are stored digitally, health care professionals can view and update patient information in real-time, from any computer with appropriate access to the facility's network. For instance, while the nurse is entering vital signs during intake, the physician can view the patient's previous diagnoses and treatments, and the medical biller can check the patient's account for any monies due. Because there is not a single paper medical chart in one physical location, multiple individuals can access the patient's record at the same time, improving coordination of care. Patient information can also be updated and accessed almost instantly, which helps with the efficiency and productivity of the provider and health care facility.

Another major benefit is that the EHR software helps guide health care professionals to input data

BOX 9.1   FEATURES OF A FULLY FUNCTIONAL EHR SYSTEM

- Store and access patient data from any location instantly
- Order tests and medications (known as computer-assisted physician order entry [CPOE])
- Suggest plans of care and treatment protocols to providers
- Print information for patients about specific diseases and treatments
- Generate care and discharge instructions specific to the patient
- Present results of laboratory and diagnostic testing
- Alert providers to drug allergies and interactions
- Prompt wellness screenings and other reminders for preventative medicine
- Assign and track tasks among various health care providers
- Facilitate messaging and communication between health care practitioners
- Generate correspondence to patients and their families
- Track authentication of the record and audit users who accessed the record
- Schedule patients
- Generate reports
- Support billing functions

From Elsevier. *Introduction to Health Services Administration.* St. Louis: Elsevier; 2018.

into the record legibly and accurately. In health care, mistaken or misread dosages, times, and other critical information can result in fatal errors—accuracy can literally be a matter of life and death. At a very basic level, the digital record in the EHR uses typeface and spellchecking rather than handwriting to reduce errors owing to misread or illegible notes. Moreover, certain safeguards exist in the EHR to ensure the data entered into the medical record are accurate and standardized. Administrative and clinical staff do not freely type into the computer system, but rather select entries through the use of dropdown menus and buttons, greatly reducing errors owing to illegible handwriting or incorrectly input information. Computer-assisted physician order entry (CPOE), which allows providers to select orders and transmit them digitally, is estimated to reduce the likelihood of medical errors by 48%—more than 17 million times every year (Radley, et al., 2013).

Additionally, most systems set a range of valid values for text entry fields to prevent staff from entering erroneous information into a patient's record. For example, the system may not allow a patient's body temperature to be entered as 201°F.

Software for EHR systems also aids providers through prompts and alerts. For instance, when entering prescriptions, the EHR can alert the provider of any contraindication, such as drug allergies or drugs the patient cannot take because of a current treatment regimen. It can flag other inappropriate orders, such as if a male patient is scheduled for a Pap smear. EHR software also helps to make sure the medical record is complete through automated reminders and prompts to fill in missing information.

More comprehensive EHR systems will include tools and applications that can help reduce potential errors and standardize delivery of health care. Using scientific evidence, patient data, and standards of care, the medical field has developed specific guidelines to follow for a given disease or disorder, which is called clinical protocols. These protocols aim to standardize the plan of care for patients using structured algorithms, which can reduce unnecessary testing and accelerate the diagnostic process. Like the information-gathering algorithms discussed in Chapter 2, these medical algorithms are included in the EHR's clinical decision support (CDS) system. The CDS recommends approaches for diagnoses of specific diseases, guides selection of the correct diagnostic tests, and assists in the treatment and monitoring of patient care. The EHR is usually linked to an information library that allows the health care professional to select and print custom educational materials to give the patient along with discharge instructions.

Another advantage of an EHR system is that it is more secure than a paper medical record. Because the content is digital, it eliminates the space needed for paper files and the security concerns that go along with having so much sensitive information in one filing room. Many facilities utilize special monitors that can only be viewed by a person facing it directly, preventing others from being able to see the information on the screen. Of course, each workstation in the medical office requires a login and password to access the EHR system. These user names and passwords are unique to every employee in the facility, and passwords are usually changed frequently. Office policy will also require staffers to log out of the system immediately or

	A	B	C	D	E	F
1	Username	Last	First	Date/Time	MRN	Action
2	TFINN	Finn	Timothy	04/24/2018 12:10	12485635401	Submitted dictation file
3	TFINN	Finn	Timothy	04/24/2018 12:12	12485635401	Played dictation file
4	PSTENNET	Stennet	Phillip	04/24/2018 14:25	12485635401	Played dictation file
5	PSTENNET	Stennet	Phillip	04/24/2018 14:28	12485635401	Countersigned dictation
6	SCODY	Cody	Scott	04/27/2018 14:03	12485635401	Edited patient demographics information
7	TFINN	Finn	Timothy	04/28/2018 7:10	12485635401	Submitted transcription file
8	SCODY	Cody	Scott	04/28/2018 11:11	12485635401	Viewed record
9	SCODY	Cody	Scott	04/28/2018 18:50	12485635401	Edited patient financial information

Fig. 9.5 The audit trail shows who accessed the medical record and when. (From Elsevier. *Introduction to Health Services Administration*. St. Louis: Elsevier; 2018.)

the terminals should log the user out automatically after a period of inactivity. Furthermore, the EHR system tracks the identity and time each user viewed the medical record, called an **audit trail**. This traces the individuals who accessed a medical record to ensure its contents are only viewed and updated by authorized persons (Fig. 9.5).

SPOTLIGHT ON SUCCESS

Usernames and Accountability

When you work in the medical setting, you will be issued a unique username with which you will log into the organization's computer system. During your orientation, you will learn about the policies for using the organization's computers, and any penalties for violating the rules.

As we discussed in Chapter 8, HIPAA regulations demand that protected health information is disclosed only to the *minimum necessary* to accomplish the intended purpose. If you are not involved with the patient's care, it is a violation of the patient's privacy to view the patient's health record. System administrators regularly check the audit trail of health care professionals to look for unauthorized access.

Never share your login information with anyone else at work and never leave a computer screen unattended when you are logged in. Anything you do in the EHR—view or access patient records, input information, make changes—is tagged with your identity. You will be responsible for any actions performed under your credentials.

The EHR also has some administrative features to help improve quality. For instance, the system can send alerts and reminders to physicians to sign and authorize notes and orders input by other health care professionals. This helps reduce the number of health records that accrediting agencies consider "deficient." Another feature can collect and report immunization data and syndromic surveillance data to public health and clinical data registries to help meet government requirements.

Health Information Exchanges

To ensure the most efficient and effective patient care and continuity of care, health care professionals need access to the patient's medical history and the ability to share patient information with other health care providers. This includes information sharing not only among the clinicians and administrative professionals in the same medical office or practice but also providers from different organizations; however, sharing patient data between different providers is not the simple and straight-forward process it could be because different health care organizations may use different software. Accessing and sharing data is not possible unless these different software systems are **interoperable** or have the ability to communicate, exchange data, and use the information that has been exchanged across clinicians, laboratories, hospital, pharmacy, and patient regardless of the EHR system. Both private and governmental agencies have recognized the benefits of widespread interoperable EHR systems. Such a network would save money spent on printing, scanning, and faxing; it would save the time it takes to mail documents; and it would reduce inefficiencies, such as duplicate tests and imaging. Despite initiatives from both public agencies and private sector groups, the United States has not yet achieved interoperability across organizational boundaries.

⟫ TAKING THE CHAPTER TO WORK

The Interoperable Record

John presents to a new physician with dry, itchy skin. He thinks it may be because of the dryer air in the winter, but the lotions he has tried do not seem to be helping. The physician reviews the patient's EHR and sees that the patient has gained 30 pounds since he was at the hospital's emergency department a year ago for a baseball injury. The physician also notes John has a family history of a thyroid condition. Using the information recorded by various providers in the patient's health record over time, the physician suspects the patient's dry skin may be caused by hypothyroidism, or an underactive thyroid, which can be hereditary and would explain his weight gain as well as skin condition. The physician orders laboratory tests and discovers values that confirm the diagnosis of hypothyroidism. Because the software at the physician's office was interoperable with the software at the hospital, the physician had the information needed to diagnose John's condition. This diagnosis was made based on the physician being able to develop a clinical picture of the patient based on his presenting condition, laboratory test results, and the documentation of his past medical and family history.

BOX 9.2 THE FIVE NEVERS OF DOCUMENTING

- Never document for someone else.
- Never give anyone your username and password.
- Never ask someone else to document for you.
- Never document false information.
- Never delete, erase, scribble over, or white out.
- Never tamper with the medical record.

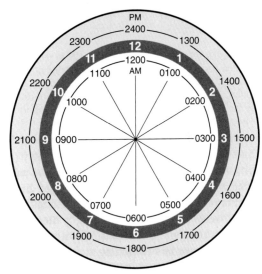

Fig. 9.6 Military time. (From LaFleur Brooks M, Gillingham EA. *Health Unit Coordinating*, ed 5. St. Louis: Saunders; 2004.)

Lastly, most EHR systems help connect patients to their providers. A public-facing side of the EHR lets patients log onto a website, often referred to as a **patient portal**. On the patient portal, users can send messages to the clinical staff and physicians. They may also view their laboratory results and track and monitor information regarding their personal health. Administratively, patients can schedule appointments, edit demographic and billing information, and request their health records be sent to a specific provider.

Documenting Guidelines

The health record is the most important communication tool in health care. The following are best practices for documenting whether you are working with paper forms and charts or typing free text into the EHR. Box 9.2 has additional tips on documentation.

Military Time

Military format is a 24-hour clock system wherein each of the 24 hours in the day are counted, rather than repeating 12 hours and separating them with the a.m. and p.m. denotation (Fig. 9.6). Further, the system eliminates the colon between the hour and the minutes to

reduce the chance that someone will misread the time. In this system, 11:00 a.m. is written as 1100; 11:15 a.m. is written as 1115; 12:00 p.m. (noon) is written as 1200, and so on. Instead of starting the hour after noon as 1:00 p.m., however, this hour is 1300, 2:00 p.m. is 1400, and on until midnight (2400), after which the day begins again with 0001. Military time helps eliminate communication mishaps because there is no question where an event happened during a.m. or p.m. hours, and it requires less writing.

Approved Abbreviations and Symbols

Abbreviations are short cuts to writing a complete word or phrase. They can save time, but can sometimes lead to confusion. Incorrect abbreviations have led to wrong dosages of medications ordered or administered to incorrect tests or therapies initiated or cancelled, and to critical errors in surgery.

TABLE 9.1 Official "Do Not Use" List

Do Not Use	Potential Problem	Use Instead
U, u (unit)	Mistaken for "0" (zero), the number "4" (four) or "cc"	Write "unit"
IU (International Unit)	Mistaken for IV (intravenous) or the number 10 (ten)	Write "International Unit"
Q.D., QD, q.d., qd (daily) Q.O.D., QOD, q.o.d, qod (every other day)	Mistaken for each other Period after the Q mistaken for "I" and the "O" mistaken for "I"	Write "daily" Write "every other day"
Trailing zero (X.0 mg)* Lack of leading zero (.X mg)	Decimal point is missed	Write X mg Write 0.X mg
MS MSO_4 and $MgSO_4$	Can mean morphine sulfate or magnesium sulfate Confused for one another	Write "morphine sulfate" Write "magnesium sulfate"

*Exception: A "trailing zero" may be used only where required to demonstrate the level of precision of the value being reported, such as for laboratory results, imaging studies that report size of lesions, or catheter/tube sizes. It may not be used in medication orders or other medication-related documentation.

The Joint Commission (TJC) recognizes the potential for errors and has developed standards regarding the use of abbreviations within health care settings. These standards were developed to improve patient safety. Table 9.1 lists the abbreviations that may not be used in any handwritten orders (including free-text computer entry) or on preprinted forms. In addition, all health care settings, both inpatient and outpatient, are required to have a policy stating which abbreviations can be used and what the abbreviation means at that institution. Failure to follow the policy can affect your performance evaluation, your job security, and, most importantly, the patient's safety. These policies may change with time, but it is your responsibility to remain current. Failure to comply with TJC standards can result in fines and loss of an institution's accreditation.

Correct Punctuation

The placement of a comma or period can completely change the message. Pay special attention to punctuation marks. Consider, for example, this note entered in the heath record:

Foley catheter removed in cardiac chair reading a magazine.

Where was the Foley catheter removed ... in the cardiac chair? It should have been documented:

Foley catheter removed. In cardiac chair reading a magazine.

It may seem a small mistake, but imagine defending yourself in court that you removed the catheter in bed and then put the patient into the chair. It is important not to leave any potential area for confusion or speculation.

The lack of a decimal point or a decimal point in the wrong place can lead to serious patient injury. For example, assume that you documented that you gave the patient 25 milligrams of a medication; however, the correct dosage was 2.5 milligrams. You may have given the correct dosage, but you documented it incorrectly. From a legal standpoint, you gave the patient 25 milligrams. The difference between those two dosages can be fatal.

Active Voice

An active voice conveys events more concisely and it does not omit who did what. The passive voice is an indirect and obscure recording. For example, "family notified," which is passive, leaves out who notified the family. "Notified family," which is in the active voice, implies that the recorder notified the family. Rather than writing "Dr. Rodriquez was contacted by the charge nurse," write "The charge nurse contacted Dr. Rodriquez."

Spelling

Errors in spelling are unacceptable. They convey unprofessionalism, laziness, and poor judgment. Electronic systems have spell checking functions and will provide suggestions for even the most unusual medical terms and medications. Spellcheckers usually do not detect instances where an incorrect word is used, however. Consider the sentence "Detected a fowl-smelling odor." Was the drainage foul smelling or was there a goose—a type of fowl—in the hospital room? The answer may seem obvious, but a prosecuting attorney might able to place doubt in the mind of jurors.

Being Concise

It is not necessary or recommended that you record lengthy narrative notes about normal events in patient care. For example, if an inpatient ate all his lunch, you can simply write, "Tolerated full lunch without problem." It would not be appropriate to write, "patient ate 1/2 a bologna sandwich, 3 bites of an orange, 6 ounces of milk, and a cup of unsweetened coffee," unless this was an unusual occurrence for the patient that required full documentation.

Being Specific

Words such as *disoriented* and *confused* are vague and can be misinterpreted. For example, a patient can be "confused" when he calls you "Brenda" and not "Bonnie." The patient can, however, still be well-oriented to person, place, and time; he is simply forgetful, not confused. The treatment and cause for confusion differs significantly from the treatment for forgetfulness.

It can be easy to be unspecific. For example, the progress note states: "Patient was uncooperative." This phrase leaves many questions in the mind of the reader, such as the following.

- What were the uncooperative actions—spitting, pushing, or fighting?
- Why was the patient uncooperative? Was he in pain? Were you giving him an injection? Was he confused?
- Did his actions affect patient care; did he refuse his pills, pull off his dressings, or refuse blood work?
- Was he uncooperative at every visit, on every shift, or just this one time?

A better sentence to communicate would be: "Patient stated that he didn't want to have any more finger sticks," and then record that the importance of blood sugar testing was explained to the patient and the provider was notified.

Be careful using subjective terms, such as "large" or "small." Use measurements when possible. For example, assume that you are working in a pediatrician's office and a mother arrives with her 6-year-old child.

The child has a laceration on her leg. Which statement communicates the best information?

- "Large laceration to left knee."
- "Three-inch laceration to left knee."

A patient may state that there was "large amount of blood," but in reality, there was only a half a cup of blood. Ask patients for clarification when they use vague terms.

Sticking to the Facts

Just state the facts when documenting. Do not put your personal assumptions or bias into the health record.

Consider this sentence: "Patient had not bathed in weeks, which caused the leg ulcer to get worse." This statement is unprofessional and presents a conclusion about the patient's bathing regimen and hygiene. Unless the patient stated that she had not taken a bath in weeks, you cannot make that assumption. A better documentation would be, "Stage 3 lower left leg ulcer noted. Patient states that she had not bathed because the shelter was closed."

It is never appropriate to use the health record to criticize other professionals or to imply staff incompetence. For example, assume that you are working in an outpatient surgical clinic and you are caring for a patient who came in for a hemorrhoidectomy. Just before discharge, he said that he "felt weak." The physician told the patient to go home and rest. In the parking lot, the patient collapsed and was brought back into the clinic. Which statement would be the best one to chart?

- Patient collapsed in parking lot. Brought back into clinic. Contacted Dr. Brown.
- Patient felt weak before discharge but was told by Dr. Brown to go home. He collapsed in parking lot.

The first statement is accurate and honest. The second statement implies friction between the team members and accuses the provider of poor judgment. An attorney for the patient would be very excited to find discrepancy or fighting among team members.

Corrections

You may accidentally record something wrong. It is important to recognize the mistake and correct it promptly. To make a correction to a paper health record or form, follow your office's policy and procedure manual. The standard method for making corrections is as follows.

- Draw a single line through the error. The error should still be legible.

- Write "mistaken entry" above or near the cross out. The term "error" is discouraged because it implies an error in care was made. You must follow your office policy.
- Make the correction as close as possible to the original entry. Be sure that it is neat and legible. Do not cram it into a small spot that cannot be read.
- Never use correction tape or fluid.
- Never completely black out the mistaken entry.

In the EHR, there are functions to make a correction that vary by software system. Typically, the user selects a function (sometimes called "amendment") and a reason for the correction, such as the information was entered for the wrong patient, the wrong time or medication was selected, and so forth. This function preserves the original note and makes the change easy to see.

Late Entries

Late entries occur for various reasons. You must follow your office policy and procedure manual to make a late entry. In the paper record, write the present date and time (in the EHR the entry will automatically be timestamped with the current time). Then, write "Entry from…" and the time and date that the information was to be entered. Record the appropriate information and authenticate the entry. Make your late entries as soon as possible.

Emergency Care

Depending on your specialty and place of employment, the type of emergencies that arise will differ. Working for a family practice physician, you may encounter an elderly patient with a heart problem or a young child with a head injury that needs emergency care. If you work in an obstetric office, you may have young women in labor or premature labor. No matter what type of emergency occurs, always treat the patient first and then document the event.

Patient Noncompliance

The health record must include factual information about patient noncompliance. Noncompliance is the failure to follow medical instructions that can lead to serious patient consequences. The information must be presented professionally. For example, it would not be appropriate to say

Patient is stupid and is not doing what he is told to do. Instead, you must document the facts.

►► TAKING THE CHAPTER TO WORK

An Error

Jennie is working in an outpatient clinic. The physician saw Jennie at the desk and asked her to give Scott James an influenza vaccine and James Smith amoxicillin 250 mg by mouth. At the same moment, the receptionist asked Jennie to come into the waiting room to triage a patient with a nosebleed. This patient needed immediate help and required about 15 minutes of care. Jennie felt rushed and went into the medication room and obtained a flu vaccine vial and the amoxicillin. Jennie asked a colleague which room "James" was in. She was told room 4. Jennie went into room 4 and gave the flu vaccine to a James Smith. Then she went into room 3 and gave Scott James the amoxicillin. These medication errors were made because Jennie did not follow numerous office policies. Neither patient suffered ill results from her mistake, but these errors never should have occurred. Jennie told the physician immediately and he examined both patients. Jennie documented the incident as follows: In James Smith's record, the administration of vaccine was documented, and in Scott James chart, the administration of the amoxicillin was documented.

A few minutes later, the physician told Jennie that it was now safe to "readminister" the correct medications. She gave the correct medications to the correct patients. Jennie documented in James Smith's chart the amoxicillin and in Scott James's chart the flu vaccine administration. After the patients went home, Jennie completed an incident report. She recorded her actions, then the physician documented his information.

The health record must always communicate the facts in an honest and truthful manner. Neither Jennie nor the physician attempted to hide or conceal the error. They completed the incident report as per policy. The failure to complete or to falsify an incident report can result in disciplinary actions.

Patient arrived for appointment with wound open. No dressing. States, "I didn't feel like putting the dressing on this morning."

Not returning for follow-up visits or the failure to keep appointments also indicates noncompliance and must be documented. If the patient fails to follow medical instructions and keep appointments and later sues the physician for malpractice, the recording of these events will be critical for the defense. If a patient cancels an appointment or fails to show, you should document the date and time of the appointment and a statement that he cancelled or did not show. Note the reason for the cancellation if known.

Poor Handwriting

Trace is nearing his one-year anniversary working as a pharmacy technician at a privately-owned, single-location drug store. The pharmacy is equipped to receive electronic prescriptions, but one local physician is still writing prescriptions by hand. With office hours only a few days a week and nearing his retirement, Dr. Seamus has not seen the value in purchasing an expensive new EHR system. The staff at the pharmacy pride themselves on being able to decipher the physician's writing when his patients come in.

This morning, a woman in her 50s comes to the pharmacy from Dr. Seamus' office with a common prescription, tramadol 150 mg. She drops it off explaining she has some errands to run and will be back later that day. Trace knows this is a typical medication for patients suffering chronic pain, such as arthritis or fibromyalgia. This is also a medication that Dr. Seamus prescribes often, and the staff at the pharmacy prepare to fill the order. Although tramadol is sometimes thought to be a "safer" opioid and the prescription is legitimate, something seems not quite right to Trace. He did not recognize this customer and the dose is rather high for an initial prescription. Trace asks the pharmacist to take another look at the prescription. The pharmacist and Trace agree that it would be wise to call Dr. Seamus' office. It was a good thing they did! The prescription was not for tramadol at all, but rather for trazodone, an antidepressant medication.

Technologies like CPOE can reduce errors caused by illegible handwriting or incorrectly input information, but their use is not yet universal. Opportunities remain for human error. In health care, being cautious and checking again is better than making an error.

CODING

Coding translates diagnoses (e.g., diseases, injuries, circumstances, and reasons for encounters) and procedures (surgical procedures, services, treatments) into a numeric or alphanumeric code. These short codes are designed to communicate the patient's health and the services she received with the highest accuracy. The codes classify information into a distinct, specific, universally understood vocabulary. Medical coding is so important that the HIPAA requires the use of specific codes for billing (Table 9.2).

Coding standardizes the communication of clinical data among health care professionals. For example, if we want to record that a patient has high blood pressure,

the diagnosis *hypertension* is translated to ICD-10-CM code **I10**, *Essential (primary) hypertension*. From just these three characters, we can tell other clinicians not only that the patient has high blood pressure, but also that the problem is not caused by some other disease or condition associated with high blood pressure, such as a thyroid problem or pregnancy. Using the code forces all providers to describe something in the same way, thus increasing clarity and reducing errors. As another example, the provider wanted to communicate that the patient received substance abuse treatment in a group counseling session and that the specific therapy offered was part of a 12-Step program. Using ICD-10-PCS, all this information is coded **HZ43ZZZ**, *Substance abuse treatment, group scounseling: the application of psychological methods to treat two or more individuals with addictive behavior, 12-Step*. Again, the use of the seven-character code HZ43ZZZ communicates the exact procedure: what was done and how. Figure 9.7 is an example of a table used to build an ICD-10-PCS code.

A Career in Medical Coding

Medical coders and billers specialize in assigning codes. They review the record to determine the specific codes to represent the patient's diagnoses and services rendered, working with providers and other staff to resolve any questions. This individual will have a knowledge of medical terminology and coding systems and most often holds a certification. The medical coder's goal is to present a complete and accurate picture of the patient's visit for both billing purposes and the generation of statistics. Even when working with EHR systems that assign codes automatically, the medical coder reviews billing claims to ensure that assigned codes meet legal and insurance requirements.

International Classification of Disease, Tenth Revision, Clinical Modification

In the health care setting, the patient's chief complaint and any diagnoses are coded with the *International Classification of Disease, 10ᵗʰ edition, Clinical Modification (ICD-10-CM)*. The ICD coding system is used by health care providers, health organizations, researchers, health information managers, medical billers and coders, and policy makers in more than 117 countries to report and monitor health data.

TABLE 9.2 Health Insurance Portability and Accountability Act Transaction Code Sets

Coding System	Description	Sample Code	Code Meaning
International Classification of Diseases, 10th edition, Clinic Modification (ICD-10-CM)	Used for chief complaints and diagnoses in all settings	A92.3	West Nile virus infection
International Classification of Diseases, 10th edition, Procedure Coding System (ICD-10-PCS)	Used for procedures in the inpatient setting	BT0B0ZZ	Radiography (x-ray) of the bladder and urethra with high osmolar contrast agent
Current Procedure Terminology (CPT®)	For physicians and other providers to code and describe medical, surgical, radiology, laboratory, and anesthesiology services. The CPT is Level I of the HCPCS	59400	Routine obstetric care including antepartum care, vaginal delivery (with or without episiotomy, and/or forceps) and postpartum care
Health Care Common Procedure Coding System (HCPCS) Level II	Nonphysician services such as ambulance services prosthetics, durable medical equipment, medications, and supplies	J0897	Injection, denosumab, 1 mg
Code on Dental Procedures and Nomenclature (CDT)	Used for dental procedures and treatments	D3348	Retreatment of previous root canal therapy—molar
National Drug Code (NDC)	A product identifier for every medication manufactured and sold for use in humans	54092-383	Adderall XR, extended release capsules labeled by Shire US Manufacturing Inc.

CPT Copyright 2018 American Medical Association. All rights reserved. CPT® is a registered trademark of the American Medical Association.

0CQ

Section	0	Medical and Surgical
Body System	C	Mouth and Throat
Operation	Q	Repair: Restoring, to the extent possible, a body part to its normal anatomic structure and function

Body Part	Approach	Device	Qualifier
0 Upper Lip 1 Lower Lip 2 Hard Palate 3 Soft Palate 4 Buccal Mucosa 5 Upper Gingiva 6 Lower Gingiva 7 Tongue N Uvula P Tonsils Q Adenoids	0 Open 3 Percutaneous X External	Z No Device	Z No Qualifier
8 Parotid Gland, Right 9 Parotid Gland, Left B Parotid Duct, Right C Parotid Duct, Left D Sublingual Gland, Right F Sublingual Gland, Left G Submaxillary Gland, Right H Submaxillary Gland, Left J Minor Salivary Gland	0 Open 3 Percutaneous	Z No Device	Z No Qualifier
M Pharynx R Epiglottis S Larynx T Vocal Cord, Right V Vocal Cord, Left	0 Open 3 Percutaneous 4 Percutaneous Endoscopic 7 Via Natural or Artificial Opening 8 Via Natural or Artificial Opening Endoscopic	Z No Device	Z No Qualifier
W Upper Tooth X Lower Tooth	0 Open X External	Z No Device	0 Single 1 Multiple 2 All

Fig. 9.7 Table for building an ICD-10-PCS code, in this case, the surgical repair of parts of the mouth or throat. The code 0CQW0Z1 would mean that multiple upper teeth were repaired.

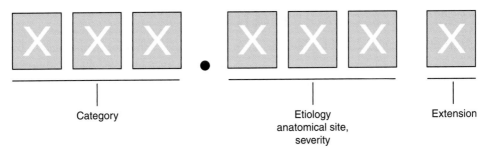

Fig. 9.8 The code format for ICD-10-CM. (From Davis. Foundations of Health Information Management, ed 5. St. Louis: Elsevier; 2020.)

The ICD has been revised and published in a series of editions to reflect changes in health care and medical services over time. The ICD is currently in its 10th revision, which increased the number of codes from 14,000 in its 9th edition (ICD-9) to more than 69,000 codes in ICD-10. This increase in codes helps health care providers better capture specificity and complexity of diseases when coding, which may support the provider's clinical decision-making to a health insurer. The structure of ICD-10-CM is organized primarily by body system and each code includes three to seven characters (Fig. 9.8).

Healthcare Common Procedure Coding System (HCPCS)

As ICD is used for coding diseases and diagnoses, the *Healthcare Common Procedure Coding System (HCPCS)*, often pronounced as "hick-picks," is used to code for treatment, procedures and other medical services. HCPCS was initially developed by the Centers for Medicare and Medicaid Services (CMS) to process Medicare claims. However, HCPCS codes are now used to represent medical procedures and services to Medicare, Medicaid, and several other third-party payers. The HCPCS code set is divided into the following two levels.

- Level I: Current Procedural Terminology (CPT)
- Level II: Codes not included in CPT, such as durable medical equipment, medications, and supplies

The *Current Procedural Terminology (CPT)* coding system, or Level I of the HCPCS, is used to code and describe medical, surgical, radiology, laboratory, and anesthesiology services; tests; evaluations; and any other procedures performed by a physician or other health care provider on a patient. For example, the casting of a broken bone is a specific treatment that would be documented using a CPT code. The CPT code was developed in 1966 by the AMA and is updated annually. There are approximately 7800 codes in the CPT coding system and each code is a five-digit number ranging from 00100 through 99499.

Level II of the HCPCS is a coding system that is used primarily to identify products, supplies, and services not included in the CPT codes, such as ambulance services and durable medical equipment, prosthetics, orthotics, and other supplies when used outside a physician's office.

CPT's Evaluation and Management Codes

In addition to codes that designate a specific procedure, CPT utilizes *evaluation and management (E/M) codes* to summarize the various levels of service provided. E/M codes are a method of representing the amount of time and skill needed to treat the patient at that particular visit. As might be expected, the higher the level of time and skill needed, the higher the payment. For example, CPT's E/M codes assign separate codes for new patients as opposed to established patients; new patients will require more time and documentation because the collection of demographic and financial information and the medical history will be more extensive and time-consuming, as will the physical examination. Using E/M codes, providers have a standard method of communicating to payers how detailed, complex, and comprehensive their services were.

CHECKING YOUR COMPREHENSION

1. What information in the health record identifies the patient?
2. What information from the health record is given to the patient at discharge?
3. What is the purpose of informed consent, and why is informed consent necessary?
4. Give an example of how the health record helps health care professionals provide care.
5. Why is the health record important for billing?
6. List three ways EHR technology improves the delivery of health care.
7. Why is it important to use correct spelling and punctuation in the health record?
8. Why do health care professionals use codes to record information?

EXPANDING CRITICAL THINKING

1. Lois was coming off her lunch break and had just returned to her seat at the reception desk when she saw her neighbor leave the urgent care center. She and her neighbor are good friends and because Lois has access to the EHR, she decides to look at her neighbor's medical record to see why she was in the office. Lois is sure she will hear all about it this weekend, so her neighbor won't mind. Why is she wrong?
2. Mrs. May wants a copy of her medical records because she is curious what the doctor is writing about her. She is afraid that her doctor has diagnosed her with a substance use disorder. Is she allowed to see her health record? Why or why not? Does she have the right to have something embarrassing changed in her health record?
3. While visiting her son, the patient's mother falls in the hospital parking lot. The CNA cleans a scrape on the woman's knee and applies a bandage. Because the woman is not a patient at the hospital, the CNA suggests it be documented in her son's health record so that there is evidence of the accident and care. Is the CNA right or wrong? Why?

Answers to Checking Your Comprehension

Chapter 1

1. Define rapport and explain its importance to health care delivery.

   Rapport is a relationship of trust and understanding. In current and future interactions with patients, rapport helps maintain the flow of communication. Full and honest disclosure during the process of communication is required for the health care professional to work toward the patient's concerns. Put another way: rapport builds trust; trust enables open and honest communication; and communication is the key to the therapeutic relationship.

2. Why is confidentiality important in health care?

   Patients must trust their providers to keep information about their health and treatment secret. Without assurances of their privacy, patients may not divulge information that is necessary for health care providers to treat their ailments and promote their well-being. Confidentiality is not only required for the ethical practice of medicine, it is required by law. Failure to maintain patient privacy is a violation of federal HIPAA legislation, which can result in termination, fines, and even imprisonment.

3. What are the five elements of communication discussed in this chapter?
   - *A message to be transmitted in a form understandable to the receiver*
   - *A sender, usually a person, to initiate and transmit the message*
   - *A channel, the method for transmitting the message—verbal, nonverbal, or written*
   - *A ready and receptive receiver to accept the message*
   - *Feedback, a response indicating whether the message was received and understood*

4. What is slang and jargon, and why should they be avoided in health care communication. Can you think of any occasions when either should be used?

Slang is the very informal words and phrases used around friends, family, and others in our social group. It should be avoided because the language you use in the workplace must be pleasant, polite, and grammatically correct. Because it is important to be professional at work, slang terms are usually not appropriate in health care. On the other hand, with some patients, using slang words may be the best or only way to help them understand their health and wellness. Jargon is speech specific to the workplace; it is often unknown by those outside the work environment, regardless of their background or level of education. You should phrase your communication appropriately without talking down to the patient.

5. Define and compare the terms kinesics and proxemics. Give two examples of each.

   These are types of nonverbal communication that pertain to body position. Kinesics is the study of body positions and movement in relation to communication, such as gestures, facial expressions, and posture. Proxemics is the study of the physical closeness tolerated by most people, the distance we prefer to be from one another.

6. What is meant by the term therapeutic touch? How is touch used in the medical profession?

   Touch is required for procedures, but it can also be used to show concern or to support a person emotionally, provided that level of intimacy is appropriate. Therapeutic touch is meant to promote healing and is a feature of many religions.

7. Explain the three steps to effective communication.

   Step 1: The preparatory, orientation, or introductory step is where the participants meet and learn their roles and responsibilities in the exchange.

   Step 2: In the working or maintenance stage, each participant works to send and receive messages and give feedback that messages were understood.

Step 3: Termination or conclusion represents the end of the exchange where the goals of the conversation are reached.

8. List five of your responsibilities in the communication process.

Answers will vary, but should include concepts such as being self-aware, knowing the patient's history, understanding the goal of the exchange, identifying barriers to communication, knowing the patient's needs, demonstrating courtesy, demonstrating compassion, using professional language, remaining open and objective, offering and asking for feedback, validating the patient's feelings, promoting independence and well-being, and offering education.

9. List four of your patient's responsibilities in the communication process.

Answers will vary, but should include concepts such as truthful and open information, a full medical history, participation in self-care, and compliance with health care directives.

10. How does sympathy differ from empathy? What is the relationship of sympathy and empathy to compassion?

Sympathy implies that you care and that are concerned for another; empathy means experiencing the same feelings as another patient. Compassion is being moved by empathy to take steps to relieve the distress of another.

Chapter 2

1. In your future profession, describe your role and responsibilities in the patient interview.

The patient interview is a conversation between a health care professional and patient with the goal of obtaining important and relevant patient information to improve the well-being of the patient. Depending on your position, you may be gathering information about the chief complaint, the history of the problem, the patient's medical history, medications the patient takes, allergies the patient has, family history, and social history. The patient interview may also include a review of systems. During the interview, you must use your tone of voice and kinesics to make the patient feel comfortable. Having a thorough and accurate patient interview provides the foundation for the patient examination, what the next steps should be, and the subsequent treatment plan.

2. Describe how you should prepare yourself and the setting for a patient interview.

The setting should be warm, inviting, and private. You should be clean, neat, and organized. You should sit at the patient's level and use body language that suggests openness.

3. Explain the difference between a subjective and objective information. Give two examples of each.

Subjective information can be experienced only by the patient. It is the patient's feelings or experience in his or her own words. Objective information is what the health care professional can see and measure. Examples of each type of information are in Table 2.1.

4. Explain the difference between an open-ended and a closed-ended question and give two examples of each type.

Open-ended questions encourage the patient to express fully any possible concerns and do not restrict an answer to "yes" or "no" responses. Some examples are:

- *"What are your symptoms?"*
- *"Who do you live with?"*
- *"Describe what happened next."*
- *"What do you like about this treatment?"*
- *"How is school going?"*
- *"How did you feel when it happened?"*

Closed-ended questions are phrased in such a way as to have a clear, direct answer from a limited set of possibilities. Some examples are:

- *How much....?" "How many....?" "How often....?*
- *How long has this been bothering you (or going on, etc.)?*
- *Does this hurt?*
- *Do you smoke?*
- *Have you eaten today?*

5. List and describe the different information-gathering tools used in patient interviews.

An algorithm is a process or a path of questions to follow, depending on the patient's answer at each step. It can prompt the healthcare professional down a general direction of questioning that may help in the patient interview. An acronym is a word or phrase to help the questioner remember questions to ask.

6. Explain the difference between hearing and listening. Discuss why active listening is so important.

Hearing is simply the sensory perception of sound; it does not require focused involvement. Listening is paying close attention to what is being said. Active listening is a communication technique using the full attention of the listener to comprehend, respond to, and remember what the speaker is communicating. All that we hear during patient interaction requires that we listen with close attention.

7. Describe the difference between the terms paraphrasing and reflecting. Explain why each is important. Give an example of each.

   Paraphrasing is when you reword what the patient stated while keeping the original meaning to verify what the patient said. A reflective response repeats what patients have said to confirm that they were heard, but gives them an opportunity to continue or complete their thought.

8. Describe the purpose of summarizing when performing a patient interview.

   Summarizing, or restating information in a briefer form, helps to highlight the main points given by the patient. It also provides the patient an opportunity to correct any information and to clarify central concerns.

Chapter 3

1. Identify the five patient education steps. Write a short explanation of each step.

   - *Assessment: defines the health care needs and concerns of the patient and family, and evaluates the patient's learning needs and readiness to learn.*
   - *Planning: the formal creation of learning goals and objectives, which helps to define expected short-term and long-term results.*
   - *Implementation: putting the teaching process in motion using one or more instructional methods.*
   - *Evaluation: the appraisal and review of the patient's learning progress during and after the patient education. Based on the evaluation, learning goals and objectives may need to be reevaluated and restructured as the patient progresses through treatment.*
   - *Documentation: the recording of the patient teaching in the medical record.*

2. Describe the characteristics of a person who is "health literate."

   A health literate person can access health information and has the capacity to understand it to make decisions about personal health care.

3. Describe the three basic learning styles.

   - *Cognitive learning style is composed of processing facts, forming conclusions, and making decisions by listening to or reading instructions or information. Examples of methods and techniques for cognitive learning are discussions groups, role playing, seminars, literature, and questions and answer sessions.*
   - *Affective learning appeals to emotions or feelings to change someone's beliefs or attitude, and to reinforce the importance of the change in concepts.*

   - *Psychomotor learning is the acquisition of a skill through participation in the skill.*

4. Differentiate the learning goal from the learning objective.

   Learning goals are broad statements about the long-term expectation of a desired result. Learning goals serve as the basis or foundation for learning objectives. Learning objectives are statements that describe the specific, measurable results. When the objectives are complete the goal is achieved.

5. List at least three instruction methods discussed in this chapter. Write a short explanation of each method.

   - *Lecture: the presentation of the information*
   - *Role-playing and demonstration: showing a procedure and having the patient repeat it*
   - *Discussion: a back-and-forth exchange of information and concepts*
   - *Patient education material (PEM): pamphlets, fact sheets, booklets, posters, and videos*
   - *Support groups: share any information, concerns, experiences, and expectations with one another*

6. List some ways to evaluate patient teaching.

   Answers will vary, but can include the teach-back method, asking open-ended questions about the material, and offering to follow up.

7. List five key components that must be included in a patient's medical record after a teaching session.

   Each step of the education process must be documented and should include the following:

   - *Patient's learning needs, learning style, and readiness to learn*
   - *Patient's knowledge of his or her condition and treatment options*
   - *Objectives and goals and what information was provided to the patient*
   - *How the information was provided to the patient, such as through discussion, demonstration, videos, or patient instruction sheet*
   - *Patient, family, and caregiver response to the patient education*
   - *Evaluation and effectives of the teaching*

   Date and time of the session if separate from regular care, such as over the phone. Include education given during routine patient care under the appropriate record entry.

   - *Copy of the signed educational material provided to the patient, when appropriate. The patient keeps the original and signs that the information has been explained adequately.*

Chapter 4

1. How does the patient's perspective in the health care system differ from the perspective of the health care professional?

   A normal day for a health care professional can include the most extraordinary things that the patient has ever experienced. Patients are undergoing stressful and anxiety-producing experiences, whereas the health care professional is having "another day at work." Besides fear for his health and perhaps his life, the patient must navigate an unfamiliar and complicated health care environment, with unfamiliar processes and many different people.

2. How do different cultural perspectives affect the delivery of health care?

   Patients from different cultures may have different ideas about what it means to be sick or well, how to make decisions about treatments and care, who should be involved in those decisions, and what those treatments should be. A person's culture may have an impact on how that person relates to and manages pain, illness, and injuries. Culture may also influence how patients feel about the health care profession versus traditional or natural healers, whether they feel they have control over their health, and whether they will follow our health care directives.

3. Explain how health insurance affects health care for minority groups.

   Blacks, Asians, and Hispanics have less access to health care services, primarily because they are less likely to have health insurance. Without insurance, persons may delay or completely forgo health care, especially preventative and follow-up care. Persons who are seen regularly for health care may be diagnosed and treated earlier, precluding major health care problems and reducing health care costs. When uninsured persons do seek care, they are more likely to visit an emergency department for treatment, even for minor injuries or ailments. This can lead to further problems. Emergency departments may not have access to a patient's medical history and, as a result, emergency physicians may order unnecessary tests. Emergency departments are not designed to provide follow-ups that promote continuity of care.

4. Explain the difference between sex and gender.

   Sex is a biological status determined by a person's DNA; it is assigned at birth based on the appearance of external genitals to distinguish between males and females. Gender is influenced by an individual's life experiences and is not set at birth. It is a psychological condition. A person determines his or her own gender identity.

5. Give examples of ways that gender-nonconforming patients can be made to feel welcome.

   Provide informational pamphlets that picture diverse patient groups; display a rainbow flag or some other symbol recognized as a welcoming symbol of diversity; address your patients with the proper pronouns, and ask them their pronouns if you are uncertain.

6. List health disparities among gay, lesbian, and bisexual patients.

   Negative attitudes of health care professionals, whether overt or perceived, may lead patients to delay or to avoid health care. LGBT youth have difficulty sharing their sexual orientation with their primary care provider. Lesbian women seek routine and preventive medical care at lower rates than the general population. Gays and lesbians have higher rates of smoking, alcohol, and other drug use, and higher rates of depression and anxiety.

7. Describe three ways religious traditions might have an impact on patient care.

   Answers will vary. Some religions may have dietary restrictions, including fasting or avoiding certain foods; Jehovah's Witnesses cannot receive blood transfusions; some religions consider pain and suffering to be spiritually enriching and may decline pain medications; and some religions may require persons to be cared for by health care providers of the same sex whenever possible.

8. List the stages of cognitive development according to Piaget.
   - Sensorimotor
   - Preoperational
   - Concrete Operational
   - Formal Operational

9. What are some things that can have an impact on your communication with older patients?

   Hearing loss is common in older adults; vision deficits can make it difficult to read medication labels or discharge instructions; and older adults may process information at a slower pace.

Chapter 5

1. What are the benefits of using a professional interpreter, as opposed to a family member?

   A trained medical interpreter is the safest and most effective way to address language barriers between patients and health care professionals. Trained interpreters are less likely to commit errors that may result in adverse clinical consequences. They have fluency in both languages and training in medical terminology, whereas the competency of a family member is unknown. Professional interpreters must adhere to the standards of practice for their professional association and complete continuing education. Using a family member, the patient may not divulge personal or embarrassing information necessary to provide care. Trained interpreters can also identify cultural differences and respond to such issues appropriately. Providing interpreted services for patients with limited English proficiency has resulted in shorter emergency department stays, fewer follow-up appointments and returns to the emergency department, fewer laboratory tests and procedures, and lower overall medical costs.

2. What are the signs a person may have a vision problem he or she has not disclosed? What are the signs of a hearing problem?

   Visually impaired patients may use aids such as a white cane (support or probing cane) or a guide dog, but the impairment may not always be obvious. Undiagnosed patients or those unwilling to accept their impairment may display more subtle signs such as tripping, not being able to find the chair in which to sit, or having difficulty reading a patient form.

   Patients who demonstrate any of the following may have a hearing impairment.

   - *Flat speech patterns with little inflection, or variation in tone. We alter and vary our speech as we hear it, raising and lowering our pitch and tone for emphasis. Hearing-impaired patients may not change their speaking tones.*
   - *Slurred or incomplete words. Patients may not be aware that they have not finished words or that the sounds were not distinct.*
   - *Frequent requests that you repeat a statement. Questioning looks or puzzled expressions after you have spoken should tell you the patient did not understand.*
   - *Apparent indifference to what you are saying. The patient may not know that you are speaking; we do not miss what we do not hear.*
   - *A tendency to dominate the conversation. Patients may not be aware when you are speaking.*

3. Consider the last time you were faced with a stressful situation, such as trying to make an important

deadline at work or having to pack up everything and move. Discuss how your body reacted during that situation. List three of your body's responses to the stress.

Answers will vary, but many people under stress experience a more rapid heartbeat, increased respiratory rate, and slowed digestion.

4. Thinking about the same stressful situation in Question #3, review the different coping mechanisms in Box 5.3. Which one did you use in the stressful situation? Discuss how it presented in the situation.

   Answers will vary.

5. In your future health care profession, discuss what steps you would take in the case of an anxious or stressed patient? Or a violent patient?

   Answers will vary. In cases of a stressed or anxious patient, you could create a relaxing environment, speak slowly and in a lower pitch. The Communication Guidelines box under the Patients and Stress heading in Chapter 5 contains more suggestions for helping patients with stress.

   These are some important steps to take if you find yourself in a highly tense or dangerous encounter with a patient:

   - *Do not let the patient come between you and the door. Always have a clear path to an escape route.*
   - *Move slowly and in full view to avoid any perceived threat to the patient.*
   - *Use caution, but firmly tell the patient that his or her actions are unacceptable.*
   - *Call for help from coworkers and the physician. If the situation is openly dangerous, a staff member must immediately call 911.*
   - *When the crisis is over, document all that happened and how it was handled.*

6. During your interview, a patient discloses she is in an abusive relationship. What specific things should you do or say?

   Always talk to patients alone and not within earshot of a partner or family member.

   If the patient does disclose abuse, thank the patient for sharing. Convey empathy for the patient who has experienced fear, anxiety, and shame. Let the patient know you will support her or him unconditionally without judgment. Ask the patient if he or she has any immediate safety concerns and discuss options. If there are no staff members trained in IPV, refer the patient to an IPV service advocate for safety planning and additional support. It is important to provide a follow-up at the patient's next medical visit.

7. List five signs or behaviors that a patient experiencing elder abuse may exhibit.

Some signs of suspected elder abuse for health care professionals are:

- *Slap marks, most pressure marks, and certain types of burns or blisters (e.g., cigarette burns). Explanations of the injury seems inconsistent with the pattern of the injury.*
- *Withdrawal from normal activities, unexplained change in alertness, or other unusual behavior may signal emotional abuse or neglect.*
- *Bruises around the breasts or genital area and unexplained sexually transmitted diseases can occur from sexual abuse.*
- *Sudden change in finances and accounts, altered wills and trusts, unusual bank withdrawals, checks written as "loans" or "gifts," and loss of property may suggest elder exploitation.*
- *Untreated bedsores, need for medical or dental care, unclean clothing, poor hygiene, overgrown hair and nails, and unusual weight loss may also signal abuse.*

8. List five signs or behaviors that a child experiencing abuse may exhibit.

There are a number of signs to child abuse, such as:

- *Previously filed reports of physical or sexual abuse of the child*
- *Documented abuse of other family members*
- *Different stories between parents and child on how an accident happened; vague or poor explanations*
- *Stories of incidents and injuries that are suspicious*
- *Child brought in for a minor illness or complaint and serious injury is found*
- *Injuries blamed on other family members*
- *Repeated visits to the emergency department for injuries*
- *Discolorations/bruising on the buttocks, back, and abdomen; bruising on a child too young to walk or crawl*
- *Elbow, wrist, and shoulder dislocations*
- *Delays in the normal growth and development patterns*
- *Erratic school attendance*
- *Poor hygiene*
- *Malnutrition*
- *Obvious dental neglect*
- *Neglected well-baby procedures (e.g., immunizations)*

Chapter 6

1. What are the unique barriers to communicating with an ill patient?

Patients who are actively sick have difficulty listening to anything other than what is happening within their body. Pain, nausea, vertigo, and other symptoms of illness make it hard to communicate beyond the most basic information needed to relieve the most disturbing concerns. Individuals under great distress are not ready to exchange or retain information. Patients may also be stressed, worried, or anxious, creating a kind of "psychological noise." There may be physical barriers to communication such as PPE. Finally, unconscious patients cannot communicate at all.

2. Explain the difference between an advance directive and a Physician Order for Life-Sustaining Treatment (POLST) form and how they work together.

An advance directive is a legal document dictating to care providers what treatments the patient wishes to receive and not receive. A POLST is a portable document containing a physician's order so that professionals know what measures to take (or forgo) in an emergency situation. They work together because the POLST stays with the patient and allows first responders to follow the instructions contained in the advance directive as they pertain to an emergent situation, wherever it happens.

3. What is the difference between acute and chronic diseases?

An acute illness has a rapid onset and is of short duration. A chronic illness develops gradually and extends over a long time (typically more than three months).

4. Explain the unique psychological stressors of patients with cancers.

Malignant cancers are fatal if untreated. Patients with cancer face many "unknowns" and much waiting between various phases of diagnosis, treatment, testing, and reevaluation of the extent of the disease. Patients and their loved ones can process this differently and at different paces. Cancer also causes opportunistic diseases and other problems that prompt patients with cancer to seek the services of many different settings.

5. List the symptoms of depression and things to ask when interviewing a patient you suspect is depressed.

A depressed person may display any of the following signs:

- *Appetite changes, either eating less with weight loss or eating more with weight gain*
- *Sleep changes, either difficulty sleeping or sleeping too much*
- *Social interaction changes, ranging from isolation to excessive*
- *Feeling worthless or guilty*
- *Fatigue, loss of energy*
- *Loss of pleasure in things once enjoyed*
- *Loss of interest in daily activities and occupations*
- *Absenteeism from work or school*
- *Difficulty thinking clearly, concentrating, or making decisions*
- *Thoughts of self-harm or suicide*

Some screening questions to ask are:

- *"How long have you been feeling this way? When did it begin?"*
- *"On a scale of 1 to 10, with 10 being the highest, how depressed would you say you currently are? What is the most depressed you have ever been?"*
- *"Is there anything that you've done or found helpful to find relief?"*
- *"Has it ever gotten to the point where you have thought of harming yourself?"*

6. How should the health care professional interview a patient she suspects has suicidal ideations?

   When interacting with patients, consider both warning signs and risk factors. If at any time you suspect a patient may be seeking to harm herself or himself, immediately discuss your concern with the physician. If the patient talks about feeling hopeless, despairing, incapable of going on in life, you can ask about the person's outlook:

   - *How does life seem to you?*
   - *Have you ever felt that life was not worth living?*
   - *Do you ever wish you could go to sleep and just not wake up?*

   Do not be afraid or hesitant to ask directly about the presence of suicidal ideation. "Are you thinking about harming (or killing) yourself?"

7. What are the physical manifestations of a patient with anxiety?

   Irritability, fatigue, sleep disturbances, nervousness, muscle aches and tension, intestinal problems, trembling, and sweating are common manifestations of a higher level of anxiety.

8. What clinical markers suggest a patient has a severe substance use disorder?

   Two or more of the following suggest a substance use disorder.

   - *The substance is taken for longer periods or in larger doses than intended.*
   - *There is a persistent desire or unsuccessful attempts to decrease the use of a substance.*
   - *Significant amount of time and energy are spent trying to get the substance or recover from its effects.*
   - *A strong craving or desire to use the substance.*
   - *Recurrent substance use resulting in a failure to complete obligations at work, school, or home.*
   - *Continued substance use despite experiencing social or interpersonal consequences.*
   - *Limiting social and/or recreational activities to the use of the substance.*
   - *Recurrent substance use in physically dangerous situations, like driving.*
   - *Continued substance use when the individual knows it is causing physical and/or psychological harm.*
   - *The development of tolerance, reduced effects following repeated use of the substance*
   - *Experiencing withdrawal symptoms following cessation of substance use*

9. What behaviors would suggest a patient is looking for drugs from the provider?

   Asking for specific controlled substances before trying other means to relieve symptoms; seeking prescription pain medications late in the day on Fridays; asking for the same controlled substances.

10. Contrast the task-centered care model with the person-centered care model.

    A task-centered model is a traditional care model based on tasks, processes, and schedules to be performed that fit the needs of the organization, such as getting patients out of bed, cleaned, dressed, and fed. Person-centered care focuses on putting the needs of the person first. Decisions are made in a way that sustains a patient's identity, comfort, attachment, inclusion, and occupation. Health care professionals who embrace person-centered care focus less on "what is done" and more on "how it is done."

11. Describe why Alzheimer's disease is a distinctive type of dementia.

    Alzheimer's disease progresses through three stages: mild (early stage), moderate (middle stage), and severe (late stage). Each stage has its own particular symptoms and related behaviors. In the early stages the patient experiences mild memory loss, but after a period of years, the patient with late-stage Alzheimer's disease loses the ability to carry on a conversation and respond to the environment.

12. Explain the difference between the behavior of someone who has bulimia nervosa and someone who has anorexia nervosa.

The patient with anorexia nervosa refrains from eating, whereas the patient with bulimia eats and then purges. Rather than avoiding the thought of food, patients with anorexia nervosa can have a food obsession, collecting recipes, watching cooking shows, hoarding food, and cooking for others. Bulimics hide both their excessive eating and their purging.

13. Identify five communication guidelines for working with a person diagnosed with autism spectrum disorder.

See the Communication Guidelines box under the Autism Spectrum Disorder heading.

14. Explain the difference between someone who "enjoys being the sick person" and someone with somatic symptom disorder.

The severe anxiety of the patient with somatic symptom disorder dominates that patient's life. They seek care frequently, become angry when diagnostics do not support their ideas about their illness, and find reasons to avoid measures that would make them well. Somatic symptom disorder persists for a period of time, usually six months or longer. Those who only occasionally escape into the sick role do not consistently demonstrate the deep-seated anxiety seen in patients with true somatic symptom disorders. The patients in the sick role may be avoiding a stressor and tend to do better once their stress level is lower.

Chapter 7

1. Explain the difference between an actual and a perceived loss. Give an example of each.

An actual loss can be seen objectively. Examples include the death of a loved one or pet, the leaving of loved ones or a physical place, and the loss of a job, a relationship, health, ability, memory, home and things, or youth. Perceived loss is usually apparent only to the one experiencing the loss, such as the loss of self-esteem, of identity, of purpose, of belonging or connection with others, of security or safety, of opportunities and of unrealized dreams.

2. Define grieving, mourning, and bereavement and how they differ.

Grief is our normal emotional response to the actual or perceived loss of something we value or of any kind of change. Mourning is the expression of grief. Bereavement is the state of having lost a loved one.

3. In the dominant U.S. culture, how have perspectives on death changed from 1900 to today? How would physicians from 1900, 1965, and today differ in their discussion of death with patients?

Compared with people in the year 1900, we are much more distant from death today. Because most people no longer die at home, it is less common to see a loved one die. Fewer people live on farms or in rural areas to witness the death of livestock.

In 1900, when physicians had few remedies and resources to save patients from disease or death, doctors, patients, and families seemed more willing to accept that death or disability was inevitable. As medical science became more effective, a physician in 1965 would commonly want to do everything possible to extend life. Today, medical practitioners empower patients and families to pursue treatment as they wish, sometimes allowing the terminally ill to die without intervention. A palliative care model attempts to comfort and relieve pain, rather than try to cure, to improve quality of life for the remainder of time a person has left.

4. What do all the theories of loss and grieving discussed in this chapter have in common? How does the dual process theory differ from other conceptualizations?

All the grief theories discussed have some component of "grief work," the idea that the grieving individual feels strong emotions toward a loss and must work through these emotions to reduce distress. The dual process model posits that a grieving person must cope with the loss on one hand, adjust to lifestyle changes on the other, and rest from both of these types of stressors at times.

5. List things you should not do when caring for a grieving patient, family member, or caregiver.

Answers will vary but may include the following.

- *Do not attempt to educate or to provide care to patients or family beyond the scope of your practice.*

- *Do not be judgmental about the reason for the patient's loss of health.*
- *Do not try to "fix" a patient's problems.*

6. Describe how a 5-year-old's understanding of death differs from an adolescent's.

   With limited or unrealistic comprehension of the finality and the inevitability of death, young children may have more difficulty working through the task of grieving. A 5-year-old would probably have questions such as, "Does it hurt?" or "Are animals there?" Some children at this age may think death is a reversible process. Developmentally, adolescents are better able to conceptualize death. They may even see it happen among their peers and understand that it can be sudden and final.

7. Describe how a young adult's understanding of death differs from that of an older adult.

   Younger adults often think they are "immortal" and often have fewer direct experiences of significant grief thus far in their lives. Older adults experience an acceleration of loss and grief in their lives, such as loss of friends, health, ability, meaning and purpose, autonomy, independence, mobility, and physical living space. Many also may have less fear of death; some may even welcome death if they feel they have lived a full life or desire to avoid any more illness, pain, or suffering.

8. List two health care specialists who can be particularly beneficial in helping patients/families/caregivers address matters of loss and grief.

   Medical social workers, chaplains, and child life specialists

9. Explain the function of hospice care and how it differs from other areas of health care.

   Hospice is a specific type of care for patients facing the end of life that focuses on pain management and emotional support. This care provides palliative comfort measures, not curative treatment.

10. List eight members of the hospice interdisciplinary team.

    Hospice interdisciplinary teams consist of providers, nurses, medical social workers, home health aides, nutritionists, pharmacists, and grief counselors, and volunteers.

Chapter 8

1. Define the term professionalism. Give three examples of professional behaviors.

   Professionalism refers to exhibiting appropriate behavior for the workplace, having the right skills, and making the right judgements. Examples will vary but can include:
   - *Honesty*
   - *Showing respect for the humanity of others*
   - *Being polite and dependable*
   - *Safeguarding patient privacy*
   - *Following ethical guidelines*
   - *Maintaining accurate and timely health records*

2. According to privacy laws, with which persons in the health care setting can you share protected health information?

   Protected health information may be shared only with those who require it for patient care (i.e., other clinicians) or as directed by the patient.

3. List three benefits of interdisciplinary communication.

   Interdisciplinary communication is beneficial because
   - *Each specialty provides a unique viewpoint and treatment plan for the patient and family.*
   - *Promotes teamwork, thus improving staff productivity and efficiency*
   - *Improves the patient care environment*
   - *Meets the requirements of various regulatory agencies*
   - *Helps to create or revise policies and procedures that affect more than one department*

4. Define the terms emergent, urgent, and nonurgent. How does provider notification vary for each setting?

   See Box 8.2. An emergent situation requires a STAT communication. The provider should be contacted non-STAT for urgent situations. The provider can be left a message in nonurgent cases.

5. What are the benefits of a meeting agenda?

   The agenda allows participants a chance to prepare for the meetings, and helps keep the meeting organized and focused.

6. How do regulatory agencies monitor health care organizations?

   Regulatory bodies set standards and monitor adherence to standards through site surveys.

7. What acronym can help you resolve conflict in the workplace? Explain each letter.

   *You can use the acronym **PEER** to work through conflicts with staff, colleagues, and others.*

- *Present the problem (explain the problem as you see it): "Today, I was trying to teach a patient how to use a home glucometer. We could hear your laughter in the hall."*
- *Explain (explain how the problem makes you feel): "I felt really embarrassed when I was talking to the patient."*
- *Effect (explain the effect the problem has on your ability to do your work): "It bothers me because I have to repeat my message and I feel that I have to apologize for the loud noise."*
- *Resolve (explain that you want to resolve this problem so that you can work together better): "I really enjoy working with you and I want us to be able to work as a team, so I would like to resolve this problem. Can you try to lower your voice when sitting at the desk?"*

8. Why are telephone skills an important part of communication?

Telephone communication is very common, and it is often the first impression the patient has of the health care organization.

9. When using email, what are the considerations for patient privacy and HIPAA regulations?

Health care professionals must be aware that much of the information they are communicating is confidential in nature. Therefore, you should always check with your supervisor on your organization's policy regarding emails to ensure compliance with the Health Insurance Portability and Accountability Act (HIPAA) guidelines. Some health care facilities may have standard privacy language that is included in all email correspondence that provides contact information in the event that the email is sent to the wrong address.

10. What occasions require a written business letter? Name three.

- *Appointment Reminder Letters*
- *Patient Billing Letters*
- *Referral Letters (referring patients to another provider)*
- *Excused Absence Letters (for students or employees to document the reason for absence from school or work)*
- *Office Announcement Letters (e.g., changes in staff, insurance, hours, or other office protocols).*

Chapter 9

1. What information is in the health record to identify the patient?

The patient is identified through demographic information, such as name, social security number, address, etc.

2. What information from the health record is given to the patient at discharge?

The discharge summary, also called a discharge report, is provided to the patient when he or she is discharged or checks out after the medical visit. The discharge summary includes the patient's diagnoses; any procedures that were performed; the patient's diagnostic studies, including laboratory and imaging; progress notes; physician's orders, consultation reports; and any discharge instructions.

3. What is the purpose of informed consent and why is informed consent necessary?

Informed consent involves a full explanation of the plan for treatment; the potential for complications, risks, and side effects; a discussion of alternate treatments, if any; and the consequences of not performing the treatment at all. The provider—and no other member of the health care team—must make sure the patient understands the treatment or procedure and answers all questions before the patient signs a consent form. Once the patient has enough information to decide to undergo the treatment, he/she can sign the form, which is maintained in his/her health record. Without consent to treat the patient, the provider could be charged with the crime of battery. Battery can mean the patient was physically harmed or injured, developed an illness because of the provider's intervention, or even felt violated because the patient did not consent to the provider's touch.

4. Give an example of how the health record helps health care professionals provide care.

Answers will vary, but should illustrate that the health record is the means by which the care of the patient is coordinated and communicated among providers. For example, by checking the record, the nurse can see that a patient has not had a flu shot this year and might suggest the vaccination.

5. Why is the health record important for billing?

The health record is used in billing to ensure that the provider is being paid for the services rendered to the patient. On the other hand, insurers or other parties paying the bill use the record to ensure they are not paying for any services that are not necessary.

6. List three ways electronic health record (EHR) technology improves the delivery of health care.
   - *The EHR allows information to be recorded and accessed instantly from any location having access, which improves care coordination and efficiency.*
   - *Through menus and the standardized data entry, it reduces errors caused by illegible handwriting or incorrect input information.*
   - *Suggests treatment plans and offer reminders for preventative care*
   - *Alerts providers of allergies or contraindications*
   - *Enhanced security of the record and a built-in audit trail*

7. Why is it important to use correct spelling and punctuation in the health record?
   Errors convey unprofessionalism, laziness, and poor judgment. Improper punctuation can change the meaning of a sentence or even make a dosage of medication fatal. These errors can be used in the courtroom to call into question the accuracy of the record.

8. Why do health care professionals use codes to record information?
   Codes are designed to communicate the patient's health and the services received with the highest accuracy. The codes classify information into a distinct, specific, universally understood vocabulary.

GLOSSARY

abuse general term for misuse or maltreatment, which may be emotional, physical, psychological, economic, and/or sexual trauma on another individual to satisfy a desire to control and have power over that individual

acronym word formed by the initial letters of a series of words

active listening communication technique using the full attention of the listener to comprehend, respond to, and remember what the speaker is communicating

activities of daily living (ADLs) self-care, such as bathing, preparing meals, cleaning, shopping, and other routines that require thought, planning, and physical motion

acute an illness with a rapid onset and short duration

ad hoc **interpreter** use of an interpreter present during a clinical encounter, such as family members, friends, untrained members of the support staff, and even strangers found in waiting rooms

addiction physiologic and/or psychological dependence on a substance beyond voluntary control

adherence to carry out the care plan as directed

advance directive legal document that provides guidance about the patient's desired treatments to sustain life when he or she becomes incapacitated

affective learning growth or change in feelings, emotions, or a mental state

agenda in a meeting, a list of what will be discussed and in what order

algorithm step-by-step procedure for solving a problem using a logical progression

Alzheimer's disease progressive disease presenting with memory, thinking, and behavioral problems that become more severe over time

anacusis type of auditory impairment with a total loss of hearing

analgesic pain relieving treatment

anorexia nervosa eating disorder in which the individual fears gaining weight, has a disturbance in the view of his or her body, and restricts food intake to lose weight even when weight is significantly low

anticipatory grief deep emotions and anxiety felt when an individual becomes aware that a loss inevitably will happen, such as in the case of a patient diagnosed with a terminal illness

asexual characteristic of having no sexual feelings

assessment collection of information about a patient's physical, mental, and emotional health

attachment theory psychological model stating that the bonds formed by the caregiver–child relationship influences personality development into adulthood, and that grief is felt when a relationship suffers an unwanted separation

audit trail feature of the electronic health record that tracks users who accessed a patient record and when they did so

authentication assumption of responsibility for the data collected

autism spectrum disorder a range of developmental conditions characterized by problems with social interactions, communication, and behavioral challenges.

benign noncancerous tumor that does not spread

bereaved person experiencing grief and mourning

bereavement state of having lost a loved one

bias tendency to favor one way of thinking

biopsy removal of a living tissue sample for visual examination

blind carbon copy (bcc) sending option used in email when the sender wants to include someone on the email for information only, but the individual's identity is not shared with other recipients

bulimia nervosa eating disorder in which the individual compulsively eats large quantities of food (binge-eating) followed by compensating for the binge through purging (vomiting, use of laxatives, and/or exercise)

bullying aggression among adolescents perpetrated by person or persons against an individual, excluding a sibling or dating partner, which is based on a power imbalance

business associate Classification under HIPAA for a contracted vendor who uses protected health information to perform a service on behalf of a covered entity.

carbon copy (cc) sending option used in email when the sender wants to include someone on the email for information only and is not expecting that individual to respond.

case conference cohesive group of interdisciplinary professionals coming together

channel means of transmitting a message

chief complaint statement made by a patient describing the most significant or serious reason for concern

chronic slowly progressing illness that lasts longer than three months

cisgender gender identity that aligns with the sex assigned at birth

clarification removal of confusion or misunderstanding

clarify to remove confusion

clinical decision support (CDS) function of the electronic health record that recommends approaches for diagnoses of specific diseases, guides selection of the correct diagnostic tests, and assists in the treatment and monitoring of patients

closed-ended question question with a limited set of possible answers

coding representation of diagnoses and health care services using alphanumeric characters

cognitive behavioral therapy (CBT) intervention for treating mental disorders that solves problems by correcting distorted thinking and helping the patient develop new coping mechanisms

cognitive learning acquisition of knowledge

colloquialism informal speech, usually relying on regionally accepted terms and pronunciations

compliance act of a patient following the instructions of the health care team

complicated grief   deep, persistent sadness accompanied by incessant and painful thoughts of the loss that interferes with the ability to function

computer-assisted physician order entry (CPOE)   software featuring decision support through which a provider selects medications and sends orders electronically

concrete operational stage   psychologist Jean Piaget's developmental stage from age 7 to age 11, during which children become more logical in thought, less egocentric, and begin to understand different viewpoints

consultation   to obtain advice or another opinion from a specialist regarding any aspect of patient care

continuity of care   communication and coordination of a patient's care among various health care professionals

continuity of care   provision of care for a patient over a period of time

contraindication   reason not to pursue a treatment

coping   contending with difficulties and overcoming them

coping mechanism   strategy to manage stress

countersignature   evidence of the supervision of a subordinate's documentation

covered entity   Classification under HIPAA for an organization that collects and manages health information, such as a provider.

cuing   inadvertently eliciting an answer by giving positive or negative feedback that signals what the questioner expects or wants to hear

cultural imposition   tendency of a person or group to believe other cultures should adhere to its values and patterns of behavior

culture   set of acceptable behaviors, beliefs, and material traits of a racial, religious, or social group

D

delirium tremens   physical withdrawal from chronic high alcohol intake with symptoms of confusion, shaking, and hallucinations

dementia   decline in mental ability caused by brain disease or injury severe enough to interfere with daily life

discharge summary   documentation of a visit given to the patient at check out

disclosure   sending of patient information

diverse   quality of being different

dual process model   theory of grieving in which the individual at times confronts, and at other times avoids, the different tasks of grieving

durable power of attorney (DPOA)   type of advance directive that allows the patient to name another individual to legally make health care decisions on the patient's behalf

dynamics   psychological background and inner workings of interpersonal relationships

dysthymia   depressed mood that lasts for at least two years

E

elder abuse   abuse, neglect, or exploitation of people over the age of 60 years, which may include physical abuse, sexual abuse, emotional abuse, neglect, abandonment, and financial abuse

electronic health record (EHR)   system that maintains patient demographic and clinical information digitally and offers computerized physician order entry, e-prescribing, and decision support

emergent   condition or situation that needs immediate attention

empathy   condition of experiencing the feelings of another

eustress   good or positive stress with beneficial emotional and physical results

evaluation   appraisal and review of the patient's learning progress during and after the patient education

F

family violence   comprehensive term that addresses abuse throughout the life cycle and includes partner abuse, child abuse, and elder abuse

feedback   return of information solicited during an exchange; usually used to verify that information was received

fight-or-flight response   body's physiologic reaction to a perceived threat consisting of the release of hormones that increases blood pressure and blood sugar and suppresses the immune system to gain a boost of energy

formal operational stage   psychologist Jean Piaget's developmental stage from age 11 to age 15, during which children think abstractly and develop full autonomy

G

gate, gating   consciously blocking the reception of sensory stimuli, such as hearing or pain

gender   psychosocial condition of being male, female, or neither of those

gender identity   one's conception of being male, female, or a nonbinary gender

genderfluid   characteristic of fluctuating between presenting as masculine, feminine, neither, or both

genderqueer   having a nonbinary gender identity

generalized anxiety disorder   a mental health disorder in which the patient suffers chronic, exaggerated worry or a sense of dread, sometimes without cause

grief   normal emotional response to the actual or perceived loss of something of value

grief work   in psychology, the notion that individuals feel strong emotions toward a loss, and must work through these emotions to reduce their distress

H

health disparity   unequal health outcome among disadvantaged populations

Health Insurance Portability and Accountability Act (HIPAA)   United States federal legislation protecting the privacy and security of health information

health literacy   patient's capacity to access and comprehend basic health information and services needed to make appropriate health decisions

health record   report of the care a patient received and the relevant facts, findings, and observations about the patient's health

holistic   considers the whole of a person, including the physiologic, intellectual, emotional, and social factors, rather than physical manifestations alone

hospice   type of care for patients facing the end of life that focuses on pain management and emotional support

I

idiom expression specific to a certain population that cannot be translated literally

implementation act of setting a plan into effect

incongruence incompatible, not in agreement, inconsistent

informed consent patient's authorization to receive treatment following the provider's discussion of various treatment options and risks

interdisciplinary combination of two or more specialties working together to meet a specific goal

interoperability capacity for different computer systems to communicate, exchange data, and use the information that has been exchanged

intimate partner violence (IPV) inclusive term that includes violence or abuse between two people, with or without marital status or sexual relationship; also referred to as domestic violence or spousal abuse

J

jargon specialized or technical language of a trade or profession

K

kinesics study of body positions and movement in relation to communication

L

leading question question that encourages or expects a certain answer

learning goal purpose toward which gaining specific knowledge or skill is directed

learning objectives observable or discernible outcome as the result of acquired knowledge or information

limited English proficiency (LEP) categorization of individuals who are not fluent in English or speak English "less than very well"

M

maintenance condition of living with incurable cancer and managing the disease to allow for an acceptable quality of life

major depressive disorder mood disorder in which the patient suffers loss of interest, sadness, and a change in functioning, among other symptoms lasting two weeks or more

malignant cancerous tumor

mandatory reporter specific professional required to report suspected abuse, neglect or violence to appropriate agencies

message communication transmitted by spoken or written word or other means from one to another

metastasis spread of cancer to sites in the body beyond the cancer's origin

minutes summary record of what took place at a meeting

mourning outward display of grief

N

nonbinary category of gender identities that are not exclusively masculine or feminine, such as identifying with both genders, neither gender, a third gender, or oscillating among genders

notice of privacy practices (NPP) plain-language document given to patients by the provider that details how a patient's information will be used and disclosed, the organization's duties to safeguard patient information, and a patient's rights concerning privacy

O

objective in the patient interview, observed and measurable information

open-ended question question for which the respondent must give a longer, free-form answer

otosclerosis hardening of the structures of the ear which interferes with the transmission of sound from the structures of the ear to the cochlear nerve to the brain, resulting in a conductive hearing impairment

P

palliative offering comfort, as in pain relief, but not bringing about a cure

paralanguage vocal expression involving rate of speech, tone, pitch, and so forth

paraphrase to restate in other words than originally transmitted, usually to make a meaning clear

pathologist medical doctor who specializes in the causes and effects of diseases

patient education process of sharing information and instruction to allow patients to gain knowledge and skills to better address their health problems and improve their wellness

patient portal website on which patients can interact and communicate with their provider, view laboratory results, and track, monitor, and send information regarding their personal

Physician Order for Life Sustaining Treatment (POLST) portable document for a terminally ill patient containing physician orders for desired treatment in the event of an emergency

prejudice opinion formed about a person, group, or situation before facts and circumstances are known

preoperational stage psychologist Jean Piaget's developmental stage from age 2 to age 7, during which children tend to be egocentric and begin to use language

presbycusis mixed auditory impairment common in older patients, literally meaning "old hearing"

professionalism skills, judgments, and behaviors that are expected in the workplace.

protected health information (PHI) under the law, any health information, such as medical history or current status, that can be linked to an individual

protocol guideline for the treatment of a disease or disorder

proxemics study of personal spatial distances and their effect on interpersonal behavior

psychomotor learning acquisition of a skill

psychotropic substance that effects an individual's brain chemistry to produce a change in thinking, emotion, or behavior (literally, "turns the mind")

R

rapport relationship, usually of mutual trust and regard

receiver in the communication process, the person or persons for whom the sender's message is intended

recovery state of abstaining from using the substance to improve health and well-being

referral formal contract between two or more health care team members to provide services to a patient

reflective response statement confirming that you received the message and leaving the patient to complete his or her thought or sentence or explore it further

relapse deteriorated condition after an improvement

release of information (ROI) authorization by the patient to disclose his or her protected health information to another person or entity

remission complete or partial disappearance of the signs and symptoms of cancer in response to treatment

remote interpreter service use of interpreters where they are not in-person, but instead provide services via phone or video

respite short interval of rest or relief

S

sender in the communication process, the individual who creates and transmits a message

sensorimotor stage psychologist Jean Piaget's developmental stage from birth to age 2, during which children learn through their interactions with the environment

sensory barrier impairment or disability of one or more senses: sight, hearing, smell, touch, taste, and spatial awareness

sex biological aspects of being male or female

sexual orientation individual's pattern of emotional, romantic, and/or sexual attractions to others

slang informal words and phrases used around friends, family, and others in our social group

spatial pertaining to a space and its relationship with things found in it

STAT requiring an immediate response

subjective that which is known or experienced only to the individual

substance use disorder (SUD) disorder in which a patient has mental, social, and/or physiologic symptoms from continued use of a substance

suicidal ideation thoughts of causing one's own death

summarize to restate in a briefer form

sympathy understanding that another is in distress

T

tolerance reduced effects following repeated use of a substance

transgender gender identity or gender expression that differs from what is typically associated with the sex assigned at birth

transition process of altering one's sex from his or her birth sex

triage process of determining the degree of sickness and placing the patient into an appropriate level of care

V

verification process of checking the accuracy of a statement

W

withdrawal symptoms following cessation of substance use

CHAPTER 1

Gumucio-Dagron A, Tufte T, eds. *Communication for social change anthology: Historical and contemporary readings.* South Orange, NJ: Denise Gray-Felder; 2006.

Singer T, Klimecki OM. Empathy and compassion. *Current Biology.* 2014;*24*:875–878.

CHAPTER 2

Baker D. *The Joint Commision's pain standards: Origins and evolution.* Oakbrook Terrace, IL: The Joint Commission; 2017.

Davidoff FD. *Who has seen a blood sugar?—Reflections on medical education.* Philadelphia, PA: American College of Physicians; 1996.

Frieden J. *Remove pain as 5th vital sign, AMA urged. Medpage Today*; 2016, June 13. Retrieved from https://www.medpagetoday.com/meetingcoverage/ama/58486; 2018, August 25.

Larson G. *9th Annual vitals wait time report released.* Retrieved from https://www.businesswire.com/news/home/20180322005683/en/9th-Annual-Vitals-Wait-Time-Report-Released; 2018, March 22.

Sklansky M. Banning the handshake from the healthcare setting. *Journal of the American Medical Association.* 2014;*311*(24):2477.

Xie Z, Or C. Associations between waiting times, service times, and patient satisfaction in an endocrinology outpatient department: A time study and questionnaire survey. *INQUIRY: The Journal of Haelth Care Organization, Provision, and Financing.* 2017. Retrieved from https://journals.sagepub.com/doi/10.1177/0046958017739527.

CHAPTER 3

Bloom BS, Engelhart MD, Furst EJ, Hill WH, Krathwohl DRA. *Taxonomy of educational objectives: The classification of educational goals. handbook 1: Cognitive domain.* New York, NY: David McKay; 1956.

Centers for Medicare and Medicaid Services. *Nation Health Expenditures Fact Sheet.* Retrieved from https://www.cms.gov/research-statistics-data-and-systems/statistics-trends-and-reports/nationalhealthexpenddata/nhe-fact-sheet.html; 2018.

Farrell AK, Simpson JA. Effects of relationship functioning on the biological experience of stress and physical health. *Current Opinion in Psychiatry.* 2016;*13*(2):49–53.

Fox S. *The social life of health information.* Retrieved from Pew Research Center website http://www.pewresearch.org/fact-tank/2014/01/15/the-social-life-of-health-information/; 2014, January 15.

Hobson K. *Why do people stop taking their meds? Cost is just one reason.* Retrieved from National Public Radio website https://www.npr.org/sections/health-shots/2017/09/08/549414152/why-do-people-stop-taking-their-meds-cost-is-just-one-reason; 2017 September 8.

Jimmy B, Jose J. Patient medication adherence: Measures in daily practice. *Oman Medical Journal.* 2011;*26*(3):155–159. https://doi.org/10.5001/omj.2011.38.

Reblin M, Uchino BN. Social and emotional support and its implication for health. *Current Opinion in Psychiatry.* 2008;*21*(2):201–205. https://doi.org/10.1097/YCO.0b013e3282f3ad89.

Scott TL, Gazmararian JA, Williams MV, Baker DW. Health literacy and preventive health care use among Medicare enrollees in a managed care organization. *Medical Care.* 2002;40(5):395–404.

U.S. Department of Health and Human Services. *Healthy People 2010.* Washington, DC: U.S. Government Printing Office; 2000. Originally developed for Ratzan SC, Parker RM. 2000. Introduction. In National Library of Medicine Current Bibliographies in Medicine: Health Literacy. Selden CR, Zorn M, Ratzan SC, Parker RM, Editors. NLM Pub. No. CBM 2000-1. Bethesda, MD: National Institutes of Health, U.S. Department of Health and Human Services.

World Health Organization. In: Sabate E, ed. *Adherence to long-term therapies: Evidence for action.* Geneva: Author; 2003.

CHAPTER 4

Administration on Aging (AoA), Administration for Community Living, U.S. Department of Health and Human Services. (2018). *2017 Profile of older americans.* Retrieved from https://www.acl.gov/sites/default/files/Aging%20and%20Disability%20in%20America/2017OlderAmericansProfile.pdf.

American Psychological Association & National Association of School Psychologists. (2015). *Resolution on gender and sexual orientation diversity in children and adolescents in schools.* Retrieved from https://www.apa.org/about/policy/orientation-diversity.

American Psychological Association. *APA dictionary of psychology.* 2nd ed. Washington, DC: Author; 2015a.

American Psychological Association. Guidelines for psychological practice with transgender and gender nonconforming people. *American Psychologist.* 2015b;*70*(9):832–864. doi.org/10.1037/a0039906.

Artiga S, Foutz J, Damico A. *Health coverage by race and ethnicity: Changes under the ACA.* Retrieved from Kaiser Family Foundation website; 2018. http://files.kff.org/attachment/Issue-Brief-Health-Coverage-by-Race-and-Ethnicity-Changes-Under-the-ACA.

Blackwell D, Villaroel MA. *Tables of summary health statistics for U.S. adults: 2016.* Retrieved from National Center for Health Statistics website; 2018. http://www.cdc.gov/nhis/SHS/tables.htm.

Carabez R, Eliason M, Martinson M. Nurses' knowledge about transgender patient care: A qualitative study. *Advances in Nursing Science.* 2016;*39*(3):257–271. https://doi.org/10.1097/ANS.0000000000000128.

Centers for Disease Control and Prevention. *National diabetes statistics report, 2017.* Atlanta, GA: Author; 2017.

Centers for Disease Control and Prevention. *HIV among African Americans.* Retrieved from https://www.cdc.gov/hiv/group/racialethnic/africanamericans/index.html; 2018, September 24.

CMS Office of Minority Health and RAND Corporation. *Racial and ethnic disparities by gender in health in health care in medical advantage.* Retrieved from https://www.cms.gov/About-CMS/Agency-Information/OMH/Downloads/Health-Disparities-Racial-and-Ethnic-Disparities-by-Gender-National-Report.pdf; 2017.

Gonzalez G, Blewett LA. National and state-specific health insurance disparities for adults in same-sex relationships. *American Journal of Public Health.* 2014;*104*(2):e95–e104. https://doi.org/10.2105/AJPH.2013.301577.

Graham G. Disparities in cardiovascular disease risk in the United States. *Current Cardiology Reviews.* 2015, August;*11*(3):238–245. https://doi.org/10.2174/1573403X11666141122220003.

Healthy People 2020. *About Healthy People.* Available at https://www.healthypeople.gov/2020/About-Healthy-People. Updated June 5, 2019. Accessed June 6, 2019.

Heslin KC, Gore JL, King WD, Fox SA. Sexual orientation and testing for prostate and colorectal cancers among men in California. *Medical Care.* 2008;*46*(12):1240–1248. https://doi.org/10.1097/MLR.0b013e31817d697f.

Steele LS, Tinmouth JM, Lu A. Regular health care use by lesbians: a path analysis of predictive factors. *Family Practice.* 2006;*23*(6):631–636. https://doi.org/10.1093/fampra/cml030.

U.S. Department of Commerce. (2018). *American Community Survey (ACS) 2012-016 ACS 5-year data profiles.* Retrieved from https://www.census.gov/programs-surveys/acs/data.html.

U.S. Department of Health and Human Services, Office of Disease Prevention and Health Promotion. (2018, September 24). *Lesbian, gay, bisexual, and transgender health.* Retrieved from https://www.healthypeople.gov/2020/topics-objectives/topic/lesbian-gay-bisexual-and-transgender-health.

U.S. Department of Health and Human Services. Bullying Prevention Training Center. Retrieved September 28, 2017, from https://www.stopbullying.gov/prevention/training-center/index.html.

CHAPTER 5

Abaza W, Lu MC. *Protecting youth from bullying: The role of the pediatrician.* Retrieved from stopbullying.gov website: https://www.stopbullying.gov/blog/2017/01/17/protecting-youth-bullying-role-pediatrician.html; 2017, January 17.

Americans With Disabilities Act of 1990, Pub. L. No. 101-336, 104 Stat. 328. (1990).

Bernstein J, Bernstein E, Dave A, Hardt E, James T, Linden J, Safi C. Trained medical interpreters in the emergency department: Effects on services, subsequent charges, and follow-up. *Journal of Immigrant Health.* 2002;*4*(4):171–176.

Diamond L, Grbic D, Genoff M, Gonzalez J, Sharaf R, Mikesell C, Gany F. Non–English-language proficiency of applicants to US residency programs. *Journal of the American Medical Association.* 2014;*312*(22):2405–2407. https://doi.org/10.1001/jama.2014.15444.

Elliott L. Barriers to screening for domestic violence. *Journal of General Internal Medicine.* 2002;*17*(2):112–116. https://doi.org/10.1046/j.1525-1497.2002.10233.x.

Fernandez A, Schillinger D, Warton EM, Adler N, Moffet HH, Schenker Y, Karter A. Language barriers, physician-patient language concordance, and glycemic control among Latinos with diabetes: The Diabetes Study of Northern California (DISTANCE). *Journal of General Internal Medicine.* 2011;*26*(2):170–176. https://doi.org/10.1007/s11606-010-1507-6.

Foden-Vencil K. *In the hospital, a bad translation can destroy a life.* Retrieved from National Public Radio website; 2014. https://www.npr.org/sections/health-shots/2014/10/27/358055673/in-the-hospital-a-bad-translation-can-destroy-a-life.

Kann L, McManus T, Harris WA, Shanklin SL, Flint KH, Hawkins J, Lowry R. Youth risk behavior surveillance—United States, 2015. *MMWR Surveillance Summary.* 2016;*65*(SS-6):67. Retrieved from https://www.cdc.gov/mmwr/volumes/65/ss/pdfs/ss6506.pdf.

Krogstad JM. *Rise in English proficiency among U.S. Hispanics is driven by the young.* Retrieved from Pew Research Center website http://www.pewresearch.org/fact-tank/2016/04/20/rise-in-english-proficiency-among-u-s-hispanics-is-driven-by-the-young/; 2016, April 20.

Lereya ST, Copeland WE, Costello EJ, Wolke D. Adult mental health consequences of peer bullying and maltreatment in childhood: Two cohorts in two countries. *The Lancet.* 2015;2(6):524–531. https://doi.org/10.1016/S2215-0366(15)00165-0.

Lo M-CM, Nguyen ET. Caring and carrying the cost: Bicultural Latina nurses' challenges and strategies for working with coethnic patients. *RSF: The Russell Sage Foundation Journal of the Social Sciences.* 2018;4(1):149–171. Retrieved from muse.jhu.edu/article/684313.

McClowery R. What family physicians can do to combat bullying. *Journal of Family Practice.* 2017;66(2):82–89. Retrieved from https://www.mdedge.com/jfponline/article/129817/pediatrics/what-family-physicians-can-do-combat-bullying/page/0/1.

Morey J, Boggero IA, Scott AB, Segerstrom SC. Current directions in stress and human immune function. *Current Opinion in Psychology.* 2015;5:13/17. https://doi.org/10.1016/j.copsyc.2015.03.007.

Chapman DP, Perry GS, Strine TW. The vital link between chronic disease and depressive disorders. *Preventing Chronic Disease.* 2005;2(1):A14. Retrieved from https://www.cdc.gov/pcd/issues/2005/jan/04_0066.htm.

National Council on Aging. (n.d.). *Elder abuse facts.* Retrieved from https://www.ncoa.org/public-policy-action/elder-justice/elder-abuse-facts/.

Occupational Health and Safety Administration. (2015). *Workplace violence in healthcare.* Retrieved from https://www.osha.gov/Publications/OSHA3826.pdf.

Perel-Levin S. *Discussing screening for elder abuse at primary health care level.* Retrieved from World Health Organization website http://www.who.int/ageing/publications/Discussing_Elder_Abuseweb.pdf; 2008.

Ramakrishnan K, Ahmad FZ. *Language diversity and English proficiency.* Retrieved from Center for American Progress website https://cdn.americanprogress.org/wp-content/uploads/2014/04/AAPI-LanguageAccess1.pdf; 2014, May 27.

Smith SG, Chen J, Basile KC, Gilbert LK, Merrick MT, Patel N, Walling M, Jain A. (2017). *The National Intimate Partner and Sexual Violence Survey (NISVS): 2010–2012 State Report.* Atlanta, GA: National Center for Injury Prevention and Control, Centers for Disease Control and Prevention. Retrieved from https://www.cdc.gov/violenceprevention/pdf/NISVS-StateReportBook.pdf.

Strayton CD, Duncan MM. Mutable influences on intimate partner abuse screening in health care settings: A synthesis of the literature. *Trauma Violence Abuse.* 2005;6(4):271–285. https://doi.org/10.1177/1524838005277439.

U.S. Census Bureau. (2017, August 31). *Newsroom: Facts for features: Hispanic heritage month 2017.* Retrieved from https://www.census.gov/newsroom/facts-for-features/2017/hispanic-heritage.html.

U.S. Department of Education, Office for Civil Rights. (2010, October 16). *Dear colleague letter: Harassment and bullying: Background, summary, and fast facts.* Retrieved from https://www2.ed.gov/about/offices/list/ocr/docs/dcl-factsheet-201010.pdf.

U.S. Department of Health & Human Services. Administration for Children and Families, Administration on Children, Youth and Families, Children's Bureau. *Child maltreatment.* 2018;2016. Retrieved from https://www.acf.hhs.gov/sites/default/files/cb/cm2016.pdf.

U.S. Department of Health and Human Services. *Bullying prevention training center.* Retrieved from https://www.stopbullying.gov/prevention/training-center/index.html; 2017, September 28.

U.S. Department of Health & Human Services, Centers for Disease Control and Prevention, National Center for HIV Viral Hepatitis STD and TB Prevention. (2011). *A guide to taking a sexual history* (CDC Publication: 99-8445). Retrieved from https://npin.cdc.gov/publication/guide-taking-sexual-history.

U.S. Department of Justice, Civil Rights Division, Disability Rights Section. (2014). *ADA requirements: Effective communication.* Retrieved from https://www.ada.gov/effective-comm.pdf.

CHAPTER 6

American Psychiatric Association. *Diagnostic and statistical manual of mental disorders: DSM-5.* Arlington, VA: Author; 2013.

American Psychiatric Association. (2017, January). *What is depression?* Retrieved from https://www.psychiatry.org/patients-families/depression/what-is-depression

Centers for Disease Control and Prevention. (2017 February 19)., *Fatal injury reports, national, regional and state, 1981–2017.* Retrieved from https://webappa.cdc.gov/sasweb/ncipc/mortrate.html

Centers for Disease Control and Prevention, National Center for HIV/AIDS, Viral Hepatitis, STD, and TB Prevention, Division of Adolescent and School Health. (2018). *Youth risk behavior survey: Data summary and trends report, 2007–2017.* Retrieved from https://www.cdc.gov/healthyyouth/data/yrbs/pdf/trendsreport.pdf

Committee to Evaluate the Supplemental Security Income Disability Program for Children with Mental Disorders; Board on the Health of Select Populations; Board on Children, Youth, and Families; Institute of Medicine. Prevalence of autism spectrum disorder. In: Boat TF, Wu JT, eds. *Mental disorders and disabilities among low-income children.* Washington, DC: National Academies Press. Retrieved from; 2015. https://www.ncbi.nlm.nih.gov/books/NBK332896/.

Fazio S, Pace D, Flinner J, Kallmyer B. The fundamentals of person-centered care for individuals with dementia. *The Gerontologist.* 2018;58(suppl_1):S10–S19. https://doi.org/10.1093/geront/gnx122.

Gliatto MF, Rai AK. Evaluation and treatment of patients with suicidal ideation. *American Family Physician*. 1999, March 15;*59*(6):1500–1506. Retrieved from https://www.aafp.org/afp/1999/0315/p1500.html.

Goriouinova NA, Mansvelder HD. Short- and long-term consequences of nicotine exposure during adolescence for prefrontal cortex neuronal network function. *Cold Spring Harbor Perspectives in Medicine*. 2012;*2*(12):a012120 https://doi.org/10.1101/cshperspect.a012120.

Hert MD, Correll CU, Bobes J, Cetkovich-Bakmas M, Cohen D, Asai I, Leucht S. Physical illness in patients with severe mental disorders. I. Prevalence, impact of medications and disparities in health care. *World Psychiatry*. 2011;*10*(1):52–77. Retrieved from https://www.ncbi.nlm.nih.gov/pmc/articles/PMC3048500/.

Jacobs DG, Baldessarini RJ, Conwell Y, Fawcett JA, Horton L, Meltzer H, Simon R. *Practice guideline for the assessment and treatment of patients with suicidal behaviors*. Retrieved from https://psychiatryonline.org/pb/assets/raw/sitewide/practice_guidelines/guidelines/suicide.pdf; 2010.

Jha P, Ramasundarahettige C, Landsman V, Rostron B, Thun M, Anderson RN, Peto R. 21st-Century hazards of smoking and benefits of cessation in the United States. *New England Journal of Medicine*. 2013;*368*:341–350. https://doi.org/10.1056/NEJMsa1211128.

Kitwood T. *Dementia reconsidered: The person comes first*. Berkshire, UK: Open University Press; 1997.

National Institute of Mental Health. *Eating disorders*. Retrieved from https://www.nimh.nih.gov/health/topics/eating-disorders/index.shtml; 2016.

National Institute of Mental Health. *Major depression*. Retrieved from https://www.nimh.nih.gov/health/statistics/major-depression.shtml; 2017.

National Institute of Mental Health. *Autism spectrum disorder (ASD)*. Retrieved from https://www.nimh.nih.gov/health/statistics/autism-spectrum-disorder-asd.shtml; 2018.

Nock M, Hwang I, Sampson N, Kessler R. Mental disorders, comorbidity and suicidal behavior: Results from the National Comorbidity Survey Replication. *Molecular Psychiatry*. 2010;*15*(8):868–876. https://doi.org/10.1038/mp.2009.29.

Slomski A. A trip on "bath salts" is cheaper than meth or cocaine but much more dangerous. *JAMA*. 2012;*308*(23):2445–2447. https://doi.org/10.1001/jama.2012.34423.

U.S. Department of Health and Human Services. (2014). *The health consequences of smoking—50 years of progress: A report of the Surgeon General*. Retrieved from https://www.cdc.gov/tobacco/data_statistics/sgr/50th-anniversary/index.htm.

United States Drug Enforcement Administration. *Slang terms and code words: A reference for law enforcement personnel (DEA Intelligence Report, Houston Division)*. Retrieved from https://ndews.umd.edu/sites/ndews.umd.edu/files/dea-drug-slang-terms-and-code-words-july2018.pdf; 2018.

United States Drug Enforcement Administration. (n.d.). *Drug scheduling: Drug schedules*. Retrieved from https://www.dea.gov/drug-scheduling

CHAPTER 7

Bowlby J. Grief and mourning in infancy and early childhood. *Psychoanalytic Study of the Child*. 1960;*15*:9–52. Retrieved from http://icpla.edu/wp-content/uploads/2012/10/Bowlby-J.-Grief-and-Mourning-in-Infancy-and-Early-Childhood-vol.15-p.9-52.pdf.

Bowlby J. *Attachment and loss: Separation, anxiety, and anger*. III, London, England: Hogarth Press; 1980.

Fuchs V. *Who shall live? Health, economics, and social choice*. New York, NY: Basic Books; 1974.

Gawande A. *Being mortal: Illness, medicine and what matters in the end*. New York, NY: Metropolitan Books; 2014.

Institute of Medicine. A profile of death and dying in America. In: Field MJ, Cassel CK, eds. *Approaching death: Improving care at the end of life*. Washington, DC: National Academies Press; 1997. Retrieved from https://www.ncbi.nlm.nih.gov/books/NBK233601/.

Kübler-Ross E. *On death and dying*. New York, NY: Macmillan; 1969.

Miniño AM. *Mortality among teenagers aged 12–19 years: United States, 1999–2006*. Retrieved from National Center for Health Statistics website https://www.cdc.gov/nchs/data/databriefs/db37.pdf; 2010.

Parkes CM. *Bereavement: Stages of grief in adult life*. London, England: Penguin Books; 1996.

Parkes CM. Bereavement in adult life. *British Medical Journal*. 1998;*316*(7134):856–859. Retrieved from https://www.ncbi.nlm.nih.gov/pmc/articles/PMC1112778/.

Price L. Doctors, don't fear the death talk with patients. *Medical Economics*. 2016;*93*(14):45.

Shear MK. Grief and mourning gone awry: Pathway and course of complicated grief. *Dialogues in Clinical Neuroscience*. 2012;*14*:119–128. Retrieved from https://www.ncbi.nlm.nih.gov/pmc/articles/PMC3384440/.

Skinner EA, Zimmer-Gembeck MJ. In: Folkman S, ed. *The Oxford handbook of stress, health, and coping*. New York, NY: Oxford University Press; 2010:35–63. Perceived control and the development of coping.

Stroebe M, Schut H. The dual process model of coping with bereavement: Rationale and description. *Death Studies*. 1999;*23*(3):197–224.

University of California, Berkeley (USA), and Max Planck Institute for Demographic Research (Germany). (n.d.). *The human mortality database*. Retrieved from www.mortality.org.

Worden JW. *Grief counseling and grief therapy: A handbook for the mental health practitioner.* 2nd ed. London, England: Routeledge; 1991.

CHAPTER 8

Davis NA. *Foundations of health information management.* 4th ed. St. Louis, MO: Elsevier; 2017.

Colvin C. Leadership, Motivation, and Conflict Management. In: Nguyen J, ed. *Introduction to health services administration.* St. Louis, MO: Elsevier; 2018.

Robertson M. Business Communication and Professionalism. In: Nguyen J, ed. *Introduction to health services administration.* St. Loius, MO: Elsevier; 2018.

CHAPTER 9

Davis NA. *Foundations of health information management.* 4th ed. St. Louis, MO: Elsevier; 2017.

Shiland B. Documentation. In: Nguyen J, ed. *Introduction to health services administration.* Elsevier: St. Louis, MO; 2018.

Radley D, Wasserman MR, Olsho LE, Shoemaker MJ, Spranca MD, Bradshaw B. Reduction in medication errors in hospitals due to adoption of computerized provider order entry systems. *Journal of the American Medical Informatics Association.* 2013;20(3):470–476. https://doi.org/10.1136/amiajnl-2012-001241.

The Joint Commission. (2018). *Facts about the official "do not use" list of abbreviations.* Retrieved from https://www.joint-commission.org/facts_about_do_not_use_list/.

U.S. Department of Health and Human Services. *Health information privacy: Notice of privacy practices for protected health information.* Retrieved July 26, 2013, from https://www.hhs.gov/hipaa/for-professionals/privacy/guidance/privacy-practices-for-protected-health-information/index.html.

Note: Page numbers followed by *f* indicate figures, *t* indicate tables, and *b* indicate boxes.